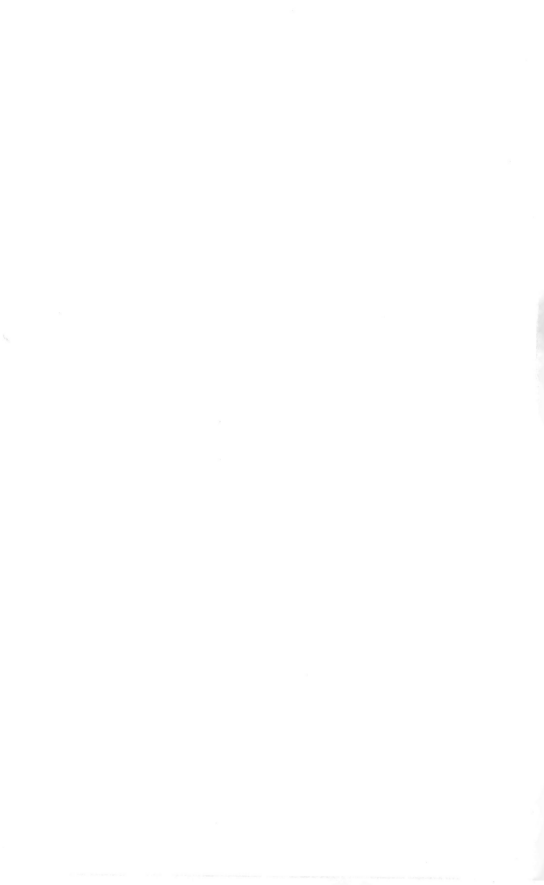

Progress in
Cancer Research and Therapy
Volume 34

TUMOR PROMOTERS: BIOLOGICAL APPROACHES FOR MECHANISTIC STUDIES AND ASSAY SYSTEMS

Progress in
Cancer Research and Therapy
Volume 34

Tumor Promoters: Biological Approaches for Mechanistic Studies and Assay Systems

EDITORS

Robert Langenbach, Ph.D.

Cellular and Genetic Toxicology Branch
National Institute of Environmental
Health Sciences
Research Triangle Park, North Carolina

Eugene Elmore, Ph.D.

Northrop Services, Inc.
Environmental Services
Research Triangle Park, North Carolina

J. Carl Barrett, Ph.D.

Laboratory of Molecular Carcinogenesis
National Institute of Environmental Health Sciences
Research Triangle Park, North Carolina

RAVEN PRESS NEW YORK

Raven Press, 1185 Avenue of the Americas, New York, New York 10036

Made in the United States of America

Library of Congress Cataloging-in-Publication Data

Tumor promoters.

    (Progress in cancer research and therapy; v. 34)
    Proceedings of a conference held Sept. 8–10, 1986
at the National Institute of Environmental Health
Sciences, Research Triangle Park, N.C.
    Includes bibliographies and index.
    1. Cocarcinogens—Congresses. 2. Carcinogenesis—
Congresses. I. Langenbach, Robert, 1942–   .
II. Elmore, Eugene. III. Barrett, J. Carl (James Carl)
IV. Series. [DNLM: 1. Carcinogens—congresses.
2. Cell Communication—congresses. 3. Cell Transfor-
mation, Neoplastic—congresses. 4. Neoplasms—etiology—
congresses. W1 PR667M v.34 / QZ 202 T9245 1986]
RC268.52.T86   1988   616.99′4071   86-43223
ISBN 0-88167-451-6

9 8 7 6 5 4 3 2 1

Progress in Cancer Research and Therapy

Vol. 35: Hormones and Cancer 3: Proceedings of the Third International Congress
Francesco Bresciani, Roger J. B. King, Marc E. Lippman, and Jean-Pierre Raynaud, editors, 1988

Vol. 34: Tumor Promoters: Biological Approaches for Mechanistic Studies and Assay Systems
Robert Langenbach, Eugene Elmore, and J. Carl Barrett, editors, 1988

Vol. 33: Methotrexate in Cancer Therapy
Kiyoji Kimura and Yeu-Ming Wang, editors, 1987

Vol. 32: Molecular Biology of Tumor Cells
Britta Wahren, Göran Holm, Sten Hammarström, and Peter Perlmann, editors, 1985

Vol. 31: Hormones and Cancer 2: Proceedings of the Second International Congress
Francesco Bresciani, Roger J.B. King, Marc E. Lippman, Moïse Namer, and Jean-Pierre Raynaud, editors, 1984

Vol. 30: Gene Transfer and Cancer
Mark L. Pearson and Nat L. Sternberg, editors, 1984

Vol. 29: Markers of Colonic Cell Differentiation
Sandra R. Wolman and Anthony J. Mastromarino, editors, 1984

Vol. 28: The Development of Target-Oriented Anticancer Drugs
Yung-Chi Cheng, Barry Goz, and Mimi Minkoff, editors, 1983

Vol. 27: Environmental Influences in the Pathogenesis of Leukemias and Lymphomas
Ian T. Magrath, Gregory T. O'Conor, and Bracha Ramot, editors, 1984

Vol. 26: Radiation Carcinogenesis: Epidemiology and Biological Significance
John D. Boice, Jr. and Joseph F. Fraumeni, editors, 1983

Vol. 25: *Steroids and Endometrial Cancer
Valerio Maria Jasonno, Italo Nenci, and Carlo Flamigni, editors, 1983

Vol. 24: Recent Clinical Developments in Gynecologic Oncology
C. Paul Morrow, John Bonnar, Timothy J. O'Brien, and William E. Gibbons, editors, 1983

Vol. 23: Maturation Factors and Cancer
Malcolm A.S. Moore, editor, 1982

Vol. 22: The Potential Role of T Cells in Cancer Therapy
Alexander Fefer and Allen L. Goldstein, editors, 1982

Vol. 21: Hybridomas in Cancer Diagnosis and Treatment
Malcolm S. Mitchell and Herbert F. Oettgen, editors, 1982

Vol. 20: *Lymphokines and Thymic Hormones: Their Potential Utilization in Cancer Therapeutics
Allen L. Goldstein and Michael A. Chirigos, editors, 1982

Vol. 19: Mediation of Cellular Immunity in Cancer by Immune Modifiers
Michael A. Chirigos, Malcolm S. Mitchell, and Michael J. Mastrangelo, editors, 1982

Vol. 18: Carcinoma of the Bladder
John G. Connolly, editor, 1981

Vol. 17: Nutrition and Cancer: Etiology and Treatment
Guy R. Newell and Neil M. Ellison, editors, 1981

Vol. 16: Augmenting Agents in Cancer Therapy
E.M. Hersch, M.A. Chirigos, and M.J. Mastrangelo, editors, 1981

Vol. 15: *Role of Medroxyprogesterone in Endocrine-Related Tumors
Stefano Iacobelli and Aurelio Di Marco, editors, 1980

Vol. 14: Hormones and Cancer
Stefano Iacobelli, R.J.B. King, Hans R. Lindner, and Marc E. Lippman, editors, 1980

Vol. 13: *Colorectal Cancer: Prevention, Epidemiology, and Screening
Sidney J. Winawer, David Schottenfield, and Paul Sherlock, editors, 1980

Vol. 12: Advances in Neuroblastoma Research
Audrey E. Evans, editor, 1980

Vol. 11: Treatment of Lung Cancer
Marcel Rozencweig and Franco Muggia, editors, 1978

Vol. 10: Hormones, Receptors, and Breast Cancer
William L. McGuire, editor, 1978

Vol. 9: Endocrine Control in Neoplasia
R.K. Sharma and W.E. Criss, editors, 1978

Vol. 8: Polyamines as Biochemical Markers of Normal and Malignant Growth
D.H. Russell and B.G.M. Durie, editors, 1978

Vol. 7: Immune Modulation and Control of Neoplasia by Adjuvant Therapy
Michael A. Chirigos, editor, 1978

Vol. 6: *Immunotherapy of Cancer: Present Status of Trials in Man
William D. Terry and Dorothy Windhorst, editors, 1978

Vol. 5: Cancer Invasion and Metastasis: Biologic Mechanisms and Therapy
Stacey B. Day, W.P. Laird Myers, Philip Stansly, Silvio Garattini, and Martin G. Lewis, editors, 1977

Vol. 4: Progesterone Receptors in Neoplastic Tissues
William L. McGuire, Jean-Pierre Raynaud, and Etienne-Emile Baulieu, editors, 1977

Vol. 3: Genetics of Human Cancer
John J. Mulvihill, Robert W. Miller, and Joseph F. Fraumeni, Jr., editors, 1977

Vol. 2: Control of Neoplasia by Modulation of the Immune System
Michael A. Chirigos, editor, 1977

Vol. 1: *Control Mechanisms in Cancer
Wayne E. Criss, Tetsuo Ono, and John R. Sabine, editors, 1976

* Out of print.

Preface

Although awareness of the role tumor promoters play in the carcinogenesis process has increased in recent years, the extent to which they contribute to human cancer is relatively unknown. Since the early studies on tumor promotion in mouse skin, the phenomenon has been extended to many other mammalian tissues and species.

This volume examines the current status of our understanding of the tissue, cellular, and molecular mechanisms of promoters and determines which approaches appear most useful for elucidating their mechanisms. An equally important goal of the research presented herein was to determine which currently available biological systems, or systems that could be developed, were most promising as short-term assays for tumor promoters.

This volume will lead oncologists to a better understanding of the promotion process and how it is involved in human carcinogenesis.

Robert Langenbach
Eugene Elmore
J. Carl Barrett

Acknowledgment

This volume presents the proceedings of a conference held at the National Institute of Environmental Health Sciences, Research Triangle Park, North Carolina, September 8–10, 1986.

Contents

Mechanisms of Tumor Promotion at the Tissue/Intercellular Level

1   Tumor Promotion—The Search for the Necessary and Sufficient
A. Sivak

11   Mechanisms of Carcinogenesis Using Mouse Skin: The Multistage
Assay Revisited
*S. M. Fischer, J. J. Reiners, Jr., B. C. Pence, C. M. Aldaz,
C. J. Conti, R. J. Morris, J. F. O'Connell, J. B. Rotstein, and
T. J. Slaga*

31   Variable Potential for Malignant Conversion of Papillomas Induced
by Initiation–Promotion Protocols
H. Hennings

39   The Conversion-Step of Multistage Tumorigenesis in NMRI-
Mouse Skin
V. Kinzel, G. Fürstenberger, and F. Marks

51   Genetic Factors Controlling Susceptibility to Skin Tumor
Promotion in Mice
J. DiGiovanni, M. Naito, and K. J. Chenicek

71   Liver Tumor Promotion: Mechanisms Revealed by Orotic Acid
*E. Laconi, S. Vasudevan, P. M. Rao, S. Rajalakshmi, and
D. S. R. Sarma*

79   Quantitative Studies on Multistage Hepatocarcinogenesis in the
Rat
H. C. Pitot and H. A. Campbell

97   Chemical and Oncogene Modulation of Gap Junctional
Intercellular Communication
J. E. Trosko and C. C. Chang

113   Disruption of Cell–Cell Channels as an Event Common to the
Potential Mechanism of Action of Some Chemicals with
Teratogenic and Carcinogenic Activity
F. Welsch

131   The Role of Selective Junctional Communication in Cell
Transformation
H. Yamasaki and D. J. Fitzgerald

149   Inhibition of Metabolic Cooperation in V79 Cells: Potential
         Correlations with Tumor Promotion
         E. Elmore, R. Langenbach, and J. S. Bohrman

161   Detection of Neoplasm Promoters in the Hepatocyte/Liver
         Epithelial Cell System
         C. C. Tong and G. M. Williams

Mechanism of Tumor Promotion at the Cellular Level

179   Chemico–Biological Interactions in the Immunologic Modulation
         of Initiated and Promoted Transformation
         C. H. Evans and J. A. DiPaolo

187   Mechanisms of Transformation and Promotion of Syrian Hamster
         Embryo Cells
         T. Sanner and E. Rivedal

201   Implications for Mechanisms of Tumor Promotion and Its
         Inhibition by Various Agents from Studies of *In Vitro*
         Transformation
         A. R. Kennedy

213   Enhancement of C3H/10T1/2 Cell Transformation by Tumor
         Promoters
         C. J. Boreiko

223   The Role of Retinoids as Inhibitors of Tumor Promotion
         J. S. Bertram

237   Comparison of Transformation Systems for Detecting Tumor
         Promoters
         A. S. Tu

247   The Potential Role of Cell Differentiation in Carcinogenesis
         E. Huberman

259   Spontaneous and Phorbol Ester Induced Chromosomal Alterations
         in Normal and Transformed Mouse Keratinocytes in Culture
         N. E. Fusenig, R. T. Petrusevska, and N. Pohlmann

275   Human Lung Cells: *In Vitro* Models for Studying Carcinogens
         *J. F. Lechner, T. Masui, M. Miyashita, J. C. Willey, R. Reddel,
         M. A. LaVeck, Y. Ke, G. H. Yoakum, P. Amstad, B. I. Gerwin,
         and C. C. Harris*

289   Effects of a Tumor Promoter on Cultures of Normal and
         Carcinogen-Treated Human Endometrial Stromal Cells:
         Evidence for Dichotomous Selection
         D. G. Kaufman and J. M. Siegfried

305 Alterations in Cellular Oncogenes During Neoplastic
      Transformation of Rat Tracheal Epithelial Cells
      C. Walker, T. Gilmer, and P. Nettesheim

Mechanism of Tumor Promotion at the Molecular/Biochemical Level

317 Multistep Carcinogenesis: Studies with Primary Fibroblasts and
      Keratinocytes
      G. P. Dotto, M. Z. Gilman, and R. A. Weinberg

331 Protein Phosphorylation and Signal Transduction in Tumor
      Promotion
      C. L. Ashendel, P. A. Baudoin, and P. L. Minor

343 The Mechanism of Action of Protein Kinase C: New Insights
      Through the Study of Inhibitors and Gene Cloning
      *C. A. O'Brian, G. M. Housey, M. D. Johnson, P. Kirschmeier,
      R. M. Liskamp, and I. B. Weinstein*

357 *Pro* Genes, a Novel Class of Genes That Specify Sensitivity to
      Induction of Neoplastic Transformation by Tumor Promoters
      M. I. Lerman and N. H. Colburn

387 Receptor and DNA Ploidy Changes During Promotion of Rat
      Liver Carcinogenesis
      K. Nelson, A. Vickers, G. I. Sunahara, and G. W. Lucier

407 TCDD Receptor: Mechanisms of Altered Growth Regulation in
      Normal and Transformed Human Keratinocytes
      *R. Osborne, J. C. Cook, K. M. Dold, L. Ross, K. Gaido, and
      W. F. Greenlee*

Overview and Future Directions

417 Reflections on the Declining Ability of the Salmonella Assay to
      Detect Rodent Carcinogens as Positive
      J. Ashby

431 Promotion and Tumor Progression
      P. Shubik

441 Tumor Promotion: A Discussion of Current Topics, Available
      Assay Systems, and Research Needs
      R. Langenbach, R. W. Tennant, and J. C. Barrett

449 Subject Index

Contributors

C. M. Aldaz
University of Texas System Cancer Center
Science Park, Research Division
Smithville, Texas 78957

Paul Amstad
Laboratory of Human Carcinogenesis
Division of Cancer Etiology
National Cancer Institute
Bethesda, Maryland 20892

John Ashby
Imperial Chemical Industries PLC
Central Toxicology Laboratory
Macclesfield, Cheshire, England

Curtis L. Ashendel
Department of Medicinal Chemistry
Purdue University
West Lafayette, Indiana 47907

J. Carl Barrett
Laboratory of Molecular Carcinogenesis
National Institute of Environmental Health Sciences
Research Triangle Park, North Carolina 27709

Phyllis A. Baudoin
Department of Medicinal Chemistry
Purdue University
West Lafayette, Indiana 47907

John S. Bertram
Cancer Research Center of Hawaii
University of Hawaii
Honolulu, Hawaii 96813

Jeffrey S. Bohrman
Division of Biomedical and Behavioral Sciences
Centers for Disease Control
National Institute for Occupational Safety and Health
Cincinnati, Ohio 45226

Craig J. Boreiko
Department of Genetic Toxicology
Chemical Industry Institute of Toxicology
Research Triangle Park, North Carolina 27709

Harold A. Campbell
Departments of Oncology and Pathology
McArdle Laboratory for Cancer Research
University of Wisconsin
Madison, Wisconsin 53706

C. C. Chang
Center for Environmental Toxicology
College of Human Medicine
Michigan State University
East Lansing, Michigan 48824

Kristine J. Chenicek
University of Texas System Cancer Center
Science Park, Research Division
Smithville, Texas 78957

N. H. Colburn
Laboratory of Viral Carcinogenesis
National Cancer Institute
Frederick, Maryland 21701

C. J. Conti
University of Texas System Cancer Center
Science Park, Research Division
Smithville, Texas 78957

J. C. Cook
Department of Cell Biology
Chemical Industry Institute of
 Toxicology
Research Triangle Park, North Carolina
27709

John DiGiovanni
University of Texas System Cancer
 Center
Science Park, Research Division
Smithville, Texas 78957

Joseph A. DiPaolo
Laboratory of Biology
Division of Cancer Etiology
National Cancer Institute
Bethesda, Maryland 20892

K. M. Dold
Department of Cell Biology
Chemical Industry Institute of
 Toxicology
Research Triangle Park, North Carolina
27709

Gian Paolo Dotta
Whitehead Institute
Nine Cambridge Center
Cambridge, Massachusetts 02142

Eugene Elmore
Cellular and Molecular Toxicology
 Program
Northrop Services, Inc.-Environmental
 Sciences
Research Triangle Park, North Carolina
27709

Charles H. Evans
Laboratory of Biology
Division of Cancer Etiology
National Cancer Institute
Bethesda, Maryland 20892

S. M. Fischer
University of Texas System Cancer
 Center
Science Park, Research Division
Smithville, Texas 78957

D. J. Fitzgerald
Division of Environmental
 Carcinogenesis
International Agency for Research on
 Cancer
69372 Lyon Cedex 08, France

G. Fürstenberger
Institute of Biochemistry
D-6900 Heidelberg, FRG

Norbert E. Fusenig
Institute of Biochemistry
German Cancer Research Center
6900 Heidelberg, FRG

K. Gaido
Department of Cell Biology
Chemical Industry Institute of
 Toxicology
Research Triangle Park, North Carolina
27709

Brenda I. Gerwin
Laboratory of Human Carcinogenesis
Division of Cancer Etiology
National Cancer Institute
Bethesda, Maryland 20892

Michael Z. Gilman
Whitehead Institute
Cambridge, Massachusetts 02142

Tona Gilmer
Laboratory of Pulmonary Pathology
National Institute for Environmental
 Health Sciences
Research Triangle Park, North Carolina
27709

W. F. Greenlee
Department of Cell Biology
Chemical Industry Institute of
 Toxicology
Research Triangle Park, North Carolina
27709

Curtis C. Harris
Laboratory of Human Carcinogenesis
Division of Cancer Etiology
National Cancer Institute
Bethesda, Maryland 20892

Henry Hennings
Laboratory of Cellular Carcinogenesis
and Tumor Promotion
National Cancer Institute
Bethesda, Maryland 20892

Gerard M. Housey
Division of Environmental Sciences
Cancer Center and Institute of Cancer
Research
Columbia University
New York, New York 10032

Eliezer Huberman
Department of Energy
Argonne National Laboratory
Argonne, Illinois 60439

Mark D. Johnson
Division of Environmental Sciences
Cancer Center and Institute of Cancer
Research
Columbia University
New York, New York 10032

David G. Kaufman
Department of Pathology
University of North Carolina
Chapel Hill, North Carolina 27514

Yang Ke
Laboratory of Human Carcinogenesis
Division of Cancer Etiology
National Cancer Institute
Bethesda, Maryland 20892

Ann R. Kennedy
Department of Cancer Biology
Harvard School of Public Health
Boston, Massachusetts 02115

V. Kinzel
German Cancer Research Center
Institute of Experimental Pathology
D-6900 Heidelberg, FRG

Paul Kirschmeier
Division of Environmental Sciences
Cancer Center and Institute of Cancer
Research
Columbia University
New York, New York 10032

E. Laconi
Department of Pathology
Medical Sciences Building
University of Toronto
Toronto, Ontario M5S 1A8, Canada

Robert Langenbach
Toxicology Research and Testing
Program
National Institute of Environmental
Health Sciences
Research Triangle Park, North Carolina
27709

Moira A. LaVeck
Laboratory of Human Carcinogenesis
Division of Cancer Etiology
National Cancer Institute
Bethesda, Maryland 20892

John F. Lechner
Laboratory of Human Carcinogenesis
Division of Cancer Etiology
National Cancer Institute
Bethesda, Maryland 20892

M. I. Lerman
Laboratory of Experimental Pathology
National Cancer Institute
Frederick, Maryland 21701

Rob M. Liskamp
Division of Environmental Sciences
Cancer Center and Institute of Cancer
Research
Columbia University
New York, New York 10032

George W. Lucier
National Institute of Environmental
Health Sciences
Research Triangle Park, North Carolina
27709

F. Marks
Institute of Biochemistry
D-6900 Heidelberg, FRG

Tohru Masui
Laboratory of Human Carcinogenesis
Division of Cancer Etiology
National Cancer Institute
Bethesda, Maryland 20892

Pamela L. Minor
Department of Medicinal Chemistry
Purdue University
West Lafayette, Indiana 47907

Masao Miyashita
Laboratory of Human Carcinogenesis
Division of Cancer Etiology
National Cancer Institute
Bethesda, Maryland 20892

R. J. Morris
University of Texas System Cancer
  Center
Science Park, Research Division
Smithville, Texas 78957

Masashi Naito
University of Texas System Cancer
  Center
Science Park, Research Division
Smithville, Texas 78957

Karen Nelson
Laboratory of Biochemical Risk
  Analysis
National Institute for Environmental
  Health Sciences
Research Triangle Park, North Carolina
  27709

Paul Nettesheim
Laboratory of Pulmonary Pathology
National Institute for Environmental
  Health Sciences
Research Triangle Park, North Carolina
  27709

Catherine A. O'Brian
Division of Environmental Sciences
Cancer Center and Institute of Cancer
  Research
Columbia University
New York, New York 10032

J. F. O'Connell
University of Texas System Cancer
  Center
Science Park, Research Division
Smithville, Texas 78957

R. Osborne
Department of Cell Biology
Chemical Industry Institute of
  Toxicology
Research Triangle Park, North Carolina
  27709

B. C. Pence
University of Texas System Cancer
  Center
Science Park, Research Division
Smithville, Texas 78957

R. T. Petrusevska
Institute of Biochemistry
German Cancer Research Center
D-6900 Heidelberg, FRG

Henry C. Pitot
McArdle Laboratory for Cancer
  Research
Departments of Oncology and Pathology
University of Wisconsin
Madison, Wisconsin 53706

N. Pohlmann
Institute of Biochemistry
German Cancer Research Center
D-6900 Heidelberg, FRG

S. Rajalakshmi
Department of Pathology
Medical Sciences Building
University of Toronto
Toronto, Ontario M5S 1A8, Canada

P. M. Rao
Department of Pathology
University of Toronto
Toronto, Ontario M5S 1A8, Canada

Roger Reddel
Laboratory of Human Carcinogenesis
Division of Cancer Etiology
National Cancer Institute
Bethesda, Maryland 20892

J. J. Reiners, Jr.
*University of Texas System Cancer
    Center*
Science Park, Research Division
Smithville, Texas 78957

Edgar Rivedal
*Laboratory for Environmental and
    Occupational Cancer*
Institute for Cancer Research
Norwegian Radium Hospital
Montebello, N-0310 Oslo 3, Norway

L. Ross
Department of Cell Biology
*Chemical Industry Park, North
    Carolina 27709*

J. B. Rotstein
*University of Texas System Cancer
    Center*
Science Park, Research Division
Smithville, Texas 78957

Tore Sanner
*Laboratory for Environmental and
    Occupational Cancer*
Institute for Cancer Research
Norwegian Radium Hospital
Montebello, N-0310 Oslo 3, Norway

D. S. R. Sarma
Department of Pathology
Medical Sciences Building
University of Toronto
Toronto, Ontario M5S 1A8, Canada

Philippe Shubik
Green College
Oxford 0X2 6HG England

Jill M. Siegfried
Carcinogenesis Section
*Environmental Health Research and
    Testing, Inc.*
*Research Triangle Park, North Carolina
    27709*

Andrew Sivak
Arthur D. Little, Inc.
Cambridge, Massachusetts 02140

T. J. Slaga
*University of Texas System Cancer
    Center*
Science Park, Research Division
Smithville, Texas 78957

Geoffrey I. Sunahara
*Laboratory of Biochemical Risk
    Analysis*
*National Institute for Environmental
    Health Sciences*
*Research Triangle Park, North Carolina
    27709*

Raymond W. Tennant
Cellular and Genetic Toxicology Branch
*National Institute of Environmental
    Health Sciences*
*Research Triangle Park, North Carolina
    27709*

Charles C. Tong
Director of Toxicology
United States Testing Company, Inc.
Hoboken, New Jersey 07030

J. E. Trosko
Center for Environmental Toxicology
College of Human Medicine
Michigan State University
East Lansing, Michigan 48824

Alice S. Tu
Arthur D. Little, Inc.
Cambridge, Massachusetts 02140

S. Vasudevan
Department of Pathology
Medical Sciences Building
University of Toronto
Toronto, Ontario M5S 1A8, Canada

Alison Vickers
Sandoz LTD, 881
CH-4002 Basel, Switzerland

Cheryl Walker
Laboratory of Pulmonary Pathology
*National Institute for Environmental
    Health Sciences*
*Research Triangle Park, North Carolina
    27709*

Robert A. Weinberg
Whitehead Institute
Cambridge, Massachusetts 02142

I. Bernard Weinstein
Division of Environmental Sciences
Cancer Center and Institute of Cancer
  Research
Columbia University
New York, New York 10032

F. Welsch
Department of Cell Biology
Chemical Industry Institute of
  Toxicology
Research Triangle Park, North Carolina
  27709

James C. Willey
Laboratory of Human Carcinogenesis
Division of Cancer Etiology
National Cancer Institute
Bethesda, Maryland 20892

Gary M. Williams
Naylor Dana Institute for Disease
  Prevention
American Health Foundation
Valhalla, New York 10595

H. Yamasaki
Division of Environmental
  Carcinogenesis
International Agency for Research on
  Cancer
69372 Lyon Cedex 08, France

George H. Yoakum
Laboratory of Human Carcinogenesis
Division of Cancer Etiology
National Cancer Institute
Bethesda, Maryland 20892

Tumor Promoters: Biological Approaches for Mechanistic Studies and Assay Systems,
edited by Robert Langenbach et al.
Raven Press, New York © 1988.

TUMOR PROMOTION - THE SEARCH FOR THE
NECESSARY AND SUFFICIENT

(Largely Referenceless Ruminations)

Dr. Andrew Sivak
Arthur D. Little, Incorporated
25 Acorn Park
Cambridge, MA 02140

The literature on tumor promotion is replete with descriptions of cellular and biochemical responses which the authors describe as necessary, but not sufficient to account for a tumor promotion response. The search for the mechanisms involved in the multistep process of carcinogensis go back to the earliest descriptions of experimental carcinogenesis studies. Indeed, Tsutsui (1) in his 1918 report of a mouse skin carcinogenesis experiment with coal tar stated:

"With tar painting, it is unquestionable that certain chemical substances in tar must be imputed as chronic chemical stimuli for the origination of carcinoma. Yet, one must not desregard mechanical lesions, since the animals often bite themselves at the painted sites, or the continued painting more or less wounds by removal of scabs."

It is clear that this early investigator already recognized the complex nature of the process of carcinogenesis. Shortly after Tsutsui's report appeared, Yamagiwa and Ichikawa (2) performed the first initiation-promotion experiment in rabbits using coal tar as an initiator and scarlet oil as promoter and concluded:

"The repetition or continuation of chronic irritation may cause a precancerous alteration in the epithelim previously normal. If the irritant continues its action, carcinoma may be the outcome."

Their conclusion needs hardly any modification to give it a contemporary ring.

Although the contemporary definitions and nomenclature for the phenomenon of tumor promotion are most often attributed to Peyton Rous (3,4), it was in fact a Dutch pathologist, H.T. Deelman(5,6,7) working at the University of Groningen, who, at least 10 years prior to Rous publications, described and defined the nature of tumor promotion based on his mouse skin carcinogenicity studies.

Among his extensive and detailed writings, several statements stand out as seminal contributions from which much of our present general view of the multistage nature of carcinogenesis derives (5):

> "The primary changes which lead to cancer must be sought in the epithelium itself."

> "We can divide the process into two phases, a first phase in which we see nothing macroscopically, and a second phase which begins locally in epithelial outgrowth, and which, sooner or later, develops into a cancer."

> The tar treatment must have an influence on the cells which can remain latent in the cells. We now see that the tumor forming attributes of the cells also can remain latent while the cells continue dividing and the original tar treatment has long been stopped."

The idea of the latency of initiated cells which have been permanently altered, and with the influence of some secondary, non-carcinogenic exposures develop into tumors, is laid out in elegant simplicity.

Though the field of study of tumor promotion in the early decades of this century was not nearly as crowded as it is today, solid work was done by a number of investigators whose names do not even appear in many historical reviews of tumor promotion (Table 1).

TABLE 1

FORGOTTEN NAMES IN TUMOR PROMOTION

J. Fibiger and F. Bang (8)	(1920)
J.A. Murray and W.H. Woglom (9)	(1921)
H.T. Deelman (5,6,7)	(1922-1929)
J.M. Twort and C.C. Twort (10)	(1939)
P.Rous and J.G. Kidd (3)	(1941)

A reading of the works of these authors remains instructive since their experimental efforts provide the basis for our now readily accepted truisms with respect to the focal nature of the lesions that develop into tumors by promotion, the reversibility of promotion by withdrawal of the promoter agent in mouse and rabbit skin experiments and the contribution of promotion to both growth and malignant progression of neoplastic lesions.

The modern era of the study of the phenomenon of tumor promotion begins with the work of Mottram (11) who started his studies in the early 1930's and of Berenblum and Shubik (12) in the mid 1940's. To be sure, the experimental design established by Berenblum and Shubik remains the standard without substantial change for mouse skin experiments to study promotion. Moreover, the development of promotion models with other organs in experimental animal systems trace their parentage directly the Berenblum-Shubik model.

Until the mid 1960's, a small, but dedicated, group of investigators (13,14,15) toiled using the mouse skin initiation-promotion system to study the chemistry of promoters, especially the phorbol esters, to identify promoters in cigarette smoke condensate and to examine the biology and biochemistry of promotion using the tools available to us at the time. Indeed, the discovery that a phorbol ester could have a dramatic effect on the expression of neoplastic properties in a cellular system (16) spawned one of the major growth industries related to the use of these remarkable plant derived chemicals in every imaginable biological system.

While the studies of that generation now seem old fashioned, the experiments that were performed by the few investigators who, at that time, recognized the importance of the concept of tumor promotion led to some very basic ideas that later were expanded and extended by others. Among these ideas were the multistep nature of promotion (conversion, promotion, progression), the discovery of "dark cells" and their possible relationship to differentiation defects, the importance of dose, frequency and interval of tumor promotion exposure for the tumor response and the observation that some agents not active as carcinogens for mouse skin could act as potent initiating agents. In addition, the studies on inhibition of initiation and promotion in the mouse skin system were the beginning of the effort in chemoprevention of cancer, which now is a significant experimental thrust in its own right in cancer research.

With the 1970's came the explosion in interest in tumor promotion driven by the development of experimental systems to study this phenomenon in the organs representing the major sites of cancer burden in humans (bladder, breast, colon, esophagus, liver, lung and stomach) and by the observation that phorbol esters would perturb almost any biological system they encountered. While the search for the sufficient factor that was rate limiting for the tumor promotion sequence to yield malignant lesions was sought assiduously, the litany of vital markers that were proposed as central to tumor promotion, largely from experiments with phorbol esters on mouse skin and in a myriad of cellular and biochemical systems, now has a somewhat hollow ring. While several of these markers are still pursued with vigor, the experimental labors of a decade or more did not identify specific causal mechanisms in tumor promotion that are related to the responses studied (ornithine decarboxylase, protease activity, lectin binding, histone phosphorylation, cyclic nuleotide metabolism, archidonic acid/prostaglandin conversions, phospholipid metabolism).

The present decade can be characterized as the bandwagon era. Whether this phenomenon is a generic one that afflicts all the experimental sciences rushing to embrace the latest fashionable methodologies, or is peculiar to the cadre of investigators studying carcinogenesis is not evident, and probably not important in the long run.

Among the responses that are presently being examined with great activity by many groups the world over are active oxygen, promoter receptors and protein kinase C, metabolic cooperation, differentiation maladjustment, enzyme altered foci, and very likely the biological bandwagon of all time, oncogenes. Though excellent, and sometimes brilliant, experimental work has been done measuring the effects of tumor promoters in the various popular systems, one can genuinely ask whether we are any closer to finding the sufficient step in tumor promotion than was Deelman in his extraordinarily insightful observations of the late 1920's.

With all the inventiveness and energy that has been applied to finding the yet elusive Rosetta stone of tumor promotion, the view must be entertained that there may be no single sufficient step in the set of events related to tumor promotion. While tumor promotion, for much of the time it has been studied, was considered to be physiologically based, and the view that there may be a genetic component would have been considered heresy at the least, our present information strongly suggests that both types of phenomena may be important. If this be the case, some courageous investigator needs to design experiments to address the role of the genes and their products as well as the role of the modulation of the operation of these gene products by tumor promoters. This is a formidable task.

Beyond the prospect that there well may be multiple sufficient factors that must operate either in a sequential or parallel array to account for the phenomenon of tumor promotion, there are several factors that have surely been minimally considered, although they both have been adequately demonstrated to be extremely important in carcinogenesis. One of these factors is an appropriate consideration of how modulation of the tumor promotion response is influenced by the immune system of the host. Although there is ample evidence that at least the phorbol esters are potent modulators of the function of a variety of cell types in the immune system, the application of this observation to explore the influence of immunological perturbation in tumor promotion studies appears to be largely ignored to the present time.

Similarly, the strong evidence that at least a number of DNA viruses play a role in the occurrence of several human and experimental animal tumors has not been seized upon to any significant degree by those exploring the mysteries of tumor promotion to probe into the role of the key biological cancer vectors.

With the fascination concerning oncogenes running at a fever pitch, there is little question that they wil be explored in considerable detail to determine their relationship to the promotion process. Yet, with the increasing complexity engendered by a growing catalog of these gene sequences and their location on almost every human chromosome (Table 2) (17) the rationalization of the role of oncogenes in the development of cancers and in their possible participation in tumor promotion will undoubtedly occupy considerable research resources over the coming years (18).

TABLE 2

<u>17 ONCOGENES ON 17 HUMAN CHROMOSOMES</u>

<u>PROTEIN KINASE</u>	<u>CHROMOSOME</u>
src	20
fps/fes	15
abl	9
yes	?
ros	?
fms	5
mos	8
raf/mil	3,4

<u>NUCLEAR PROTEINS</u>	
N-myc	2
myc	8
fos	14
myb	6
B-lym	1

<u>GTP-ASE</u>	
H-ras	11,X
N-ras	1
K-ras	6,12

<u>PDGF</u>	
sis	22

<u>EGF RECEPTOR</u>	
erb-B	7

With all the fervor of activity in attempting to sort out the mechainisms of tumor promotion, there remain a number of unanswered questions, which are not new and have been articulated in reviews over the last decade (19,20,21,22,23). Some of these are:

.   Beyond the few reasonably sure examples of promotion in humans (lung-asbestos/smoking; breast-hormones), how extensive is promotion as a factor in human cancer burden?

.   Are there animal models for promotion that have relevance for the human situation?

.   Has the omni-pharmacological activity of the phorbol esters raised false expectations about some universality of mechanisms of promotion from organ to organ and species to species?

.   What is the relationship between the detailed molecular parameters being studied and the actual pathological cancer lesion.

A final factor which receives too little attention looks back to the beginnings of the craft of experimental carcinogenesis. When no other tools were available to analyze the events associated with tumor formation and progression other than a tissue section and a microscope, the thoroughness and elegance of description of the cellular and tissue configurations in the development of neoplastic lesions is truly impressive. As our tools have led us to increasingly reductionist approaches to probing the phenomena associated with cancer induction, consideration of the maladjustment of the three dimensional architecture that is the essence of the carcinogenic sequence has diminished. Ultimately, whatever cellular or molecular mysteries are revealed by the powerful analytical means at our disposal now and in the future, they must be related back to the architectural responses of the relevant tissues, if the mechanisms of carcinogen, in general, and tumor promotion, in particular are to yield the understanding that can lead to prevention and inhibition of human cancers.

8   *THE SEARCH FOR THE NECESSARY AND SUFFICIENT*

REFERENCES

1.   Tsutsui, H. Kurze inhaltsangabe der Originalaufsatze. Uber das kunstlich erzeugte Cancroid bei der Maus. Gann 12:17-21 (1918).

2.   Yamagiwa, K., K. Ichikawa. Experimental study of the pathogenesis of carcinoma. J. Cancer Res. 3:1-21 (1918).

3.   Rous, P. J.G. Kidd. Conditional neoplasms and subthreshold neoplastic states: A study of the tar tumors of rabbits. J. Exp. Med. 73:365-390 (1941).

4.   Friedewald, W.F., P. Rous. The initiating and promoting elements in tumor productin. J. Exp. Med. 80:101-126 (1944).

5.   Deelman, H.T., J.P. van Erp. Beobachtungen and experimentallen Tumorwachstum. Z. Krebsforch 24:86-98 (1927).

6.   Deelman, H.T. Uber die histogenese des Teerkrebses. Z. Krebsforsch 19:125-170 (1922).

7.   Deelman, H.T. Das Pracarcinom. Zeitschrift fur Krebsforschung 29:307-319 (1929).

8.   Fibinger, F., R. Bang. Production experimentale du cancer goudron chez la souris blanche. C.R.Soc. Biol 83:157 (1920).

9.   Murray, J.A., W.H. Woglom. Expeimrental tar cancer in mice: Seventh Scientific Report of the Imperial Cancer Research Fund, 1921.

10.   Twort, J.M., C.C. Twort. Comparative activity of some carcinogenic hydrocarbons. Am. J. Cancer 35:80-85, 1939.

11.   Mottram, J.C. A developing factor in experimental blastogenesis. J. Path. Bact. 56:181-187 (1944).

12.   Berenblum, I., P. Shubik. A new quantitative approach to the study of the stages of chemical carcinogenesis in the mouse's skin. Brit. J. Cancer 1:383-391 (1947).

13. Boutwell, R.K. Some biological aspects of skin carcingenesis. Progr. Exp. Tumor Res. 4:207-250 (1964).

14. Hecker, E. Cocarinogenic principles from the seed oil of croton tiglium and other euphorbiacae. Cancer Res., 28:2338-2348 (1968).

15. Van Duuren, B.L. Tumor-promoting agents in two-stage carcinogenesis. Prog. Exp. Tumor Res. 11:31 (1969).

16. Sivak, A., B.L. Van Duuren. Phenotypic expression of transformation: Inductin in cell culture by a phorbol ester. Science 157:1443-1444 (1967).

17. Weiss, R.A., C.J. Marshall. DNA in medicine - Oncogenes. The Lancet, 1138-1142, November (1984).

18. Balmain, A. Transforming ras oncogenes and multistage carcinogenesis. Br. J.Cancer 51:1-7 (1985).

19. Berenblum, I. Guest Editorial: Established principlea and unresolved problems in carcinogenesis. J. Nat. Cancer Inst. 60:723-726 (1978).

20. Sivak, A. Mechanisms of tumor promotion and cocarcinogenesis: A summary from one point of view, in Mechanisms of Cocarcinogenesis and Tumor Promotion, ed. T.J.Slaga, A. Sivak and R.K. Boutwell, Raven Press, New York, p. 553-564 (1978).

21. Becker, F.F. Presidential Address: Recent concepts of intiation and promotion in carcinogenesis. Amer. Assoc. of Pathologists 105:3-9 (1981).

22. Weinstein, I.B. Carcinogenesis asa multistage process-experimental evidence. Printed from: Host Factors in Human CarcinogenesisB. Armstrong, H. Bartsch.Lyon (IARC Scientific Publications No. 39), 1982.

23. Cairns, J. The origin of human cancers. Nature 289:353-357 (1981).

Tumor Promoters: Biological Approaches for
Mechanistic Studies and Assay Systems,
edited by Robert Langenbach et al.
Raven Press, New York © 1988.

Mechanisms of Carcinogenesis Using Mouse Skin:
The Multistage Assay Revisited

S.M. Fischer, J.J. Reiners, Jr., B.C. Pence, C.M. Aldaz, C.J.
Conti, R.J. Morris, J.F. O'Connell, J.B. Rotstein and T.J. Slaga

University of Texas System Cancer Center
Science Park - Research Division
Smithville, Texas 78957

Available information suggests that chemical carcinogenesis
is a multistage process with one of the best studied models in
this regard being the mouse skin. Figure 1 summarizes the operational protocols used to achieve skin tumors; these protocols
provide mechanistic and working definitions for the various
stages. Skin tumors can be induced by direct or indirect acting
carcinogens, either as the result of the application of a single
large dose or smaller fractionated doses. This by definition is
referred to as complete carcinogenesis. Tumors can also be induced by the application of a subthreshold dose of a carcinogen
(initiation stage) followed by repetitive treatment with a noncarcinogenic tumor promoter. The initiation stage requires only a
single application of either a direct or indirect acting carcinogen and is an essentially irreversible process. The promotion
stage on the other hand is brought about only by repetitive
treatments after initiation and is initially reversible, later
becoming irreversible. Two-stage carcinogenesis, i.e., initiation and promotion has been previously extensively reviewed
(45). The promotion stage can be further subdivided such that
agents can be classified as complete or first vs. second stage
promoters (40,41). In addition, agents have been identified
(16,30,38) which enhance the conversion or progression of benign
tumors (papillomas) to malignant tumors (carcinomas).

The value of a multistage carcinogenesis system such as the
mouse skin system is two-fold: first as a bioassay system and
secondly, as a system in which to elucidate the mechanisms of
action of carcinogens, promoters and progressors.

Mouse skin as a bioassay system

The mouse skin system can be used not only to determine the
tumor initiating and promoting activities of a compound but if the
agent is given repeatedly by itself one can also determine if it

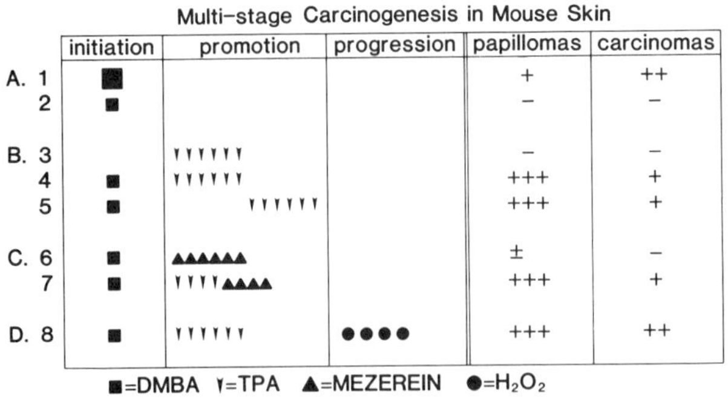

Multi-stage Carcinogenesis in Mouse Skin

	initiation	promotion	progression	papillomas	carcinomas
A. 1	■			+	++
2	■			−	−
B. 3		ΥΥΥΥΥΥ		−	−
4	■	ΥΥΥΥΥΥ		+++	+
5	■	ΥΥΥΥΥΥ		+++	+
C. 6	■	▲▲▲▲▲▲		±	−
7	■	ΥΥΥΥ▲▲▲		+++	+
D. 8	■	ΥΥΥΥΥΥ	●●●●	+++	++

■=DMBA Υ=TPA ▲=MEZEREIN ●=H₂O₂

Figure 1

is a complete carcinogen; i.e., if it has both tumor initiating and promoting activity. Additionally, if an agent is given concurrently with a known complete carcinogen or a tumor initiator it can also be determined if the agent has co-carcinogenic or co-initiating activity or even possibly anti-carcinogenic activity. Likewise some agents may display co-promoting activity when used in the appropriate protocols. This system is therefore an important model for bioassaying the carcinogenic potentials of many diverse compounds. While tissue-specificity remains the major disadvantage of the skin system, which is also true for other model systems, the list of agents that have initiating and/or promoting activity is quite lengthy. Table 1 provides a catalogue (that is by no means complete) of known mouse skin tumor promoters. Although the phorbol esters are the most potent and most widely used, a variety of structurally dissimilar compounds have been shown to have promoting activity. The value in identifying diverse agents as promoters lies not only in possible applicability to the human situation but also that structure-function studies may provide information useful for predicting whether or not an agent has promoting activity.

In using the mouse skin system as a bioassay tool for identifying the carcinogenic or promoting properties of an agent it must be kept in mind that extreme differences in susceptibilities between strains and stocks of mice exist with regard to certain classes of compounds. The most notable example is a comparison of SENCAR and C57Bl/6J mice. As demonstrated by Reiners et al. (34,35) and shown in Table 2, TPA is an excellent promoter in the SENCAR but has little activity in the C57Bl/6J mice. This is most likely not due to significant differences in initiation since (a) the C57Bl/6J are more sensitive than SENCAR to complete skin carcinogenesis protocols using either 7,12 dimethylbenz[a]anthracene (DMBA) or benzo(a)pyrene (B(a)P) and (b) since benzoyl peroxide is an effective promoter in both mice. The difference in susceptibility to phorbol ester promotion is proving to be beneficial both

TABLE 1. <u>Mouse skin tumor promoters</u>

A. Complete Promoters[d]	Potency
Croton oil.	Strong
Certain phorbol esters found in croton oil.	Strong
Some synthetic phorbol esters	Strong
Certain euphorbia latices	Strong
Anthralin	Moderate
Certain fatty acids and fatty acid methyl esters. . . .	Weak
Certain long chain alkanes.	Weak
A number of phenolic compounds.	Weak
Surface active agents (sodium lauryl sulfate, Tween 60)	Weak
Citrus oils	Weak
Methyl ethyl ketone peroxide.	Weak[b]
Extracts of unburned tobacco.	Moderate
Tobacco smoke condensate.	Moderate
Iodoacetic acid	Weak
1-Fluoro-2,4-dinitrobenzene	Moderate
Benzo(e)pyrene.	Moderate
Benzoyl peroxide.	Moderate
7-Bromomethylbenz(a)anthacene	Strong
Dihydroteleocidin B[1].	Strong
Aplysiatoxin.	Strong[c]
Lyngbyatoxin A.	Strong[c]

B. First Stage Promoters	
TPA	Strong
4-O-Me TPA.	Moderate
A 23187	Moderate

C. Second Stage Promoters	
Mezerein.	Strong
RPA	Strong[d]

[a] See Slaga et al. (1983), Mech. of Tumor Promotion, vol.1, for individual references except where noted.
[b] Logani et al. (1984) Fd. Chem. Toxic. 22:879-882.
[c] See Fujiki and Sugimura (1983), Cancer Surveys, vol 2; pp. 539.
[d] In NMRI mice.

in studies on the genetics of promotion, as will be discussed in detail by John DiGiovanni in a later chapter, and in studies on the mechanisms of tumor promoter action. Since the development and availability of mouse strains selectively bred for suscepti- bility or resistance to skin carcinogenesis should allow the performance of meaningful experiments with regard to mechanisms, we have recently developed an inbred strain of the outbred stock of SENCAR mouse (14). Furthermore, in many situations, particu- larly tissue transplantation studies, an inbred strain is more useful than an outbred stock. The SENCAR mouse has been ranked along with the DBA/2 as one of the more sensitive mice with respect to TPA-promotion (8). The inbred strain, designated SSIN, was selected through a 10-generation challenge-selection protocol of DMBA-initiation and TPA-promotion (14). These animals are now past the 20th generation and are considered inbred based on tail skin grafting histocompatability. A comparison of these mice with the outbred SENCAR indicates that the SSIN are much more sensitive to phorbol esters than the parental stock. A typical tumor experiment is shown in Figure 2 in which the increased sensitivity is particularly notable at the lower doses of TPA. Continuing work on the genotypes/phenotypes confering sensitivity or resistance to carcinogens or promoters will be very helpful in elucidating the mechanisms of action of these agents.

TABLE 2.   Influence of genetic background, tumor protocol and agents used for initiation and promotion on skin tumor development

Stock or Strain	Protocol	Initiator	Promoter	Relative no. tumors	
				Paps	Carcinomas
SENCAR	complete	DMBA	---	++++	++
		BP	---	+	+
				+++++	
	two-stage	DMBA	TPA	+++++	+
		BP	TPA	++++++	+
				++++	
		DMBA	BzPo	++++	+
C57B1/6J	complete	DMBA	---	++++	++++
		BP	---	-	+++++
	two-stage	DMBA	TPA	+	+
		BP	TPA	+	-
		DMBA	BzPo	+	++
		BP	BzPo	-	+++

Data from Reiners et al. (35).
BzPo = benzoyl peroxide

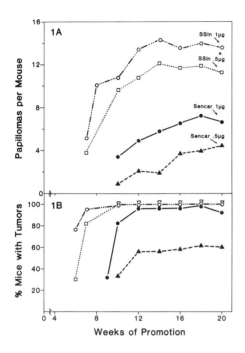

Figure 2. Comparison of the tumor response between the inbred (SSIN) and outbred SENCAR. Groups of 30 mice were initiated with 10 nmol DMBA and promoted with TPA twice weekly at the doses shown. Data from Fischer et al. (14).

Mouse Skin for Mechanism Studies

The mouse skin system is extremely useful in addressing the questions of how tumor promoters carry-out their promoting activity and whether there are common mechanisms of action for structurally diverse promoting agents. Multistage promotion is particularly valuable because comparisons of the biological effects of complete and partial promoters (i.e., TPA and mezerein) can be made with the hope of distinguishing between the common and unique features of each. In addition the repertoire of inhibitors with known activities, i.e., antioxidants or protease inhibitors, continue to be useful in elucidating the sequence of biochemical events apparently needed for the promoting process. This aspect has been most thoroughly studied and reviewed by Slaga et al. (39-45).

One of the important questions in chemical carcinogenesis is the identification of the target cell that becomes initiated. Effective initiators, such as the polycyclic hydrocarbons, have in common the capacity for covalent binding to DNA and the ability to cause an essentially irreversible alteration of the genome. In fact, one characteristic of initiation is that very similar tumor responses are evoked regardless of whether promotion is begun 1 week or 1 year after initiation. This suggests that an epidermal stem cell is the ultimate target for chemical carcinogens (43,44).

Morris et al. (26,27) have recently described evidence that a population of epidermal cells with the requisite characteristics of stem cells retains carcinogen for at least one month after a single application while the amplifying population and postmitotic maturing keratinocytes are lost from the skin due to turnover and terminal differentiation. An epidermal stem cell is a good candidate for an initiated cell because of its stem cell characteristics: i.e., it is a small slowly cycling population occupying a characteristic position within the tissue architecture and capable of clonogenic regeneration, continuous self-renewal and the production of progeny that terminally differentiate.

Toward this end Morris et al. (unpublished data) have developed an in vitro assay for identifying and quantitating clonogenic epidermal cells. This assay has been used to quantitate the number of clonogenic cells during two-stage carcinogenesis. It would be predicted that initiation would not alter the number of clonogenic cells isolated from mice at various times after initiation. On the other hand, application of tumor promoters would be expected to expand the population of initiated cells but not normal stem cells. The data from the clonogenic cell assay (Table 3) strongly suggests that this is the case.

The possibility that these putative stem cells are selected for during TPA promotion comes also from the work of Morris et al. (26). The kinetics of the mitotic responses to TPA of these putative stem cells was compared to the amplifying or maturing classes of basal cells in the epidermis of adult mice. Through the use of ^{3}H-thymidine labeling at specified times before or

TABLE 3. Colony formation by epidermal cells during two-stage carcinogenesis

Number of Promoting Treatments	Number of Colonies per 10,000 Viable Epidermal Cells Initiator/Promoting Agent				
	Nor/Nor	Ace/Ace	Ace/TPA	DMBA/Ace	DMBA/TPA
1	32 ± 5.1	31 ± 2.7	43 ± 2.4	37 ± 1.3	47 ± 3.1
4	33 ± 2.1	30 ± 6.4	32 ± 4.9	27 ± 4.5	57 ± 7.5
5	-	39 ± 4.0	34 ± 2.8	47 ± 3.5	62 ± 6.2
12	45 ± 3.0	54 ± 4.1	62 ± 7.1	56 ± 6.3	101 ± 7.9

CD-1 mice were initiated with either 200 nmol DMBA, nothing (Nor) or acetone (Ace) and twice weekly promotion with 17 nmol TPA or acetone started 1 week later. Cells were harvested 4 weeks after the last promotion treatment and plated on a Swiss 3T3 cell feeder layer in collagen coated dishes. Colonies were counted after 2 to 3 weeks.

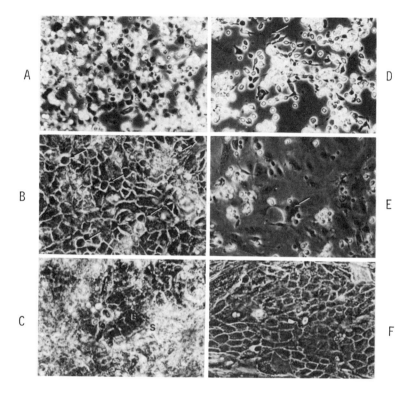

Figure 3. <u>Primary cultures of adult murine epidermal cells</u>
<u>(200 x)</u>. A, control cultures 48 hr after plating; B, control
cultures after 7 days; C, control cultures after two weeks; D,
24 hr old cultures treated for 24 hr with 0.1 µg/ml TPA; E,
7 day TPA-treated cultures; F, two week TPA-treated culture.

after TPA it was shown that the putative stem population, located
at the center of the proliferative units, undergo mitosis within
22 h of TPA treatment while the "maturing" cells in the basal
layer labeled 4 days earlier with ^{3}H-thymidine did not respond
with mitosis but continued to differentiate and undergo displacement to the suprabasal layers.

Additional evidence that populations of basal cells exist
which respond differently to TPA comes from recent <u>in vitro</u>
studies by Morris et al. (28). When primary cultures of normal
adult epidermal cells, grown in high calcium medium, are treated
with TPA, it was observed that within one day approximately 70%
of the cells detach from the dish. Of the remaining cells, most
undergo morphological changes such as elongation that have been
previously reported by others. A small population of cells,

however, remains morphologically unaltered by TPA treatment. After one or two weeks, nests of small basal cells formed and expanded until the dish became confluent and indistinguishable from the control cultures. Studies using cells from carcinogen-treated mice are currently underway to determine if differences in behavior and perhaps in vitro promotion can be demonstrated.

The means by which phorbol esters, the most commonly used and most extensively studied tumor promoters, cause promotion remains unknown although much progress has been made in recent years. Table 4 provides a list of possible mechanisms; these are not necessarily mutually exclusive processes and in fact all are probably involved to varying degrees. Since some of these processes, notably protein kinase c, will be described in detail in later chapters, discussion will be restricted primarily to the involvement of reactive oxygens.

TABLE 4. Some Possible Mechanisms of Tumor Promotion

1. Altered expression of specific genes involved in the regulation of growth and/or differentiation; i.e., growth factors, polyamines.

2. Oncogene activation and/or expression: ^{H}ras, c-myc, etc.

3. "Promotion Receptor": protein kinase c

4. Free radical involvement; inflammatory products

Ultimately, direct or indirect selection for a given population of keratinocytes, probably the initiated stem cells.

A substantial amount of evidence has been accumulating that suggests that the generation of reactive oxygen species, particularly superoxide anion and hydroxyl radical, may be involved in tumor promotion. The most direct evidence of free radical involvement comes from the work of Slaga et al. (46) in which free radical generating compounds such as benzoyl peroxide were shown to be complete tumor promoters. The involvement of free radicals in promotion is suggested by the somewhat more indirect evidence from studies using various antioxidants as inhibitors of promotion; butylated hydroxyanisole, vitamins E and C, dimethyl sulfoxide, and the superoxide dismutase (SOD) mimetic copper(II)-[diisopropylsalicylate]$_2$ referred to as CuDIPS have all been shown to inhibit promotion (reviewed in ref. 19,22,48). In addition CuDIPS and butylated hydroxyanisole were also shown to inhibit TPA-induced ornithine decarboxylase activity as described by Kensler and Trush (19) and Kozumbo et al.(21). Solanki et al. (47) found that application of TPA to mouse skin caused a substantial decrease in the level of SOD and catalase, the major detoxification enzymes for superoxide and H_2O_2 respectively. De Chatelet et al. (7) was among the first to demonstrate that treatment of polymorphonuclear leukocytes with TPA results in superoxide anion production. Antipromoters such as dexamethasone, retinoids and protease inhibitors were shown by Witz et al. (49) and Kensler and Trush (18) to counteract this effect.

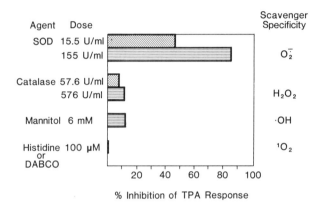

Figure 4. <u>Effect of modifiers of reactive oxygen on TPA-induced oxidants in epidermal cells.</u> Mouse epidermal cells were used in a chemiluminescence assay; the cpm at the peak of the response were used to determine the percentage of the TPA-alone response. Data from Fischer et al. (11).

An important and as yet unresolved question in mouse skin tumor promotion is the contribution of the inflammatory process and in particular the infiltrating macrophages and neutrophils. Since such leukocytes are part of the inflammatory state induced by TPA treatment, their ability to generate free radicals may contribute to the promotion process. A key question therefore is whether such radical generation is restricted to leukocytes or whether epidermal cells may also produce oxidants in response to TPA. We recently were able to demonstrate (11) through chemiluminescence (CL) assays that TPA does in fact induce the production of oxidants from murine epidermal cells. This response is cell number and TPA-dose dependent and a correlation was found between the extent of oxidant production and a series of phorbol esters with different promoting abilities. Based on the use of specific radical scavengers or inhibitors, the principal oxidant is believed to be superoxide anion, as shown in Figure 3. Many known antipromoters inhibited the production of this oxidant by TPA, most notably the retinoids, antioxidants and inhibitors of the

lipoxygenase pathway of arachidonic acid metabolism. These latter inhibitors suggested that at least a major part of the TPA-
induced response was via lipoxygenase metabolism of liberated
arachidonate. This introduces the question of the mechanism of
arachidonate release from phospholipids. Free arachidonate can
result from either phospholipase A_2 or phospholipase C activity
followed by diacylglcerol lipase action. This latter pathway,
illustrated in Figure 5, is of particular interest since TPA
both competes for diacylglycerol (DAG) binding and activation of
protein kinase c (29) and increases DAG production, presumably
through phospholipase C activation (17). Based on the ability

Figure 5. <u>Phospholipid-protein kinase c model</u>

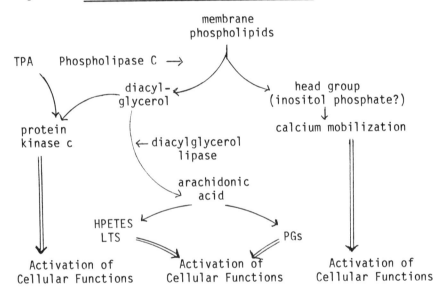

of these two phospholipases to release arachidonate (which has
been demonstrated in epidermal cells prelabeled with ^{14}C-arcachi-
donate), it was predicted that both phospholipases should also
generate oxidants. However, it was found (12) that only phospholipase C, and in particular that isolated from C. perfringens,
produced an oxidant response, as shown in Figure 6. This oxidant
is also believed to be superoxide anion and is inhibited by the
same inhibitors that inhibit the TPA response. The specificity
of this response to phospholipase C has led us to the hypothesis
that specific phospholipid metabolism may be involved in the
TPA-induced oxidant response in mouse epidermal cells. A causal
relationship of this oxidant respone to TPA mediated events is
suggested by the finding that the induction of ODC by TPA may be
mediated in part by reactive oxygens. This is indicated by
experiments on cultured epidermal cells in which ODC was induced

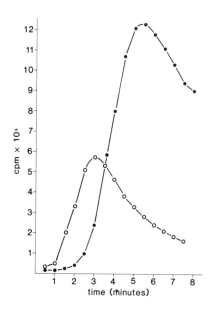

Figure 6. Kinetics of the chemi-luminescence response to either TPA or phospholipase C. Mouse epidermal cells were isolated and treated with either 100 ng/ml TPA (●) or 1 unit/ml phospholipase C (○), as described by Fischer et al. (12).

following treatment with xanthine oxidase and xanthine, an enzyme-substrate system that produces superoxide anion (Figure 7). In addition, ODC induction by either TPA or the xanthine oxidase system can be inhibited by inclusion of SOD in the cultures (unpublished data). This is in agreement with the in vivo inhibition of TPA-induced ODC by antioxidants shown by Kozumbo et al. (22).

Another approach to the issue of reactive oxygen involvement in promotion is the question of whether there are qualitative or quantitative differences in oxidant production in epidermal cells from TPA promotion sensitive vs. resistant mice. As shown in Figure 8 the level of oxidants generated by TPA stimulation of cells from C57Bl/6J mice is considerably less than from either SENCAR or particularly SSIN (13). Similar differences have also

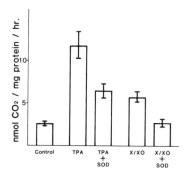

Figure 7. Induction of ornithine decarboxylase by superoxide anion. Primary cultures of mouse epidermal cells were treated with TPA, xanthine and xanthine oxidase (O_2^- generating system), with or without SOD.

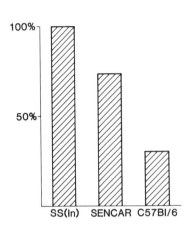

Figure 8.   Strain differences in the ability of TPA to induce oxidant generation in epidermal cells. Freshly isolated mouse epidermal cells were treated with 1 ɲg/ml TPA and the chemiluminescence determined. Data from SSIN arbitrarily set at 100%. Data from Fischer et al. (13).

been reported by Lewis and Adams (23) for H_2O_2 production from peritoneal macrophages from these animals. Collectively these data strongly suggest that TPA-induced oxidant production mediates essential events in tumor promotion.

Very recently, Reiners et al. (36) have found that topical application of TPA elevates xanthine oxidase activity in mouse skin. As shown in Figure 9, maximal elevation occurs 48-96 h after TPA and remains elevated for up to 11 days. Xanthine dehydrogenase (XD) and xanthine oxidase (XO) are purine catabolism enzymes responsible for the conversion of hypoxanthine to xanthine and xanthine to uric acid. As a dehydrogenase XD uses NAD as an oxidant whereas XO uses O_2 as an oxidant resulting in the production of superoxide anion. XD can be converted to XO both in vivo and in vitro by proteolysis, sulfhydryl modifying reagents and heat. It is of interest that elevated XO activity is associated with several pathological conditions including intestinal ischemia, and ethanol associated myocardial and hepatic toxicity. Such elevation of XO is believed to be a causative factor of the cytotoxicity since the XD/XO inhibitor allopurinol can eliminate or lessen the severity of the tissue injury. The mediator of this toxicity is probably superoxide or its reduction products.

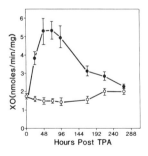

Figure 9.   Kinetics of TPA-stimulated elevation of xanthine oxidase activity in mouse epidermis. Mice were sacrificed at given times after topical treatment with either acetone (o) or 2 ɲg TPA (o) as described by Reiners et al. (36).

TABLE 5. Elevation of xanthine oxidase (xo) in murine epidemis
         by TPA and its analogs[d]

Treatment	Dose (µg)	% control XO activity[b]
Acetone	---	100.0
TPA	1.0	188.7 ± 8.4[c]
	2.0	291.6 ± 11.7[c]
Phorbol	20.0	94.3 ± 6.0
4-0-Me TPA	20.0	100.7 ± 4.6
Phorbol dibenzoate	10.0	178.9 ± 7.0[c]
Mezerein	1.0	259.8 ± 22.7[c]
	2.0	292.3 ± 41.0[c]

[a] Data from Reiners et al. (36).
[b] Epidermal homogenates were prepared from the dorsal skins of
     mice 48 h post-treatment. Values represent the mean ± S.E.M.
     from duplicate determinations of samples from at least 4
     mice.
[c] Significantly different from acetone treated animals.

The role of XO induction in tumor promotion is speculative
at this time. Reiners et al. (36) reported that the promoting
activities of a series of phorbol esters correlated with their
abilities to induce epidermal XO activity. While the first stage
promoter 4-0-methyl TPA had no effect, the second stage promoter
mezerein was a very effective inducer, as shown in Table 5. The
kinetics of XO induction following TPA treatment parallel the
kinetics of epidermal hyperplasia and keratinocyte differentiation following a single topical application of TPA. This suggests that XO induction may be a marker for epidermal hyperplasia
and/or differentiation. Elevated XO activity may possibly be part
of the means by which TPA enhances terminal differentiation (37).

The possible biological consequences of overproduction of
reactive oxygen, referred to as the prooxidant state by Cerutti
(4), are variable, dependent on the type of cell and mechanism of
induction. Major reactions include (a) lipid peroxidation which
can result in such diverse effects as decreased receptor binding,
inhibition of Na-K ATPase, alteration in respiratory function,
etc., (b) activation or inactivation of enzymes, i.e. guanylate
cyclase is activated by hydroperoxides and (c) chromosome aberrations or DNA damage, resulting in changes in gene expression.

This latter, chromosomal aberrations, is of particular interest with respect to the clastogenic factor-inducing activity
of TPA in human lymphocytes reported by Emerit and Cerutti (10)

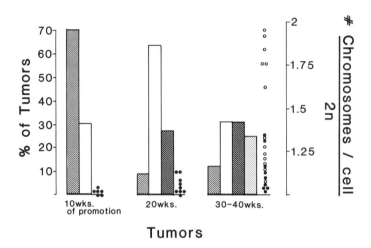

Tumors

Figure 10.   Histopathologic grading and aneuploidy index of
mouse skin tumors. Tumor classification (left ordinate) as
follows:▨ , regular papilloma - a well differentiated hyperplastic lesion with no or very few atypical cells in the basal layer;
□ , moderately dysplastic papilloma - lesions with atypical cells
in the basal and some in the suprabasal layers up to one-third
of the thickness of the epithelium;▦ , severely diplastic papilloma - over two thirds of the thickness of the epithelium occupied by atypical cells;▨ , intrapapillomatous carcinoma - marked
atypia in all layers and lack of differentiation patterns in the
surface. Aneuploidy index (right ordinate) gives the distribution
of chromosome numbers in tumors at given times during promotion.
●, papillomas; o, carcinomas. Data from Aldaz et al. (3) and
Conti et al. (6).

and more pertinently to the alterations seen during mouse skin
tumor development by Dzarlieva and Fusenig (9) and Conti et al.
(6). The biological significance of aneuploidy in cancer has
been recently reviewed by Ohimura and Barrett (33); they concluded
that the principal effects of aneuploidy are genetic disbalance,
phenotypic expression of recessive mutations and changes in
genetic stability. The work of Conti et al.(6) and Aldaz et al.
(1-3) indicates that a high level of chromosomal instability is
characteristic of chemically induced papillomas from the very
early stages. While it is not clear whether this instability is
related either to an event that occurs during initiation or to
the action of tumor promoters (TPA), the reported clastogenicity
(10) and induction of aneuploidy (9) by TPA alone strongly
implicates TPA as causal to the observed instability. Conti et
al. (6) recently presented evidence suggesting that the aneuploid

cells present in the very early papillomas eventually displace the diploid stem line. They have further suggested that the genomic imbalance produced by aneuploidy may be related to the malignant conversion of the benign papillomas. Aldaz et al. (2,3) have recently expanded these observations through a systematic histopathological study of papillomas from different stages of promotion in order to correlate the pathology or extent of cellular atypia with the extent of chromosomal abnormalities. They found that with increasing time of promotion the papillomas shift from diploid, well-differentiated hyperplastic lesions to moderately aneuploid and moderately dyplastic and eventually by 40 weeks of promotion to severe dysplasia with all papillomas showing aneuploidy (Figure 10). These results support their hypothesis that most, if not all, papillomas are truly premalignant lesions in different stages of evolution in the progression toward malignancy. Experimental data from two-stage tumor experiments also indicates that carcinoma incidence almost never reaches a plateau by the time the experiments are terminated.

One complicating feature of progression from papilloma to carcinoma is that the rate of change is variable from one tumor to another. Aldaz et al. (3) have suggested that possibly random chromosomal changes occur constantly in papillomas and carcinomas and that it is by chance that a specific change occurs that confers a selective advantage to a particular clone of cells. This rate of change in progression to a carcinoma can be experimentally increased by the topical application of a number of agents. Hennings et al. (16) and O'Connell et al. (31,32) reported the number of carcinomas but not papillomas increased after limited applications of the tumor initiators N'methyl-N-nitro-nitrosoguanidine (MNNG) and ethyl nitrosuridine (ENU), but not by TPA to mice in the plateau stage of papilloma development. This progression stage of skin carcinogenesis is the least studied and least understood of the stages. Benzoyl peroxide or H_2O_2 can also be used as progressors as described recently by O'Connell et al. (32) and Rotstein et al. (38). As shown in Table 6, the greater the number of benzoyl peroxide applications the higher the carcinoma incidence (38). Because of the limited period of treatment with the progressor agent and due to the latency until carcinomas appear, protocols of this type are amenable to studies of inhibitors of the progression stage.

The mechanisms involved in progression in the mouse skin system are unclear. The carcinogens such as ENU and MNNG that act as progressors are genotoxic compounds and as such may induce mutations and/or increased chromosomal instability leading more rapidly to aneuploidy. In additon to chromosomal alterations, squamous cell carcinomas exhibit a number of changes in gene expression including the lack of high molecular weight keratins (20) and filaggrin (25) as well as the appearance of gamma glutamyl transferase (5). One alternative hypothesis for the cells present in the very early papillomas eventually displace the diploid stem line. They have further suggested that the genomic imbalance produced by aneuploidy may be related to the malignant conversion of the benign papillomas. Aldaz et al. (2,3) have recently expanded these observations through a systematic histopathological study of papillomas from different stages of promotion in order to correlate the pathology or extent of cellular atypia with the extent of chromosomal abnormalities. They found that with increasing time of promotion the papillomas shift from diploid, well-differentiated hyperplastic lesions to moderately aneuploid and moderately dyplastic and eventually by 40 weeks of promotion to severe dysplasia with all papillomas showing aneuploidy (Figure 10). These results support their hypothesis that most, if not all, papillomas are truly premalignant lesions in different stages of evolution in the progression toward malignancy. Experimental data from two-stage tumor experiments also indicates that carcinoma incidence almost never reaches a plateau by the time the experiments are terminated.

One complicating feature of progression from papilloma to carcinoma is that the rate of change is variable from one tumor to another. Aldaz et al. (3) have suggested that possibly random chromosomal changes occur constantly in papillomas and carcinomas and that it is by chance that a specific change occurs that confers a selective advantage to a particular clone of cells. This rate of change in progression to a carcinoma can be experimentally increased by the topical application of a number of agents. Hennings et al. (16) demonstrated following TPA promotion that repetitive treatment with N'methyl-N-nitro-nitrosoguanidine(MNNG) increased papilloma and carcinoma incidence. O'connell et al. (31) reported that the number of carcinomas but not papillomas increased after only limited applications of the initiators MNNG and ethylnitrosourea (ENU), but not by TPA,to mice in the plateau stage of papilloma development. Benzoyl peroxide or H_2O_2 can also be used as progressors as described recently by O'Connell et al. (32) and Rotstein et al. (38). As shown in Table 6, the greater the number of benzoyl peroxide applications the higher the carcinoma incidence (38). Because of the limited number of treatments required with the progressor agent and due to the latency until carcinomas appear, protocols of this type are amenable to studies of inhibitors of the progression stage.

The mechanisms involved in progression in the mouse skin system are unclear. The carcinogens such as ENU and MNNG that act as progressors are genotoxic compounds and as such may induce mutations and/or increased chromosomal instability leading more rapidly to aneuploidy. In additon to chromosomal alterations, squamous cell carcinomas exhibit a number of changes in gene expression including the lack of high molecular weight keratins (20) and filaggrin (25) as well as the appearance of gamma glutamyl transferase (5). One alternative hypothesis for the

TABLE 6. Effects on carcinoma incidence of H_2O_2 and
benzoyl peroxide[a]

Agent	Incidence[b] (%)	% Mice with Carcinomas[c]
Acetone	27/337 (8.0)	41
H_2O_2 (290 nmol)	41/382 (10.7)	64
(880 nmol)	40/397 (12.3)	68
BzPo[d] (83 μmol)		
4 weeks	32/408 (7.8)	61
12 weeks	38/442 (8.6)	74
20 weeks	65/431 (15.1)	81

[a] data from Rotstein et al. (38)
[b] cumulative no. carcinomas/no. papillomas at start
[c] after 20 weeks of progression
[d] BzPo = benzoyl peroxide

action of progressors is related to their high degree of cytotoxicity. In this model, highly cytotoxic agents may (a) selectively or nonselectively kill some cells within a tumor and thus
allow the growth of more malignant cells and/or (b) increase
terminal differentiation of normal cells and thus reduce the
constraints against expansion along the border between normal
and tumor tissue.

Clearly, the progression stage of skin carcinogenesis is the
least studied and least understood of the stages. Protocols
designed to include the progression stage may be useful for
assessing the carcinogenic risk of environmental chemicals. The
need to evaluate chemicals for activity during the progression
stage is underscored by the high potency of benzoyl peroxide and
H_2O_2 in enhancing progression. By contrast, neither agent is
active as a tumor initiator or complete carcinogen and they are
only moderately (benzoyl peroxide) or weakly (H_2O_2) active as
tumor promoters. Consequently, the potency of a tumor promoter
during the first or second stage of promotion does not correlate
with its potency as a progressing agent.

Summary

Multi-stage chemical carcinogenesis in the mouse skin offers
a valuable model system that is useful both as a bioassay system
to test for the tumor initiating, promoting and/or progressing
activity of an agent, and useful for studies designed to elucidate the mechanisms of action of carcinogens, promoters and

progressors. With respect to this last aspect, significant progress has been made toward identifying the target cell that becomes initiated; future work on the biological responses of these cells to tumor promoters should expand our knowledge of early events in the promotion process. A role for reactive oxygens in promotion is strongly suggested; the function of these reactive species remains to be elucidated but at least one TPA-elicited event, the induction of ODC, may be mediated by such oxidants. Whether the chromosome aberrations observed as early as the small papilloma stage are due to reactive oxygens or other TPA-induced events (or perhaps set in motion by initiators) remains to be determined. Finally, the recent identification of agents that enhance the conversion of benign to malignant tumors sets the stage for future studies on the mechanisms of such conversion which will increase our understanding of the cancer process considerably. Ultimately, with increasing knowledge of the biological processes involved in the development of neoplasia, we can hope to someday be able to design rational approaches to interfering with these processes in order to prevent the formation of malignancies.

References

1. Aldaz, C.M., Conti, C.J., Klein-Szanto, A.J.P., and Slaga, T.J. (1986): Cancer Genet. Cytogenet., 20:223-229.
2. Aldaz, C.M., Conti, C.J., O'Connell, J., Yuspa, S.H., Klein-Szanto, A.J.P., and Slaga, T.J. (1986): Cancer Res., 46:3565-3568.
3. Aldaz, C.M., Conti, C.J., Klein-Szanto, A.J.P., and Slaga, T.J. (submitted).
4. Cerutti, P.A. (1985): Science, 227:375-381.
5. Chiba, M., Maley, M.A., and Klein-Szanto, A.J.P. (1986) Cancer Res, 46:259-263.
6. Conti, C.J., Aldaz, C.M., O'Connell, J., Klein-Szanto, A.J.P., and Slaga, T.J. (1986): Carcinogenesis 7:1845-1848.
7. DeChalelet, L.R., Shirley, P.S., and Johnston, R.B. (1976): Blood, 47:545-554.
8. DiGiovanni, J., Prichett, W.P., Decina, P.C., and Diamond, L. (1984): Carcinogenesis, 5:1493-1498.
9. Dzarlieva, R.T. and Fusenig, N.E. (1982): Cancer Lett., 16: 7-17.
10. Emerit, I.E. and Cerutti, P.A. (1981): Nature, 293:144-146.
11. Fischer, S.M. and Adams, L.M. (1985): Cancer Res., 45:3130-3136.
12. Fischer, S.M., Baldwin, J.B., and Adams, L.M. (1985): Biochem. Biophys. Res. Commun., 131:1103-1108.
13. Fischer, S.M., Baldwin, J.B., and Adams, L.M. (1986): Carcinogenesis, 7:915-918.
14. Fischer, S.M., O'Connell, J., Conti, C.J., Tacker, K.C., Fries, J.W., Patrick, K.E., Adams, L.M., and Slaga, T.J., Carcinogenesis (in press).

15. Fujiki, H. and Sugimura, T. (1983): In: Cancer Surveys, vol. 2, edited by T.J. Slaga, and R. Montesano, pp. 539. Oxford Univ. Press, London.
16. Hennings, H., Shores, R., Wenk, M.L., Spangler, E.F., Tarene, R., and Yuspa, S.H. (1983): Nature, 304:67-69.
17. Jeng, A.Y., Lichti, U., Strickland, J.E., and Blumberg (1985): Cancer Res., 45:5714-5721.
18. Kensler, T.W. and Trush, M.A. (1981): Cancer Res., 41: 216-222.
19. Kensler, T.W. and Trush, M.A. (1984): Environ. Mut., 6: 593-616.
20. Klein-Szanto, A.J.P., Nelson, K.G., Shah, Y, and Slaga, T.J. (1983): J. Natl. Cancer Inst., 70:161-168.
21. Kozumbo, W.J., Seed, J.L., and Kensler, T.W. (1983): Cancer Res., 43:2555-2559.
22. Kozumbo, W.J., Seed, J.L., and Kensler, T.W. (1985): Chem.-Biol. Interactions, 54:3061-3066.
23. Lewis, J.G. and Adams, D.O. (1986): Proc. Amer. Assoc. Cancer Res., 27:146.
24. Logani, M.K., Sambuco, C.P., Forbes, P.D., and Davies, R.E. (1984): Fd. Chem. Toxic, 22:879-882.
25. Mamrack, M.D., Klein-Szanto, A.J.P. and Reiners, J.J. and Slaga, T.J. (1984): Cancer Res., 44:2634-2641.
26. Morris, R.J., Fischer, S.M., and Slaga, T.J. (1985) J. Invest. Dermatol. 34:277-281.
27. Morris, R.J., Fischer, S.M., and Slaga, T.J. (1986): Cancer Res., 46:3061-3066.
28. Morris, R.J., Tacker, K.C., Baldwin, J.K., Fischer, S.M., Slaga, T.J.: Cancer Lett (in press).
29. Nishizuka, Y. (1984): Nature, 308:693-698.
30. O'Connell, J.F., Klein-Szanto, A.J.P., DiGiovanni, D.M., Fries, J.W., and Slaga, T.J. (1986a): Cancer Lett. 30:269-274.
31. O'Connell, J.F., Klein-Szanto, A.J.P., DiGiovanni, D.M., Fries, J.W., and Slaga, T.J. (1986b): Cancer Res., 46: 2863-2865.
32. O'Connell, J.F., Rotstein, J.B., and Slaga, T.J. (1986): Banbury Report (in press).
33. Orimura, M. and Barrett, J.C. (1986): Environ. Mut., 8: 129-159.
34. Reiners, J.J., Davidson, K., Nelson, K., Mamrack, M., and Slaga, T.J. (1983): In: Organ and Species Specificity in Chemical Carcinogenesis, vol 24, Basic Life Sciences, edited by R. Langenbach, S. Nesnow, and J.M. Rice, pp. 173-186. Plenum Press, N.Y.
35. Reiners, J.J., Nesnow, S., and Slaga, T.J. (1984): Carcinogenesis, 5:301-307.
36. Reiners, J.J., Pence, B.C., Barcus, M.C.S., and Cantu, A. (1986): Cancer Res. (in press).
37. Reiners, J.J. and Slaga, T.J. (1983): Cell 32:247.

38. Rotstein, J., O'Connell, J., and Slaga, T. (1986): Proc. Amer. Assoc. Cancer Res., 27:143.

39. Slaga, T.J. and Fischer, S.M. (1983): Prog. in Exper. Tumor Res., 26:85-109.

40. Slaga, T.J., Fischer, S.M., Nelson, K.G., and Gleason, G.L. (1980a): Proc. Natl. Acad. Sci. U.S.A., 77:3659-3663.

41. Slaga, T.J., Fischer, S.M., Nelson, K.G., and Major, S. (1980b): Proc. Natl. Acad. Sci. U.S.A., 77:2251-2254.

42. Slaga, T.J., Fischer, S.M., Triplett, L.L., and Nesnow, S. (1972): J. Environ. Pathol. Toxicol. 4:1025-1041.

43. Slaga, T.J., Fischer, S.M., Weeks, C.E., and Klein-Szanto, A.J.P. (1980): In: Biochemistry of Normal and Abnormal Epidermal Differentiation, vol 10, Current Problems in Dermatology, edited by J.A. Bernstein and M. Seiji, pp. 193-218. S. Karger, Basel.

44. Slaga, T.J., Fischer, S.M., Weeks, C.E., Klein-Szanto, A.J.P., and Reiners, J.J. (1982): J. Cell. Biochem., 18:99-119.

45. Slaga, T.J., Sivak, A., and Boutwell, R.K., editors (1977): Carcinogenesis: A Comprehensive Survey, Vol. 2. Raven Press, NY.

46. Slaga, T.J., Klein-Szanto, A.J.P., Triplett, L.L., Yotti, L.P., and Trosko, J.E. (1981): Science, 213:1023-1025.

47. Solanki, V., Rana, R.S., and Slaga, T.J. (1981): Carcinogenesis, 2:1141-1146.

48. Troll, W. and Weisner, R. (1985): Ann. Rev. Pharmacol. Toxicol., 25:509-528.

49. Witz, G., Goldstein, B.D., Amoruso, M., Stone, D.S. and Troll, W. (1980): Biochem. Biophys. Res. Commun. 97:883-888.

Tumor Promoters: Biological Approaches for
Mechanistic Studies and Assay Systems,
edited by Robert Langenbach et al.
Raven Press, New York © 1988.

VARIABLE POTENTIAL FOR MALIGNANT CONVERSION OF PAPILLOMAS INDUCED BY INITIATION-PROMOTION PROTOCOLS

Henry Hennings

Laboratory of Cellular Carcinogenesis and Tumor
Promotion, National Cancer Institute,
Bethesda, MD 20892

MULTISTAGE CARCINOGENESIS IN MOUSE SKIN

Results of studies utilizing the initiation-promotion model of carcinogenesis in mouse skin have provided the basis for many of the generally accepted hypotheses regarding mechanisms of carcinogenesis (1,2,6). Multiple stages have been defined operationally. The first stage, initiation, can be accomplished by a single exposure to a low dose of carcinogen, such as 7,12-dimethylbenz-[a]anthracene (DMBA). Initiation causes a permanent alteration in some epidermal cells, which are termed "initiated". Without subsequent treatment with a tumor promoter, these initiated cells do not develop into tumors. Promotion of initiated skin to produce multiple benign papillomas is accomplished by repeated topical treatments with a promoting agent such as 12-0-tetradecanoyl-phorbol-13-acetate (TPA). Promotion is effective even when promoter exposure is delayed for several months after initiation, indicating that the initiator-induced change is heritable. The effects of individual promoter treatments are reversible. That is, papillomas do not develop after insufficient exposure of initiated skin to promoters or if the interval between treatments is prolonged. The stage in which papillomas progress to squamous cell carcinomas has been termed "malignant conversion" (9). This process, which proceeds spontaneously at a low frequency, is unaffected by further TPA treatments after papilloma appearance (9). However, treatment of papilloma-bearing mice with tumor initiators (9) or other agents (13) greatly increases the frequency of conversion of benign to malignant tumors.

The irreversibility of both initiation and malignant conversion suggests a genetic mechanism for these stages. The reversibility of promotion, on the other hand, indicates an epigenetic mechanism. The selection for the growth of the cells with altered developmental potential, the initiated cells, during tumor promotion may involve changes in gene expression, differentiation and proliferation. The induction of terminal differentiation of normal epidermal cells by the promoter, combined with the inability of initiated cells to respond to this stimulus (7), could

31

accomplish the selective growth of initiated cells (16), resulting in a papilloma. Alternatively, some promoters could act by selective toxicity, in which initiated cells can survive a higher dose of the promoter than the surrounding normal epidermal cells (5). The high rate of proliferation in promoter-treated epidermis and in papillomas may facilitate the subsequent irreversible changes necessary for conversion to malignancy.

The stages of initiation, resulting in initiated cells, promotion, resulting in benign lesions (papillomas), and malignant conversion, in which benign tumors convert to malignant tumors (carcinomas), are illustrated in Figure 1. Progression of papillomas to metastatic carcinomas involves at least 2 stages, malignant conversion followed by a metastatic change. As indicated in Figure 1, at least two types of initiated cells are hypothesized (14), based on the types of papillomas which develop after promotion by TPA. Two types of papillomas can be identified in initiation-promotion experiments: those which regress and do not convert to carcinomas and those which persist and can potentially convert to carcinomas spontaneously (3,8). Experimental evidence supporting the heterogeneity of papillomas, as well as protocols for producing persistent papillomas, will be presented in the next section. The characteristics of the malignant conversion stage which distinguish it from the stage of promotion will be discussed in the last section.

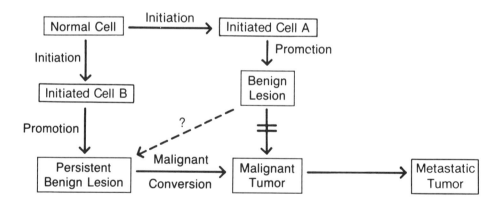

FIG. 1. Stages in carcinogenesis.

PAPILLOMAS ARE HETEROGENEOUS IN THEIR POTENTIAL FOR CONVERSION TO CARCINOMAS

To assess whether the duration of promoter treatment might have a differential effect on development of papillomas and carcinomas, SENCAR mice initiated with DMBA were promoted with TPA for 5, 10, 20, or 40 weeks. With 10, 20 or 40 weeks of promotion, a peak papilloma incidence at 15-20 weeks was followed by a 35-40% decrease by Week 28 (8). With promotion for 5 weeks, a much lower papilloma response was found, but these papillomas persisted (8). Figure 2 shows the total numbers of papillomas and carcinomas which developed in each group, as well as the Percent Conversion (Total papillomas/total carcinomas x 100). Surprisingly, the mice promoted for only 5 weeks developed as many carcinomas as the mice promoted for 10 weeks or longer. Thus, the percent conversion of papillomas to carcinomas was 3-4 fold higher in the group promoted for 5 weeks (Figure 2). This result suggests that the papillomas induced by TPA exposure from Week 6-40 are not at risk for spontaneous malignant conversion. Those papillomas which will convert to malignancy are promoted by the first 5 TPA treatments.

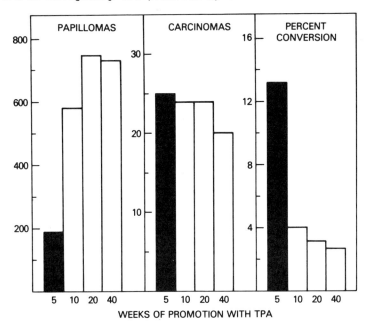

Fig. 2. Short-term promotion with TPA induces papillomas with a high conversion frequency. Groups of 30 SENCAR mice were initiated by 20 μg DMBA and promoted with 2 μg TPA for either 5, 10, 20 or 40 weeks. The total number of papillomas and carcinomas which developed by Week 52 and the percent conversion of papillomas to carcinomas are plotted.

Papillomas can be induced by a two-stage promotion protocol, in which initiation by DMBA is followed one week later by a short exposure to TPA (Stage 1), followed by repeated treatment with a Stage 2 promoter such as mezerein (15). To evaluate the potential of these papillomas for spontaneous conversion to carcinomas, the yields of papillomas and carcinomas were determined in groups of DMBA-initiated SENCAR mice promoted as follows: 1) TPA alone; 2) mezerein alone; or 3) TPA (twice in Week 1) followed by mezerein. As shown in Table 1, similar numbers of carcinomas developed in the 3 groups, even though the total number of papillomas varied from 205 with mezerein promotion to 624 with TPA promotion. The 10.7% conversion in the mice promoted by mezerein alone was clearly higher than the 3.2-3.7% conversion in mice promoted by TPA alone or by TPA followed by mezerein. The papillomas resulting from mezerein promotion are considerably more likely to progress to carcinomas than those promoted by TPA or TPA followed by mezerein (8). That is, promotion by mezerein alone preferentially induces those papillomas with a high risk for conversion. In analogy to the result with short-term (5 week) TPA promotion (8), the papillomas promoted by mezerein alone do not regress (not shown).

TABLE 1. Malignant conversion frequency of papillomas induced by TPA, mezerein or TPA followed by mezerein[a]

Group	Promotion	Total Papillomas	Total Carcinomas	Percent Conversion
1	TPA	624	20	3.2
2	Mezerein	205	22	10.7
3	TPA/Mezerein	403	15	3.7

[a]Three groups of 25 SENCAR mice were initiated with a single application of DMBA (20 µg/0.2 ml acetone) at Time 0. Group 1 was treated with TPA (2 µg/0.2 ml acetone, once/week) from Week 2-31. Group 2 was exposed to mezerein (4 µg/0.2 ml acetone, twice/week) from Week 2-31. In Group 3, Stage 1 promotion by TPA (2 µg twice, at Days 7 and 10 after initiation) was followed by Stage 2 promotion with mezerein (4 µg, twice/week) from Week 2-31. The total number of papillomas and carcinomas which developed in the 72 weeks of the experiment are shown.

In CD-1 mice, as in most strains of mice (3), many papillomas regress when TPA treatments are stopped. DMBA-initiated mice promoted for 12 weeks with TPA were divided into 2 groups. In the first, weekly treatments with TPA were continued; in the second, mice were exposed similarly to acetone solvent (8). In the absence of continued TPA, papillomas regressed from a peak value of 13.7/mouse at Week 16 to 8.7/mouse by Week 28. With continued TPA, 18.5 papillomas/mouse were present at Week 28. Carcinomas developed sooner in the group with continued TPA, but the final carcinoma yield at Week 60 was similar in the 2 groups (8). Thus, the TPA-dependent [conditional (4)] papillomas are at low risk for conversion to carcinomas. This result also emphasizes that exposure of papilloma-bearing mice to TPA does not increase the frequency of malignant conversion of the papillomas (9).

MALIGNANT CONVERSION IS DISTINCT FROM PHORBOL ESTER-INDUCED TUMOR PROMOTION

Three-stage carcinogenesis (initiation-promotion-malignant conversion) has been demonstrated in SENCAR (9) and CD-1 (10) mice. The rationale for these experiments was as follows: Papillomas were induced by DMBA initiation (Stage I) followed by limited (10-12 weeks) TPA promotion (Stage II). These papilloma-bearing mice were then utilized to test tumor initiators, tumor promoters, or other agents for their effect on the conversion of papillomas to carcinomas. Treatment in Stage III with tumor initiators such as 4-nitroquinoline-N-oxide or urethane increased both the rate of appearance and the final yield of carcinomas (9,10). As mentioned in the preceding section, treatment in Stage III with TPA did not increase the final carcinoma incidence compared to acetone, although carcinomas developed somewhat earlier in TPA-treated mice (9,10). While TPA is ineffective in Stage III of carcinogenesis protocols, TPA promotion resulting in papillomas is necessary for the efficient induction of carcinomas. DMBA initiation and acetone solvent (rather than TPA) exposure for 12 weeks in Stage II, followed by urethane in Stage III resulted in only 3 papillomas and no carcinomas in 40 mice (10). Thus, a papilloma stage appears to be required for carcinoma development by this protocol. It has been suggested that a single critical mutation is sufficient for initiation while 2 or more relevant mutations are required for malignant tumor formation (4,15). If a papilloma represents the clonal expansion of an initiated cell (11), the role of TPA in carcinoma development may be to enlarge the size of the target cell population for the second mutation (9). This action of TPA is consistent with the reversibility of TPA promotion.

Two known inhibitors of TPA promotion (15), fluocinolone acetonide (FA) and retinoic acid (RA), were tested for their effects on papilloma and carcinoma incidence when given to CD-1 mice in either Stage II or Stage III. After DMBA initiation, treatment with FA 30 minutes prior to each TPA treatment in Stage II inhibited papilloma development by almost 90% (Table 2). When these mice were treated with urethane in Stage III, a similar decrease in carcinoma yield was seen. Retinoic acid in Stage II was less effective (many papillomas developed after Week 12), but the 30% reduction in number of papillomas corresponded closely with the reduction in number of carcinomas. When either FA or RA were given to papilloma-bearing mice in Stage III, neither papilloma nor carcinoma development was inhibited. Thus, these inhibitors of TPA promotion do not inhibit malignant conversion.

These results suggest the necessity of a papilloma stage in the development of carcinomas in initiation-promotion or initiation-promotion-conversion experiments. In the experiment shown in Table 2, the 5% conversion in the control group was unaffected by FA or RA treatment (Table 2). Thus, FA and RA in Stage II appear to inhibit equally the development of papillomas at high or low risk of conversion to carcinomas.

TABLE 2.   Effects of FA and RA on papilloma and carcinoma development in a three-stage carcinogenesis experiment[a]

Inhibitor Treatment	Total Papillomas	Total Carcinomas	Percent Conversion
None	480	24	5.0
FA in Stage II	64	4	6.3
RA in Stage II	328	16	4.9
FA in Stage III	392	23	5.9
RA in Stage III	491	18	3.7

[a]Groups of 40 Charles River CD-1 mice were initiated with 50 μg DMBA (Stage I) and promoted with 10 μg TPA once per week for 12 weeks (Stage II). Weekly i.p. injections of 20 mg urethane (Stage III) were begun at Week 13 and continued through Week 40. The inhibitors FA (1 μg/0.2 ml acetone) and RA (5.1 μg/10.2 ml acetone) were applied topically 30 min before each weekly TPA treatment in Stage II or 30 min before each urethane injection in Stage III. The cumulative papilloma and carcinoma incidences are shown at the time the experiment ended at Week 52.

CONCLUSIONS AND SUMMARY

Evidence has been presented to demonstrate the heterogeneity of papillomas. The papillomas most easily promoted, by either a weak promoter or short-term treatment with a strong promoter, are at high risk for spontaneous conversion to carcinomas. These papillomas do not regress. TPA-dependent papillomas and other papillomas which regress are at very low risk for malignant conversion. Because of papilloma heterogeneity, papilloma multiplicity alone is often invalid as an endpoint in multistage carcinogenesis experiments.

Malignant conversion of DMBA-initiated, TPA-promoted papillomas is unaffected by continued TPA exposure. Treatment of papilloma-bearing mice with tumor initiators such as urethane or 4-NQO increases both the rate of carcinoma formation and, apparently, the final carcinoma incidence. Inhibitors of TPA promotion do not inhibit malignant conversion. Therefore, the malignant conversion stage in the carcinogenesis process is clearly distinct from promotion by phorbol esters.

REFERENCES

1. Boutwell, R.K. (1974): CRC Crit. Rev. Toxicol., 2:419-443.
2. Burns, F., Albert, R., Altshuler, B., and Morris, E. (1983): Environ. Health Perspec., 50:309-320.
3. Burns, F.J., Vanderlaan, M., Sivak, A., and Albert, R.E. (1976): Cancer Res., 36:1422-1426.
4. Burns, F.J., Vanderlaan, M., Snyder, E., and Albert, R.E. (1978): In: Carcinogenesis, Vol. 2. Mechanisms of Tumor, Promotion and Cocarcinogenesis, edited by T. J. Slaga, A. Sivak, and R.K. Boutwell, pp. 91-96. Raven Press, New York.
5. Hartley, J.A., Gibson, N.W., Zwelling, L.A., and Yuspa, S.H. (1985): Cancer Res., 45:4864-4870.
6. Hennings, H. (1984): In: Pathophysiology of Dermatologic Diseases, edited by N.A. Soter and H.P. Baden, pp. 389-404. McGraw-Hill, New York.
7. Hennings, H., Michael, D., Lichti, U., and Yuspa, S.H. (1987): J. Invest. Dermatol., 88:60-65.
8. Hennings, H., Shores, R., Mitchell, P., Spangler, E.F., and Yuspa, S.H. (1985): Carcinogenesis 6: 1607-1610.
9. Hennings, H., Shores, R., Wenk, M.L., Spangler, E.F., Tarone, R., and Yuspa, S.H. (1983): Nature, 304:67-69
10. Hennings, H. Spangler, E.F., Shores, R., Mitchell, P., Devor, D., Shamsuddin, A.K.M., Elgjo, K.M., and Yuspa, S.H. (1986): Env. Health Perspec. 68:69-74.
11. Hennings, H. and Yuspa, S.H. (1985): J. Natl. Cancer Inst. 74:735-740.
12. Moolgavkar, S.H. and Knudson, A.G. (1981): J. Natl. Cancer Inst., 66:1037-1052.
13. O'Connell, J.F., Klein-Szanto, A.J.P., DiGiovanni, D.M., Fries, J.W., and Slaga, T.J. (1986): Cancer Res., 46:2863-2865.
14. Scribner, J.D., Scribner, N.K., McKnight, B., and Mottet, N.K. (1983): Cancer Res., 43:2034-2041.
15. Slaga, T.J., Fischer, S.M., Nelson, K., and Gleason, G.L. (1980): Proc. Natl. Acad. Sci. USA, 77:3659-3663.
16. Yuspa, S.H., Ben, T., Hennings, H., and Lichti, U. (1982): Cancer Res., 42:2344-2349.

Tumor Promoters: Biological Approaches for Mechanistic Studies and Assay Systems,
edited by Robert Langenbach et al.
Raven Press, New York © 1988.

THE CONVERSION-STEP OF MULTISTAGE TUMORIGENESIS IN

NMRI-MOUSE SKIN

V. Kinzel[1], G. Fürstenberger[2], and F. Marks[2]

German Cancer Research Center, Institute of Experimental
Pathology[1] and Institute of Biochemistry[2],
Im Neuenheimer Feld 280, D-6900 Heidelberg
Federal Republic of Germany

INTRODUCTION

Tumorigenesis in mouse skin can be effected by a subthreshold dose of a carcinogen (initiation) followed by repeated treatment with a tumor promoter (1,20). After a latency period papillomas appear first, later on a distinct but smaller number of carcinomas follows. Since a further promoter treatment beyond a certain length of time does not increase further the subsequent appearance of carcinomas (12) papilloma formation as it reaches the plateau can be taken as endpoint of tumor promotion i.e. of two-stage tumorigenesis in mouse skin.

The process of promotion itself has been further subdivided by Boutwell (3) into two operationally defined stages. Stage I of promotion is effected in initiated skin by a few treatments with crotonoil (insufficient to elicit tumor formation) followed by application of non-promoting turpentine for effecting stage II of promotion. Stage I was called conversion, stage II propagation (3). These observations were confirmed by Slaga et al. using Sencar mice and the diterpene ester mezerein as a propagating agent (25).

At the same time Fürstenberger et al. (5) succeeded in transforming the "full promotor" TPA (12-0-tetradecanoylphorbol-13-acetate) into a "second stage promoter" (propagating agent), by exchanging the tetradecanoyl residue of the molecule by a retinoyl residue (26). Using this compound "two-stage promotion" in NMRI mice could be effected by a single application of TPA onto initiated skin followed by chronical treatment with the "disarmed" promoter RPA (12-0-retinoylphorbol-13-acetate).

Abbreviations:
DMBA   7,12-dimethylbenz(a)anthracene
RPA   12-0-retinoylphorbol-13-acetate
TPA   12-0-tetradecanoylphorbol-13-acetate

RPA is as mitogenic and irritant but more than an order of magnitude less active in eliciting tumor growth when applied onto initiated NMRI mouse skin (5).

The effectiveness of TPA in stage I of promotion has two important properties: (i) Treatment of skin with RPA for effecting stage II does not need to follow the TPA treatment immediately but can be delayed for several weeks (11) thus indicating that TPA causes in skin long lasting effects; (ii) these long lasting effects of TPA do not require initiation since TPA given several weeks prior to DMBA is as effective as TPA given after DMBA (7). This observation has meanwhile been confirmed by others using Sencar mice (22). These results indicate that the effects of TPA in stage I represent a discrete and unique step in tumorigenesis which is independent of initiation. Since the term promotion, however, is strictly defined as completion of tumorigenesis i.e. restricted to events which have to occur after initiation we have proposed (7) to replace the term stage I by the term CONVERSION thereby following the nomenclature originally used by Boutwell (3) but with an extended meaning. Accordingly the term PROMOTION should be used only for events following initiation which were formerly called stage II of promotion.

As conversion in mouse skin represents a discrete step of tumorigenesis it should be possible to distinguish it mechanistically from initiation as well as from promotion. In order to become able to approach the biological nature of conversion on a cellular and molecular level it is also necessary to define and to characterize circumstances leading to conversion.

MATERIALS AND METHODS

Materials

The phorbol ester TPA was a generous gift from Dr. E. Hecker (German Cancer Research Center), RPA was prepared by Dr. B. Sorg as reported (26). The phorbol esters were dissolved in analytical grade acetone from Merck (Darmstadt) and kept at -70°C in dark bottles until use. Solutions were protected from direct light during handling. DMBA was obtained from Sigma (Munich). Cycloheximide was obtained from Serva (Heidelberg).

Animals

Female NMRI mice (outbred strain from the Zentralinstitut für Versuchstiere, Hannover, FRG) at the age of 8 weeks were assigned by random distribution to experimental groups of 20 animals. They were kept at 22°C ± 2°C under specific pathogen-free conditions (five animals per cage, each individually marked), with an artificial day/night rhythm (12 h each), and were fed Altromin standard food pellets (Altromin, Lage, FRG) with sterile water available ad libitum.

Tumorigenesis experiments

For systemical initiation, DMBA (200 nmol/g body weight) was dissolved in sesame oil and applied intragastrically by means of a stomach tube. For topical initiation, DMBA (100 nmol/animal) was applied in 100 µl acetone to the back skin by means of a pipette. Both initiation protocols yield similar numbers of papillomas elicited by twice weekly treatment with 10 nmol TPA (see also ref. 23). For effecting conversion animals received either 1 or 2 applications of TPA (20 nmol) in acetone or acetone for control relative to DMBA as indicated in the text. Two weeks after DMBA treatment all groups of mice received once or twice weekly 10 nmol of RPA dissolved in 100 µl of acetone. The number of animals with tumors (tumor incidence) and the number of tumors per animal (tumor yield) were recorded weekly, starting at week 8 of RPA treatment. RPA treatment was continued for 20 weeks and then stopped. A single treatment weekly with 10 nmol RPA was as effective as two treatments per week with 10 nmol RPA each. After 20 weeks of RPA treatment in the first case tumor incidence was 67%, tumor yield 5 papillomas per animal; in the second case tumor incidence was 79%, tumor yield 5 papillomas per animal.

For statistical analysis of the tumor yield, the Kruskal-Wallis test was used (17).

RESULTS AND DISCUSSION

Characterization of Conversion

The convertogenic activity of a single application of 20 nmol TPA either given 3 weeks prior to or 1 week after initiation by DMBA (200 nmol per g body weight intragastrically) and promotion by twice weekly application of 10 nmol RPA is shown in Figure 1.

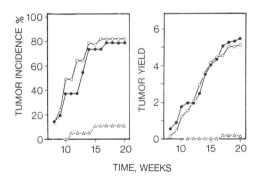

TIME, WEEKS

Figure 1: Conversion effected prior and after initiation; TPA after DMBA (●), TPA prior to DMBA (○), no TPA (▲); (for further details see Materials and Methods as well as text)

RPA-treatment alone is almost inactive in eliciting tumor development in initiated mouse skin.
    Having determined the convertogenic activity of a single dose
of TPA or two in NMRI-mice (see refs. 5,11) it is possible to
approach a comparison of conversion with initiation on the one
hand and with promotion on the other hand. The most prominent
and well known features of initiators such as DMBA are twofold:
(i) the effectiveness of papilloma formation after subsequent
"full promotion"* with TPA depends on the dose of the initiator
DMBA; splitting one dose of DMBA into 10, 5 or 2 applications
yields almost superimposed data. This means that initiating
doses of DMBA work additively yielding linear dose-response
relations. (ii) The action of a single application of DMBA in
NMRI-mouse skin appears to be irreversible; whether full promotion by repeated application of TPA is started 4 weeks after
initiation or is delayed for 40 weeks, degree of papilloma formation and incidence are almost identical (18).
    The NMRI skin system is completely converted by 4 applications
of TPA if compared with a full promotion (10 nmol TPA twice
weekly for 20 weeks) as shown in Table 1 (see also ref. 5). Conversion by TPA therefore appears to be a saturable phenomenon.

TABLE 1. Tumor yield after 1 to 4 TPA treatments in a two-stage
          promotion protocol compared with full promotion

Treatment (after initiation with DMBA)	Tumor yield at week 18 of promotion
TPA 1 x 20 nmol; RPA 10 nmol twice weekly	3.8
TPA 2 x 20 nmol; RPA 10 nmol twice weekly	5.9
TPA 4 x 20 nmol; RPA 10 nmol twice weekly	10.8
acetone; RPA 10 nmol twice weekly	0.6
TPA 10 nmol twice weekly	9.6

Seven-week-old female NMRI mice (16 animals/group) were topically initiated followed 1 week later by 1 to 4 applications
of 20 nmol of TPA applied twice weekly. Beginning with the
third week after initiation the treatment was continued with
RPA for additional 18 weeks as indicated. At the end of the
experiment ≥ 94 % of the mice were alive. Tumor promoting
activity was measured as yield (no. of tumors per no. of
survivors.).

    These experiments were done with the usual 3 to 4 day inter-
val between the applications of 20 nmol TPA. By varying this
regimen of treatment it may become possible to reach saturation

---

*In contrast to the conversion/promotion approach (i.e. initial
TPA treatment followed by chronical RPA treatment) the classical approach i.e. chronical TPA treatment alone, is called
"full promotion".

of conversion even by less than 4 applications of TPA. The analysis of the convertogenic action of more than one dose of TPA
may be complicated by a number of problems, particularly by the
cytotoxicity of larger doses and by superimposed tissue responses
such as irritation and mitogenesis induced by TPA. There may be
a particularly sensitive phase for conversion (14) which makes
it difficult to find the right timing or interval between more
than one dose of TPA. This consideration gains support by data
reported by Takigawa et al. (27) who have shown that the effectiveness of two TPA applications on the degree of ornithine decarboxylase induction depends very much on the length of the
interval between the two treatments. Their results range from a
complete inhibition to a severalfold stimulation over that induced by a single dose of TPA. Presently we try to find a suitable spacing between two TPA applications.

In "full promotion" effected by repeated treatment with TPA,
conversion probably is elicited by the first few treatments with
TPA. Later on, the mitogenic and irritant activities of TPA seem
to be required to effect promotion.

The question regarding the duration of the converted state has
been addressed earlier; by varying the interval between conversion (effected by two treatments with 20 nmol TPA) and the start
of promotion (effected by repeated treatment with RPA) from 1 to
24 weeks it was shown in NMRI mouse skin that the converted state
is slowly reversible with a half life of 10 to 12 weeks (7).

The slow reversibility of the converted state of mouse skin
is contrasted by the fast reversibility of the promoting effect
of RPA as shown in Figure 2a (see also ref. 8). If the frequency
of RPA treatment is decreased from one application per week to
one per two weeks the papilloma yield decreases from 4.5 to 1
per animal, thus indicating that the half life of the promoting
effect is less than 2 weeks. Similar observations have been made

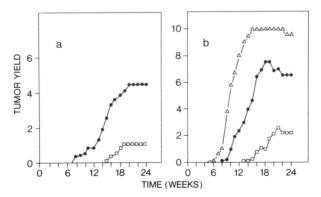

Figure 2: Reversibility of the promoting effect of RPA (a) and
of TPA (b) in NMRI mouse skin: treatment with 10 nmol
twice weekly (Δ), once weekly (●), once in two weeks
(□) (for details see text and Materials and Methods).

for "full promotion" experiments (see footnote) whereby a decrease of the frequency of crotonoil application (3) or of TPA
application (Fig. 2b) results in a reduced tumor formation.

If the frequency but not the total number of applications of
promoters such as RPA determines the degree of papilloma formation, then the effectivity of RPA is certainly not additive in
the sense DMBA is for initiation.

Our results indicate that conversion differs from both initiation and promotion as far as the "memory" of skin for the
different effects is concerned. Unlike the irreversibility of
initiation conversion by TPA is slowly reversible. In addition,
the effect of TPA appears to be saturable pointing to a high
probability of the converted state to take place. Promotion, on
the other hand, exhibits a faster reversibility than conversion.
Promoting compounds, in addition, do not act additively.

A summary of the different types of "memory" for the effects
of the different compounds eliciting multistage tumorigenesis in
NMRI mouse skin is shown schematically in Figure 3.

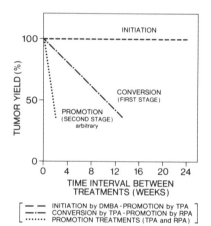

Figure 3: Schematic illustration of different types of "memory"
          in multistage tumorigenesis in NMRI mouse skin.

This scheme indicates that the biological processes under-
laying each step of tumorigenesis differ basically. It must be
concluded that conversion represents a mechanistically unique
step of multistage tumorigenesis in NMRI mouse skin.

Circumstances leading to Conversion

1. Principles for the application of modulators of conversion:

As a consequence of the unique nature of conversion it is
imperative to define and to characterize the circumstances
leading to conversion. The fact that conversion can be effected
to a large degree by a single application of TPA (Figure 1) facilitates the application of potential modulators of conversion.

A meaningful interpretation of a modulating effect depends critically on proper controls in order to exclude toxic side effects. Moreover, the action of a modulator should be reversible, i.e. should not influence a subsequent conversion in the absence of the modulator. Consequently, 2 types of control experiments have been designed as shown in Figure 4 schematically (the necessary groups without modulator have not been sketched therein).

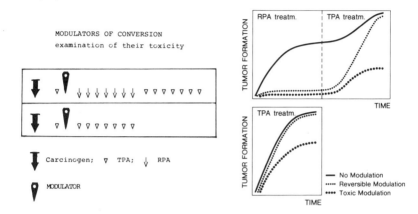

Figure 4: Evaluation of the mode of action of modulators.
Left: Schemata of treatment, Right: possible results
Upper panels: type I of control experiment
Lower panels: Type II of control experiment (for details see text).

As shown in this figure, a potential modulator of conversion is applied once before, after or simultaneously with TPA and promotion is subsequently effected by repeated RPA treatment. In the first type of experiment an inhibition of tumor development seen after promotion (at week 20) could be due to a toxic effect e.g. killing of initiated and converted cells by the modulating agent, or could be due to a reversible action of the modulator. Therefore, the remaining potential of the skin to form tumors is challenged by post-treatment with TPA (twice weekly) over an additional 15-20 week period. If the modulator was not toxic, TPA-post-treatment should result in papilloma incidence and yield which merges with the data from the control animals which have been treated in the same way except that they have not received the modulator. The second type of experiment shown in Figure 4 is identical with type I except that RPA-treatment has been omitted. Such a "full promotion" experiment takes only half as long as a type I experiment and, although it does not yield information on the modulators influence on conversion, it is especially suited to determine the validity of a modulator for the purpose envisaged. Modulator doses which have decreased tumor formation at the end of both types of experiments may be regarded as toxic and, therefore, should not be used for the investigation of conversion.

For mechanistic considerations it might be interesting to apply a modulator at different periods around a single application of TPA. Then, of course, the toxicity of a modulator may vary depending on the TPA-induced alteration of the status of the skin, i.e. during induction phase of mitogenesis. Therefore, it is required to rule out toxicity of a modulator for each time point relative to application of TPA.

Another important approach allowing to verify the validity of an inhibitor is to overcome its inhibitory effect by adding the agent the formation of which is supposedly impaired. An example for this is the inhibition of conversion by indomethacin which can be reversed by simultaneous application of $PGF_{2\alpha}$ (9).

2. Mapping of circumstances leading to conversion

Role of Protein Synthesis and Mitogenesis. In view of the fact that all phorbolesters exhibiting convertogenic (plus promoting) efficacy are mitogenic but not all mitogenic phorbolesters have a convertogenic capacity, the question for the role of mitogenesis in conversion must be raised. The observation that the skin of neonatal mice is refractory to both, the TPA-induced epidermal hyperproliferation and the convertogenic activity (10) indicates that TPA-induced conversion requires as a necessary element the concomitant induction of hyperproliferation and hyperplasia.

It has been reported by O'Brien et al. (21) that cycloheximide applied shortly before TPA inhibits the induction of polyamine-biosynthetic enzymes such as ornithine and S-adenosyl-L-methionine decarboxylase which are thought to play a role in the induction of hyperproliferative processes in mouse skin. To investigate the role of protein synthesis in conversion, we injected a non-toxic dose of cycloheximide (75 mg/kg body weight) to a

TABLE 2.   Influence of cycloheximide on conversion

treatment	tumor incidence(%)/yield
TPA	79/5.0
acetone	8/0.2
TPA -1 hr cyclh.	33/1.7
TPA +6 hr cyclh.	59/3.4
TPA +12 hr cyclh.	71/4.7

Eight-week-old female NMRI mice (20 animals/group) were intragastrically initiated with a single dose of DMBA (200 nmol/g body weight) followed 1 week later by one application of 20 nmol TPA (or of acetone for control). At the times indicated 3 groups received a single dose of cycloheximide (75 mg/kg body weight). Beginning with the third week after initiation all groups were treated twice weekly with 10 nmol RPA for additional 20 weeks. At the end of the experiment ≥ 85% of the mice were alive.

number of different groups of DMBA-initiated NMRI mice at various times relative to a single application of TPA. The duration
of inhibition by cycloheximide of epidermal protein synthesis in
NMRI-mice is rather short lasting (19). The animals were further
treated with RPA for 20 weeks. Table 2 shows that cycloheximide
given 1 hour before TPA effectively inhibits conversion. Delayed
application of cycloheximide influences conversion only weakly.

Role of Arachidonic Acid Metabolism. The question regarding
the role of arachidonic acid metabolism for conversion has been
addressed earlier (9). The inhibitor of cyclooxygenase activity,
indomethacin, abolishes conversion to a large degree if locally
applied onto mouse skin 3 hours after TPA. This inhibition can
be prevented by application of $PGF_{2\alpha}$ simultaneously with indomethacin (9). The arachidonic acid analogue eicosatetraynoic
acid (ETYA), an inhibitor of both, cyclooxygenase and lipoxygenase activities, prevents conversion almost completely if it is
applied either shortly before TPA or 18 hours after TPA (6). The
inhibitory action of ETYA at 18 hours is not accompanied by an
inhibition of the TPA-stimulated DNA synthesis occurring at this
time (6).

Role of DNA Replication. In order to approach the role of
DNA-replication for conversion, a non-toxic dose of hydroxyurea
has been used as a modulator (13,14). The published data show
that hydroxyurea inhibits conversion almost completely if given
18 hours after TPA. The degree of inhibition of tumor formation
is correlated with the percentage of cells stimulated by TPA to
undergo DNA-replication. These experiments seem to indicate (i)
that the process of conversion takes place rather rapidly, (ii)
that "fixation" of conversion requires ongoing DNA synthesis.
This could mean that TPA by its mitogenic activity generates a
large population of target cells which are most susceptible for
the convertogenic action of TPA.

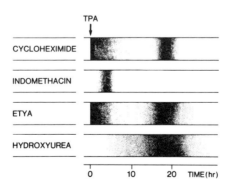

Figure 5: Time courses of inhibition of conversion by the var-
          ious modulators indicated.

A schematical summary map of the susceptibility of conversion to various modulators tested during approx. 24 hours is shown in Figure 5.

In view of the strong and rapid convertogenic effect of a single TPA dose and under the consideration that complete conversion can be achieved by a few TPA treatments one may speculate that TPA leads to conversion on the first interaction with a cell, provided this cell is in a susceptible phase. It has indeed been shown that a single dose of TPA induces a number of chromosome alterations in mouse keratinocytes during one cell cycle (4, and contribution by Dr. N. Fusenig to this conference). They most probably occur during or after S-phase and may parallel the radiomimetic activity of TPA on the cell cycle of HeLa cells described earlier (15,16). Even though such TPA-induced chromosome alterations may not be reversible they may represent the peak of an iceberg of more subtile alterations in the genome. Most interestingly, the almost non-convertogenic tumor promoter RPA does not show this effect on chromosomes (4).

CONCLUSION

The data shown here and published elsewhere indicate that papilloma-formation in NMRI-mouse skin can be effected by 3 mechanistically independent but complementary steps as outlined in the following scheme:

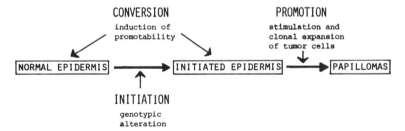

The conversion state i.e. the induction of promotability can be induced by TPA in normal as well as in initiated skin. In contrast to initiation which is thought to be due to a genotypic alteration, presumably a somatic mutation (2,24), conversion may represent a long lasting but reversible alteration of the expression of certain genes. The corresponding gene products in concert with the genotypic alteration induced by initiation, finally result in the neoplastic phenotype. The "cooperation" of the initiated and the converted state is independent of the order by which both have been effected. As the converted state decreases the dose level of the critical products may fall below that necessary for the expression of the neoplastic phenotype. Such cells then exhibit the normal phenotype of an epidermal cell even though they are initiated. In the initiated plus converted state the cells have the capacity to develop a tumor provided the normal surrounding tissue permits it. Permission is elicited by treatment of the skin with promoters such as RPA resulting in a selective clonal expansion of the neoplastic cell as proposed by Yuspa (28) leading to visible tumors.

Any explanation of the mechanism of TPA induced conversion on a cellular or molecular level has to deal with the following circumstances:

(1.) a rather fast establishment and the saturation of conversion
(2.) the slow reversibility of conversion
(3.) and the additional fact, not discussed in this paper, namely that TPA can be replaced by wounding for effecting conversion

ACKNOWLEDGEMENT

We thank H. Loehrke for his suggestions regarding the control of the toxicity of modulators. The work was supported by the Deutsche Forschungsgemeinschaft.

REFERENCES

1. Berenblum, I., and Shubik, P. (1947): Brit J. Cancer, 1: 383-391.
2. Bizub, D., Wood, A.W., and Skalka, A.M. (1986): Proc. Natl. Acad. Sci. USA, 83: 6048-6052.
3. Boutwell, R.K. (1964): Progr. Exp. Tumor Res., 4: 207-250.
4. Dzarlieva-Petrusevska, R.T., and Fusenig, N. (1986): Cancer Letters, 30: 62s.
5. Fürstenberger, G., Berry, D.L., Sorg, B., and Marks, F. (1981): Proc. Natl. Acad. Sci. USA, 78: 7722-7726.
6. Fürstenberger, G., Gschwendt, M., Hagedorn, H., and Marks, F. (1986): Proceedings of the 1986 International Conference on Prostaglandins and Cancer, Springer Verlag, Heidelberg, in press.
7. Fürstenberger, G., Kinzel, V., Schwarz, M., and Marks, F. (1985): Science, 230: 76-78.
8. Fürstenberger, G., and Marks, F. (1983): J. Invest. Dermatol., 81: 157s-161s.
9. Fürstenberger, G., and Marks, F. (1985): In: Arachidonic Acid Metabolism and Tumor Promotion, edited by S.M. Fischer and T.J. Slaga, pp 50-72 Martinus Nijhoff Publishing, Boston
10. Fürstenberger, G., Schweizer, J., and Marks, F. (1985): Carcinogenesis 6: 289-294.
11. Fürstenberger, G., Sorg, B., and Marks, F. (1983): Science, 220: 89-91.
12. Hennings, H., Shores, R., Wenk, M.L., Spangler, E.F., Tarone, R., and Yuspa, S.H. (1983): Nature (London), 304: 67-69.
13. Kinzel, V., Fürstenberger, G., Loehrke, H., and Marks, F. (1986): Carcinogenesis, 7: 779-782.

14. Kinzel, V., Loehrke, H., Goerttler, K., Fürstenberger, G., and Marks, F. (1984): Proc. Natl. Acad. Sci. USA, 81: 5858-5862.
15. Kinzel, V., Richards, J., and Stöhr, M. (1980): Science, 210: 429-431.
16. Kinzel, V., Richards, J., and Stöhr, M. (1981): Cancer Res., 41: 300-305.
17. Kruskal, W.H., and Wallis, W.A. (1952): J. Am. Stat. Assoc., 47: 583-621.
18. Loehrke, H., Schweizer, J., Dederer, E., Hesse, B., Rosenkranz, G., and Goerttler, K. (1983): Carcinogenesis, 4: 771-775.
19. Marks, F., and Fürstenberger, G. (1980): Hoppe Seyler's Z. Physiol. Chem. 361: 1641-1650.
20. Mottram, J.C. (1944): J. Pathol. Bact., 56: 181-187.
21. O'Brien, T.G., Simsiman, R.C., and Boutwell, R.K. (1975): Cancer Res., 35: 1662-1670.
22. Ordman, A.B., Cleaveland, J.S., and Boutwell, R.K. (1985): Cancer Letters, 29: 79-84.
23. Pyerin, W.G., Oberender, H.A., and Hecker, E. (1980): Cancer Letters, 10: 155-162.
24. Quintanilla, M., Brown, K., Ramsden, M., and Balmain, A. (1986): Nature (London) 322: 78-80.
25. Slaga, T.J., Fischer, S.M., Nelson, K., and Gleason, G.L. (1980): Proc. Natl. Acad. Sci. USA, 77: 3659-3663.
26. Sorg, B., Fürstenberger, G., Berry, D.L., Hecker, E., and Marks, F. (1982): J. Lipid Res., 23: 443-447.
27. Takigawa, M., Simsiman, R.C., and Boutwell, R.K. (1986): Cancer Res., 46: 106-112.
28. Yuspa, S.H. (1984): In: Cellular Interactions by Environmental Tumor Promoters, edited by H. Fujiki et al., pp. 315-326. Japan Sc. Soc. Press, Tokyo. VNU Science Press, Utrecht.

Tumor Promoters: Biological Approaches for Mechanistic Studies and Assay Systems,
edited by Robert Langenbach et al.
Raven Press, New York © 1988.

GENETIC FACTORS CONTROLLING SUSCEPTIBILITY TO SKIN TUMOR

PROMOTION IN MICE

John DiGiovanni, Masashi Naito, and Kristine J. Chenicek

The University of Texas System Cancer Center
Science Park-Research Division
P.O. Box 389
Smithville, Texas 78957

INTRODUCTION

It has been known for many years that skin carcinogenesis in mice can occur by a two-stage process (reviewed in 1 and 2). Recently, the two-stage initiation-promotion system of chemical carcinogenesis has been demonstrated in a number of other tissues and animal species including liver, bladder, colon, esophagus, mammary gland, and stomach of mice and rats and also cells in culture (reviewed in 3 and 4) showing the generality of this phenomenon.

Initiation is accomplished by topical application of a single dose of a skin carcinogen such as 7,12-dimethylbenz(a)anthracene (DMBA), and is essentially irreversible. An initiating dose of a carcinogen per se will not lead to the development of visible tumors. Visible tumors will result only following repeated applications of a tumor promoter such as 12-O-tetradecanoyl-phorbol-13-acetate (TPA), to the initiated skin (1,2). Complete carcinogenesis protocols involve the administration of a single large dose or repeated applications of smaller doses of a carcinogen. For example, multiple papillomas and carcinomas can be produced on the backs of sensitive mice following a single application of as little as 600-800 nmol of DMBA (5). Presumably, both the initiating and promoting components are present under these experimental conditions.

Mouse skin is generally considered most sensitive to epidermal carcinogenesis by either the complete carcinogenesis protocol or by the initiation-promotion protocol (6-8). Other species such as the rat, hamster, and rabbit are less sensitive, and the guinea pig is very resistant (7,8). Furthermore, the spectrum of induced tumors differs dramatically depending on the species studied (7,8). In general, the mouse is the only species in which the major skin tumors induced after topical treatment with initiators and promoters are papillomas and squamous cell carcinomas. In addition to these species differences, there are marked strain differences with respect to epidermal carcinogenesis.

TABLE 1. Sensitivity to Complete Carcinogenesis and Initiation-Promotion in Various Stocks and Strains of Mice[d]

Mouse Stock or Strain	Relative Sensitivity	
	Complete Carcinogenesis	Initiation-Promotion
SENCAR	+++++	+++++
DBA/2	+	+++
CD-1	+++	+++
ICR/Ha	+++	+++
C3H	++	++
Balb/c	++	+
C57BL/6	+++++	±

[d]Rankings apply only to studies where polycyclic aromatic hydrocarbons (PAH) were used as complete carcinogens or initiators and phorbol esters (croton oil or TPA) were used as promoters. The relative response is indicated by the number of +'s with +++++ being most responsive and ± being little or no response.

Table 1 ranks some of the commonly employed mouse stocks and strains used in epidermal carcinogenesis studies for their sensitivity to complete carcinogenesis and initiation-promotion. This ranking is based on available data in the literature as well as unpublished studies from our laboratories and should be considered somewhat tentative at the present time. However, the differences between SENCAR, CD-1, Balb/c, and C57BL/6 mice have been reasonably well documented (8-11). It should be immediately apparent that certain mouse strains are much more sensitive to one type of treatment protocol than another. For example, C57BL/6 mice are quite refractory to the initiation-promotion regimen when TPA is used as the promoter, however, this mouse strain is highly sensitive to complete carcinogenesis with either DMBA or benzo(a)pyrene [B(a)P](11). Furthermore, the inbred strain DBA/2 is very sensitive to skin tumor promotion by phorbol esters and under defined experimental conditions is quite sensitive to the initiation-promotion regimen (12, and see discussion below).

PROMOTION AS A DETERMINANT IN GENETIC DIFFERENCES TO EPIDERMAL
CARCINOGENESIS

A number of studies have attempted to determine the basis for
altered susceptibility to epidermal carcinogenesis (as well as
carcinogenesis in other tissues) between mouse strains. A considerable body of literature exists regarding susceptibility to
polycyclic aromatic hydrocarbon (PAH)-induced tumorigenesis and
its association with genetic differences in responsiveness to
PAH enzyme inducers (reviewed in 13 and 14). In general, aryl
hydrocarbon hydroxylase (AHH, EC 1.14.14.2), the enzyme system
responsible for oxidizing PAH carcinogens, is present and inducible in the tissues of various inbred strains of mice to different
extents (15,16). Numerous studies have suggested a positive
correlation between the level of AHH (both basal and induced) and
susceptibility to tumorigenesis by PAH (17-25). On the other
hand, other investigators have failed to establish a correlation
between levels of tissue monooxygenase activity (basal or induced)
and tumorigenesis by PAH (26-28, and see below). Previous
work from our laboratory (29,30 and J. DiGiovanni, unpublished
studies) demonstrated that the patterns as well as the rates of
metabolite formation from DMBA were very similar in the epidermis
from SENCAR, CD-1, and Balb/c mice. The level of hydrocarbon
DNA-adduct formation was also similar in these mice. Reiners
et al. (11) demonstrated that there was little difference between
the ability of keratinocytes from SENCAR, Balb/c, and C57BL/6
mice to activate DMBA to mutagenic metabolites and DBA/2 mice
were slightly less effective in this regard.

In general, there is a good correlation between the amount of
covalently bound PAH to epidermal DNA in an individual mouse
strain and the mouse skin tumor response in the same strain (31-
33). However, as noted above when comparisons are made between
mouse strains for DNA-binding of a given PAH skin carcinogen and
the final tumor response, no correlation is apparent. Phillips
et al. (32) found no qualitative difference in the formation of
B(a)P DNA-adducts and no quantitative differences in total DNA
binding with B(a)P in the skins of Swiss, C57BL/6 or DBA/2 mice.
Similar results were obtained by these authors using DMBA as well
(32). Ashurst and Cohen (34) described in detail the formation
of B(a)P DNA-adducts in the skin of the same inbred strains of
mice (i.e., Swiss, C57BL/6, and DBA/2). No apparent strain
differences in the formation of B[a]P DNA-adducts at one time
point (24 hr) was observed. Abbott et al. (35,36) using similar
mouse strains showed that little or no differences existed with
respect to DNA-adduct formation or removal using the skin carcinogen 15,16-dihydro-11-methylcyclopenta[a]phenanthren-17-one.
Although there is the possibility that an undetected metabolite
of the PAH used in these studies was responsible for the tumor
response, the major metabolites of both DMBA and B(a)P appear to
be qualitatively similar in mouse strains that vary in their

response to skin carcinogenesis by PAH (23,30,29,37). All of the above data suggest that certain aspects of initiation with PAH are qualitatively similar in mouse stocks and strains that differ in their sensitivity to epidermal carcinogenesis. In addition, these data have led to the suggestion that the primary determinant in strain differences to epidermal chemical carcinogenesis is at the level of tumor promotion (11,12,38). Table 2 briefly summarizes the evidence supporting the conclusion that genetic differences in sensitivity to two-stage skin carcinogenesis are primarily a result of differences in response to promoter treatment. It should be emphasized that some aspects of the initiation process may differ between different stocks and strains of mice. However, due to the irreversible nature of the initiation process, differences at the level of initiation can, in many cases, be overcome under defined experimental conditions and appear to play a lesser role in determining overall sensitivity to two-stage carcinogenesis.

Table 2. Evidence that Genetically Determined Sensitivity to Two-Stage Skin Carcinogenesis is Primarily at the Level of Tumor Promotion.

1) Ability of epidermis to metabolize skin carcinogens such as B(a)P or DMBA does not vary dramatically between different stocks and strains of mice.
2) The formation and removal of hydrocarbon DNA-adducts is similar in the epidermis of various stocks and strains of mice.
3) Mice initiated with direct acting carcinogens or UV-light in general show the same distribution in susceptibility to two-stage epidermal carcinogenesis.
4) Mouse strains and stocks vary widely in their hyperplasiogenic response following topical exposure to phorbol ester skin tumor promoters.

GENETICS OF SUSCEPTIBILITY TO SKIN TUMOR PROMOTION BY PHORBOL ESTERS

Of the many effects produced by the phorbol esters after topical application to the skins of mice, the induction of epidermal hyperplasia, ornithine decarboxylase (ODC) activity followed by increased polyamine levels, and dark basal keratinocytes correlate most closely with skin tumor promotion (reviewed in 2-4). Marked species and strain differences have been observed in the hyperplasiogenic response to TPA as noted in Table 2. For example, in sensitive stocks and strains of mice there is a potentiation of the hyperplasiogenic response to TPA following repetitive applications compared with a single application (39), whereas, hamster skin appears to adapt to repetitive TPA treatments (40). Interest-

ingly, after multiple treatments with TPA, hamster skin no longer
displays a hyperplasiogenic response (40). This species is also
very resistant to two-stage epidermal carcinogenesis (7). Sisskin
et al.(39) compared various mouse strains for the extent of
epidermal hyperplasia induced by single or multiple applications
of TPA. Both CD-1 mice, which are relatively sensitive to
initiation-promotion (see Table 1), and DBA/2 mice responded
with slight hyperplasia after a single application of TPA and
with potentiation of hyperplasia after multiple applications.
C57BL/6 mice displayed slight hyperplasia after both single and
multiple treatments with TPA, and Balb/c mice responded with
hyperplasia after a single application but became somewhat
refractory to TPA-induced hyperplasia after multiple applications. These same authors suggested, based on their observations, that DBA/2 mice might actually be sensitive to TPA promotion.

TABLE 3. Susceptibility of SENCAR, C57BL/6, and DBA/2 Mice to
Initiation-Promotion and Complete Carcinogenesis[d]

Mouse Stock or Strain	Initiator or Complete Carcinogen[b,c]	Papillomas per Mouse	% of Mice with Papillomas
SENCAR	DMBA (10nmol)[b]	10.30	100%
	MNNG (2 μmol)[b]	3.31	83%
	DMBA (50 nmol, complete)[c]	2.09	66%
C57BL/6	DMBA (400 nmol)[b]	.04	4%
	MNNG (2 μmol)[b]	.10	10%
	DMBA (400 nmol, complete)[c]	2.20	90%
DBA/2	DMBA (400 nmol)[b]	5.71	94%
	MNNG (2 μmol)[b]	3.60	90%
	DMBA (400 nmol, complete)[c]	0.41	37%

[d]30 female mice were used for each experimental group.
[b]Groups of mice were initiated with either DMBA (doses as
shown) or MNNG (2μmol) and one week later promoted with
twice weekly applications of 6.8 nmol TPA. Tumor data is given
at 15 weeks of promotion and represents maximal tumor responses
achieved under the experimental conditions employed.
[c]Groups of mice were treated once weekly with the dose of DMBA
indicated. Tumor data is given after 22 weeks of treatment.

Table 3 illustrates the results of initiation-promotion
experiments from our laboratory which demonstrated that DBA/2
mice are in fact quite sensitive to tumor promotion by TPA.
This is especially apparent when a direct acting carcinogen
such as N-methy-N'-nitro-N-nitrosoguanidine (MNNG) is used as
the initiating agent.

These data suggested that DBA/2 mice were as sensitive as
SENCAR mice to skin tumor promotion by TPA under conditions
where tumor initiation is the same or similar in both strains.
Thus, our data suggest an explanation for the conflicting
literature dealing with DBA/2 mice and their resistance to
epidermal carcinogenesis. The susceptibility of the DBA/2
mouse to skin tumor-initiation is dependent on the dose of
hydrocarbon [e.g., DMBA or B(a)P] used. At low initiating
doses of hydrocarbons that require metabolic activation for
their tumor-initiating activity, the genetic differences at
the Ah locus between the DBA/2 mouse and other mouse strains
(such as C57BL/6 or SENCAR) play a major role in the initiation
process. There appears, however, to be a threshold dose above
which differences with respect to metabolism of hydrocarbons
are minimized in DBA/2 mice. Thus, in the studies by Phillips
et al.(32,33), Ashurst and Cohen (34), and Abbott and coworkers
(35,36) discussed above, high initiating doses were used to
measure covalent binding to DNA in these strains and few, if
any, differences were noted. Our data indicate that when
similar high initiating doses of DMBA are utilized, DBA/2 mice
are highly sensitive to two-stage carcinogenesis using TPA
promotion. Furthermore, if one uses a direct acting initiating
agent, and eliminates the need for metabolic activation, DBA/2
mice appear as sensitive as SENCAR mice to skin tumor promotion
by TPA at the doses utilized in these studies.

Also shown in Table 3 is the susceptibility of SENCAR,
C57BL/6, and DBA/2 mice to a short-term complete carcinogenesis
protocol. The DBA/2 mouse, although sensitive, is less sensitive to complete carcinogenesis by DMBA since both the SENCAR
and C57BL/6 mice already had developed carcinomas (data not
shown) by 20 weeks. These data confirm the studies of Reiners
et al. (11) that C57BL/6 mice are quite sensitive to complete
carcinogenesis, but essentially resistant to tumor promotion by
TPA. In light of the marked resistance of C57BL/6 and relative
sensitivity of DBA/2 mice to TPA promotion we began examining
the genetic basis for susceptibility to phorbol ester tumor
promotion in these inbred mice.

Table 4 summarizes the sensitivity of reciprocal F_1 crosses
between C57BL/6 and DBA/2 mice. B6D2F_1 and D2B6F_1 mice showed
a response similar to the DBA/2 parent in this initiation-
promotion regimen suggesting that susceptibility to TPA promotion was inherited as a dominant trait under the conditions of
our original experimental protocol (12). Furthermore, the
fact that the reciprocal F_1 generations responded similarly
indicates that cytoplasmic genetic determinants are probably
not involved in determining susceptibility in DBA/2 mice. To
study the involvement of the X-chromosome in determining
susceptibiliby to phorbol ester promotion of DBA/2 mice, we
are currently examining the sensitivity of male B6D2F_1 mice

TABLE 4. Sensitivity of C57BL/6, DBA/2, B6D2F$_1$, and D2B6F$_1$ Mice to TPA Promotion[a]

Mouse Stock or Strain	Papillomas per Mouse	% of Mice with Papillomas
C57BL/6	0.11	11
DBA/2	4.37	100
B6D2F$_1$	4.64	94
D2B6F$_1$	5.00	100

[a] 30 female mice were used for each experimental group except the D2B6F$_1$ group which consisted of approximately equal numbers of males and females. One week after initiation with 400 nmol DMBA, mice received twice weekly applications of 6.8 nmol TPA. Data are presented after 24 weeks of promotion and represent the maximal tumor response achieved under the experimental conditions employed.

to various doses of TPA. It should be noted that extensive dose-response experiments for TPA promotion currently in progress have detected slight differences between the F$_1$ mice (both the B6D2F$_1$ and D2B6F$_1$) and the DBA/2 parental strain (i.e., the F$_1$ mice are less sensitive than DBA/2 mice at lower dose levels of TPA). These data may suggest that inheritance of susceptibility to TPA promotion in F$_1$ hybrids between DBA/2 and C57BL/6 mice does not segregate in a true autosomal dominant manner. The results of these latter experiments when completed will be published in more detail elsewhere.

ROLE OF HYPERPLASIA, DARK BASAL KERATINOCYTES, AND INFLAMMATION IN SUSCEPTIBILITY TO PHORBOL ESTER SKIN TUMOR PROMOTION

As noted above the induction of epidermal hyperplasia and dark basal keratinocytes are closely associated with the promoting ability of various phorbol esters as well as other types of tumor promoters (reviewed in 2-4). In addition, a correlation exists between the ability to respond with a sustained epidermal hyperplasia and genetically controlled susceptibility to TPA promotion in various stocks and strains of mice (39). We have been examining the response of B6D2F$_1$ mice to TPA induced hyperplasia, dark basal keratinocyte production, and inflammation. The inflammatory response to TPA is characterized by erythema, edema, and a marked leukocyte infiltration into the dermis which can be readily scored (41). A recent report demonstrated that the inflammatory response in C57BL/6 mice was markedly reduced in comparison to SENCAR mice (42,43). The goal of our experiments has been to determine which parameter(s) are most

closely linked with the inherited susceptibility to TPA promotion.

Figure 1 illustrates the response of DBA/2, B6D2F$_1$, and
C57BL/6 mice to 4 applications of 6.8 nmol TPA given over a two
week period. The dose and treatment protocol was similar to
that used in the tumor experiments shown in Tables 3 and 4 and
the animals were sacrificed 48 hr after the last treatment. As
noted previously (39), C57BL/6 and DBA/2 mice differ significantly in their hyperplasiogenic response to TPA (see also
panel a of Figure 1). Interestingly, the B6D2F$_1$ hybrid gave a
hyperplasia response intermediate between the two parental
strains. At the 6.8 nmol dose of TPA, the percentage of dark
basal keratinocytes induced in C57BL/6 mice was 5-fold less
than in DBA/2 mice (panel b, Figure 1). Again, the response of
the B6D2F$_1$ hybrid was intermediate between the sensitive and
resistant parental strains. Finally, determination of the
number of polymorphonuclear leukocytes (PMNL's) infiltrating
the dermis indicated a similar response in DBA/2 and B6D2F$_1$
whereas the magnitude of the response was considerably less in
C57BL/6 mice (panel c, Figure 1).

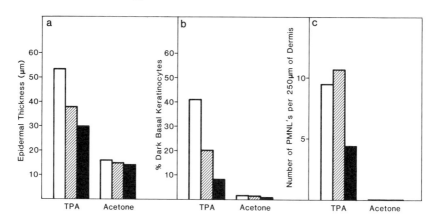

Figure 1: Morphological changes in skin from female DBA/2,
B6D2F$_1$, and C57BL/6 mice following repetitive applications of
6.8 nmol TPA. Seven week old female DBA/2, C57BL/6, and B6D2F$_1$
mice were treated twice-weekly with either 6.8 nmol TPA or
acetone (0.2 ml) for two weeks. Forty-eight hours after the
last treatment mice were sacrificed and the skins removed and
processed for histological analyses. Each value in the figure
represents an average of at least 12 observations per mouse
from 2 mice. Panel a, epidermal thickness in microns; panel b,
percentage of dark basal keratinocytes; and panel c, number of
polymorphonuclear leukocytes per 250 microns of the dermis.
☐, DBA/2; ▨, B6D2F$_1$; ▆, C57BL/6.

The data in Figure 1 demonstrate that all three parameters displayed good correlations with susceptibility in these mouse stocks or strains. The induction of dark basal keratinocytes appeared to be the most sensitive parameter for observing the genetic differences in susceptibility of DBA/2, B6D2F$_1$, and C57BL/6 mice to TPA promotion. This latter point is based primarily on the observation that the magnitude of the difference between sensitive and resistant strains was greatest for dark cell induction.

RESPONSE OF MOUSE STRAINS AND STOCKS TO OTHER CLASSES OF TUMOR PROMOTERS

Skin tumor promotion and the phenomenon of tumor promotion in general has been studied primarily with the phorbol esters (2-4). The promotion response to phorbol esters appears to be mediated in part by interaction of this class of compounds with protein kinase C (PKC)(44,45). A number of compounds which differ in chemical structure but induce many of the same cellular and biochemical responses as the phorbol esters include the indole alkaloids (e.g., teleocidin) and the polyacetates (e.g., aplysiatoxin) (46). Despite differences in chemical structure with phorbol esters these compounds appear to interact with the phorbol ester receptor and thus exhibit a similar mechanism of action (46). Many other classes of compounds possess skin tumor promoting activity, for example, free radical generating peroxides (e.g., benzoyl peroxide)(47), certain polycyclic hydrocarbons with weak tumor-initiating activity [e.g., benzo(e)pyrene and 7-bromomethylbenz(a)-anthracene](48,49) and several anthrone derivatives such as anthralin and chrysarobin (50,51). These latter derivatives, which do not appear to interact with the phorbol ester receptor, are considered the next most potent skin tumor promoters after the phorbol esters (and other compounds capable of interacting with PKC)(2-4,46). Current evidence suggests that this class of promoters works through an initial mechanism different than the phorbol esters (51).

It is of interest, then, to determine whether genetic factors controlling susceptibility in various inbred mouse strains to phorbol esters also control susceptibility to other classes of tumor promoters. As noted above, C57BL/6 mice, although refractory to two-stage carcinogenesis and skin tumor promotion by TPA, are quite sensitive to complete carcinogenesis protocols with B(a)P and DMBA. Interestingly, C57BL/6 mice are sensitive to two-stage carcinogenesis if benzoyl peroxide is used as the promoter (11). We have found that another class of tumor promoter, the anthrones (50,51), are capable of promoting skin tumors in C57BL/6 mice. In this regard, 1,8-dihydroxy-3-methyl-9-anthrone (chrysarobin) is an effective skin tumor promoter

in both SENCAR and C57BL/6 mice (Table 5). The ability of
benzoyl peroxide (20 mg/mouse) and chrysarobin (220 nmol/mouse)
to induce epidermal hyperplasia and dark basal keratinocytes in
C57BL/6 and DBA/2 mice also has been examined (M. Naito and J.
DiGiovanni, unpublished studies). These histology experiments
were conducted under conditions similar to those which mimicked
the treatment protocol used in the tumor experiments for both
compounds (11 and Table 5). A significant hyperplasiogenic and
dark cell response was observed in both mouse strains using
both compounds. Interestingly, no differences in hyperplasiogenic or dark cell response were detected between the two
strains with either compound. These data correlate very well
with the tumor experiments and suggest that C57BL/6 mice may
be peculiar in their resistance to phorbol ester skin tumor
promotion.

It should be emphasized that the current data available do
not allow us to ascertain whether C57BL/6 mice are of equal or
lower sensitivity to organic peroxide and anthrone tumor promotion compared to SENCAR (or DBA/2) mice. This is admittedly
due to the fact that in the studies by Reiners et al. (11)

Table 5. Ability of Chrysarobin to Function as a Tumor Promoter
in SENCAR and C57BL/6 Mice[a]

Promoter	SENCAR		C57BL/6	
(dose)	Papillomas/ Mouse	% with Papillomas	Papillomas/ Mouse	% with Papillomas
TPA (6.8 nmol)	10.6	97	0.07	7
Chrysarobin (220 nmol)	3.4	76	1.35	72

[a]30 female mice were used for each experimental group. Animals
were initiated with DMBA as follows: SENCAR, 10 nmol; C57BL/6,
400 nmol. One week later mice began receiving twice weekly
applications of promoter. Values in the table represent the
average number of papillomas per mouse and the % of mice with
one or more papillomas after 21 (TPA) and 31 (chrysarobin)
weeks of promotion.

and the study presented in Table 5, different initiating doses
of DMBA were used in SENCAR mice (10 nmol) compared with C57BL/6
mice (400 nmol). The reasons for using such a high initiating
dose in the C57BL/6 mice was to insure that initiation had
taken place in this strain (see reference 12 for a further
discussion). Bock and Burns (52) presented data suggesting
that C57/st mice were less sensitive to anthralin than Swiss
mice initiated with the same dose of DMBA, although small numbers of animals were used in the experimental groups of this

study. Ideally, strain comparisons for sensitivity to tumor promotion by various classes of agents potentially exhibiting different mechanisms of action should use direct acting agents such as MNNG for the initiation stage. B6C3F$_1$ mice initiated with MNNG and promoted with either TPA or benzoyl peroxide have been shown to be considerably less sensitive to both agents compared with SENCAR mice (Dr. Skip Easton, National Toxicology Program, personal communication). CD-1 mice appear to be less sensitive than SENCAR mice to the promoting effects of 7-bromo-methylbenz(a)anthracene (53) and UV-light (54). The important question of cross sensitivity/resistance to other classes of tumor promoters deserves further investigation in a variety of stocks and strains of mice.

Poland et al. (55 and reviewed in 56) have demonstrated that 2,3,7,8-tetrachlorodibenzo-p-dioxin (TCDD) is capable of promoting skin tumors in mice. This response, however, appears only in mice that are homozygous for the hr locus (i.e., hr/hr or hairless mice) and thus capable of responding with a sustained epidermal hyperplasia following topical application of TCDD. The ability of TCDD to promote skin tumors in hairless mice is associated with the Ah locus in that the structure-activity relationships for binding to the cytosolic Ah-receptor in hairless mice (hr/hr) follows closely the ability of a given congener of TCDD to promote skin tumors in these mice. TCDD appears to promote skin tumors in hr/hr mice by first interacting with the cytosol receptor, leading to a pleiotropic response which includes the induction of a number of enzymes and also includes the induction of a sustained hyperplasia in the skin of these mice.

These findings further support the hypothesis that tumor promotion is a major determinant in genetic differences with respect to epidermal carcinogenesis. The susceptibility of C57BL/6 mice (and possibly other strains) to different classes of promoters support the hypothesis that these compounds (i.e., benzoyl peroxide and chrysarobin) may work through different mechanisms than the phorbol esters. A similar conclusion may be drawn from the studies with TCDD and TPA promotion in HRS/J haired vs. hairless mice (55,56). In this regard, the fact that hairless mice respond to both TCDD and TPA whereas haired mice respond only to TPA implies different initial mechanisms for these two compounds. Finally, the data point out the importance of studies to determine the cross sensitivity and/or resistance of various mouse strains to different classes of tumor promoters. If multiple genes are involved in controlling susceptibility to phorbol ester skin tumor promotion (and other classes of promoters) then multiple mechanisms may account for the sensitivity/resistance among various inbred strains and outbred stocks of mice.

GENETIC DIFFERENCES IN RESPONSE TO FIRST AND SECOND STAGE PROMOTERS

Boutwell (1) showed that the process of skin tumor promotion could be divided into two steps, which he referred to as "conversion and propagation", using a limited number of croton oil treatments followed by repetitive applications of turpentine (1) or skin wounding (57). These original studies by Boutwell were conducted in STS female mice (the progenitors of the current SENCAR outbred mouse). Slaga et al. (58), using a similar scheme and SENCAR mice, demonstrated that mezerein was inactive as a complete promoter but a good second stage promoter when preceded by a limited number of TPA applications. Furstenberger et al. (59) using an inbred mouse strain called NMRI showed that 12-0-retinoylphorbol-13-acetate (RPA) was inactive as a complete promoter but was quite effective as a second stage promoter. Of interest to the present discussion is the fact that mezerein was reported to be a weak complete promoter in NMRI mice (59) but not SENCAR (as noted above), whereas RPA was found to be a moderate skin tumor promoter in SENCAR mice (60). In addition, skin wounding appeared to act as a stage II promoting stimulus in STS mice (57) whereas in SENCAR (2) and NMRI (61) mice it has been reported to be a stage I promoting stimulus.

The above studies indicate significant differences in the way STS, SENCAR, and NMRI mice respond to first and second stage promoters. The NMRI mouse is somewhat less sensitive to TPA as a complete promoter when compared with SENCAR mice (59). Thus, higher doses of TPA are commonly used in NMRI mice. Perhaps NMRI mice are less sensitive to the toxic actions of mezerein than SENCAR mice. Hennings and Yuspa (62) have suggested that mezerein is in fact a weak complete promoter in SENCAR mice and that epidermal toxicity plays a role in limiting the promoting actions of this compound. In our hands, mezerein also appears to be a weak complete promoter in SENCAR mice (J. DiGiovanni and M.W. Ewing, unpublished studies). Further work characterizing the response(s) of various strains and stocks of mice to the different types and classes of promoting agents including putative first and second stage promoters (and hence the underlying genetic factors controlling these differences) will be necessary to fully understand the process of tumor promotion in general and the nature of multiple stages of promotion.

MECHANISM(S) FOR ALTERED SENSITIVITY TO PHORBOL ESTER SKIN TUMOR PROMOTION

A number of possible mechanisms that might explain the genetic differences in response to phorbol ester skin tumor promotion have been explored. Firstly, since the phorbol ester and phorbol ester-like compounds appear to work at least in part through interaction with PKC, genetic differences might be related to differences in number or affinity of receptors. To date, however, significant differences in phorbol ester receptor number or affinity have not been observed in mice that differ in their response to TPA (63,64). Furthermore, the levels of epidermal PKC are not significantly different in SENCAR and C57BL/6 mice (65) or in other organs such as brain, spleen, lung, and heart between DBA/2 and C57BL/6 (66). We have examined the number and affinity of phorbol ester binding sites in brain particulate fractions from DBA/2 and C57BL/6 mice and have found similar values in both mouse strains (J. DiGiovanni and K.J. Chenicek, unpublished studies). All of these studies are consistent with a number of additional investigations showing similar phorbol ester binding characteristics in cultured cell variants which are altered in their responsiveness to phorbol esters (reviewed in 45). It is important to point out, however, that recent studies suggest the possibility of phorbol ester receptor heterogeneity (reviewed in 45). Therefore, until we have a better understanding of the existence and possible importance of multiple phorbol ester receptors, we cannot rule out the possibility that some aspect of phorbol ester receptor interaction is involved in genetic differences in sensitivity to tumor promotion. If there is cross sensitivity/ resistance to other classes of tumor promoters that may not work through the phorbol ester receptor then this would be strong evidence against involvement of the phorbol ester receptor in genetically mediated differences to skin tumor promotion. Clearly, the C57BL/6 strain can respond to other classes of promoters. Whether this will hold for the other stocks and strains of mice remains to be determined.

Another possible mechanism for the strain differences in sensitivity to phorbol esters could reside in their ability to metabolize these compounds. It is clear that TPA does not require metabolic activation for its promoting action in mouse skin. The major metabolic pathways for TPA in mouse skin involve formation of monoesters and the parent phorbol molecule (67,68). Interestingly, when mouse skin is treated with TPA prior to isolation of epidermal homogenates, metabolism is enhanced (67). To date, metabolism studies with TPA have not been performed in the skin of C57BL/6 or DBA/2 mice. Reiners et al. (11) have suggested that "since the skin of CD-1 mice and Syrian hamsters are similar in their ability to clear and metabolize TPA, it is unlikely that differences in metabolism can account for differences in response to TPA promotion". Barret and coworkers (69) have also provided convincing evidence that species differences in responsiveness to phorbol esters are not related to the ability or inability to deacylate TPA. It therefore appears unlikely that differences in the pharmacokinetics of TPA in mouse skin can explain the strain differences in response to TPA promotion. It should be pointed out that the differences between strains are apparent primarily after multiple applications of TPA (e.g., hyperplasia). The possibility exists that some aspect of the absorption, distribution, metabolism or elimination of TPA from the skin changes after multiple but not single treatments in the various mouse stocks and strains. Furthermore, Shoyab et al. (70) have identified a tissue esterase capable of rapidly metabolizing TPA. These investigators reported that the enzyme is apparently present in skin from hamsters (a species relatively resistant to TPA) whereas it was virtually absent from the skin of mice. The extent to which this enzyme is induced or elevated after high doses or repetitive treatments with TPA on mouse skin is unknown. It should also be stressed that the reported stock and strain differences in response to putative stage I and stage II promoters could reside in the genetically determined differences in pharmacokinetics of the various types of compounds in the skins of these mice. The above ideas related to metabolic differerences have not been adequately explored. Finally, the same argument regarding cross sensitivity/resistance to other classes of tumor promoters discussed above would rule out any mechanism related to phorbol ester metabolism.

A role for inflammation and inflammatory processes in tumor promotion is supported by a variety of studies (reviewed in 2 and 71). Clearly, the C57BL/6 mouse displays a markedly reduced inflammatory response after exposure to TPA compared with SENCAR (42,43) and DBA/2 mice (J. DiGiovanni, M. Naito, and K.J. Chenicek, unpublished studies and Figure 1). It has been suggested that oxygen radicals (O_2^-, $OH\cdot$) produced during inflammatory processes may play an important role in skin tumor promotion (reviewed in 72). Lewis and Adams (42,43) have recently demonstrated that the sensitivity of SENCAR and C57BL/6 mice to TPA promotion correlates with the ability of TPA to attract inflammatory cells to the skin as well as stimulate oxygen radical production in macrophages. Furthermore, the release of oxidized metabolites of arachidonic acid stimulated by TPA was greatly enhanced in macrophages from SENCAR vs. C57BL/6 mice. Fischer et al. (72) have shown that TPA can induce oxidant production directly in mouse epidermal cells in an in vitro system measured by the technique of chemiluminescence. When the response was compared between SSIn (a new inbred SENCAR mouse), SENCAR, and C57BL/6 mice, a good correlation was observed between sensitivity to TPA promotion and oxidant production by the isolated epidermal cells. The role of oxidant production by inflammatory cells and/or epidermal keratinocytes in the process of tumor promotion remains to be answered. However, these genetic differences provide support for an important role that certainly requires further investigation.

A comparison of the relative differences in some of the morphological and biochemical responses induced by TPA in sen-

sitive (SENCAR, DBA/2) and resistant (C57BL/6) mice is summarized in Table 6.

SUMMARY AND CONCLUSIONS

The availability of inbred mouse strains, differing widely
in their susceptibility to multistage skin carcinogenesis,
provide useful models for studying the genetic factors involved
and further advance our understanding of the biochemical and
molecular events associated with this process. The process of
skin tumor-initiation appears to be somewhat similar in various
strains and stocks of mice, and the majority of data in the
literature suggests that differences in response to skin tumor
promoters is a major determinant in controlling susceptibility
to multistage skin carcinogenesis. A model system has been
developed for examining the genetics of susceptibility to skin
tumor promotion. Some progress has been made in determining
the mode of inheritance of susceptibility to phorbol ester
skin tumor promotion. In an inbred mouse strain that is sensitive to TPA promotion (i.e., DBA/2), susceptibility of offspring generated with a known resistant parent (C57BL/6) appears
to segregate in a semi-dominant manner. Further work is in
progress to determine the number of genes involved in this
process.

Table 6. Relative Differences in Morphological and Biochemical
Responses Induced by TPA in the Skin of Sensitive (SENCAR,
DBA/2) and Resistant (C57BL/6) Mice

	Skin Response	SENCAR	DBA/2	C57BL/6	Reference
1.	Hyperplasia	++++	++++	++	9,39,Figure 1
2.	Inflammation	++++	++++	+	42,43,Figure 1
3.	Induction of Dark Cells	++++	++++	+	9,Figure 1
4.	Oxidant Production in Epidermal Cells	++++	ND[a]	+	73
5.	Stimulation of ODC Activity	++++	++++	++	9,Footnote[b]
6.	Presence, Number and Affinity of TPA Receptors	+	+	+	63,64,Footnote[b]
7.	Protein Kinase C Activity and Activation by TPA	+	ND[a]	+	65

[a]Parameter not determined in this mouse strain.
[b]Unpublished studies.

While the mechanism for altered sensitivity to phorbol ester skin tumor promotion is not known, the ability of animals to respond with a sustained hyperplasia, dark cell induction, and an inflammatory response following repetitive TPA application correlate closely with tumor promotion sensitivity. Some important questions that remain to be answered include, 1) Is there cross sensitivity/resistance to all classes of skin tumor promoters among various stocks and strains of mice; 2) What is the genetic basis for altered responsiveness to stage-specific skin tumor promoting agents; and 3) What is the biochemical/ molecular basis for altered sensitivity to phorbol ester (and possibly other classes) skin tumor promoters. The answers to these and other questions will be necessary for us to better understand the process of skin tumor promotion. In addition, such information is essential if better assays are to be developed for detecting potential promoting substances.

ACKNOWLEDGEMENTS

Original research was supported by PHS grant CA 38871 from the National Cancer Institute, U.S. Department of Health and Human Services. The authors thank Joyce Mayhugh for her help in preparing this manuscript.

REFERENCES

1. Boutwell, R.K. (1964): Prog. Exp. Tumor Res., 4:207-250.
2. Slaga, T.J. (1984): In: Mechanisms of Tumor Promotion, Vol. II, Tumor Promotion and Skin Carcinogenesis, edited by T.J. Slaga, pp. 1-16, CRC Press, Inc., Boca Raton, FL.
3. Slaga, T.J. (1983): Environ. Health Prespect., 50:3-14.
4. Diamond L., O'Brien, T.G., and Baird, W.M. (1980): Adv. Cancer Res., 32:1-74.
5. Slaga, T.J., Bowden, G.T., Scribner, J.D., and Boutwell, R.K. (1974): J. Natl. Cancer Inst., 53:1337-1340.
6. Shubik, P. (1950): Cancer Res., 10:13-17.
7. Goerttler, K., Loehrke, H., Schweizer, J., and Hesse, B. (1982): In: Cocarcinogenesis and Biological Effects of Tumor Promoters, Carcinogenesis, Vol. 7, edited by E. Hecker, N.E. Fusenig, W. Kunz, F. Marks, and H.W. Thielmann, pp. 75-83, Raven Press, New York.
8. Slaga, T.J., and Fischer, S.M. (1983): Prog. Exp. Tumor Res., 26: 85-109.
9. Reiners, J., Davidson, K., Nelson, K., Mamrack, M., and Slaga, T.J. (1983): In: Organ and Species Specificity in Chemical Carcinogenesis, edited by R. Langenbach, S. Nesnow, and J.M, Rice, pp. 173-188, Plenum Press, New York.
10. Hennings, H., Devor, D., Wenk, M., Slaga, T.J., Farmer, B., Colburn, N., Bowden, G.T., Elgio, K., and Yuspa, S.H.

(1981): Cancer Res., 41:773-779.

11. Reiners, J.J., Nesnow, S., and Slaga, T.J. (1984): Carcinogenesis, 5:301-307.

12. DiGiovanni, J., Prichett, W.P., Decina, P.C., and Diamond L. (1984): Carcinogenesis, 5:1493-1498.

13. Nebert, D.W., Atlas, S.A., Guenthner, T.M., and Kouri, R.E. (1978): In: Polycyclic Hydrocarbons and Cancer, Vol. 3 edited by, H.V. Gelboin and P.O.P. Ts'o, pp. 346-390, Academic Press, New York.

14. Nebert. D.W. (1980): J. Natl. Cancer Inst., 64:1279-1290.

15. Robinson, J.R., Considine, N., and Nebert, D.W. (1974): J. Biol. Chem., 249:5851-5859.

16. Nebert, D.W., Robinson, J.R., Niwa, A., Kumaki, K., and Poland, A.P. (1975): J. Cell Physiol., 85:393-414.

17. Kinoshita, N., and Gelboin, H.V. (1972): Cancer Res., 32:1329-1339.

18. Kouri, R.E., Ratrie, H., and Whitmore, C.E. (1974): Int. J. Cancer, 13:714-720.

19. Kouri, R.E. (1976): In: Carcinogenesis, A Comprehensive Survey, Vol. 1, Chemistry, Metabolism and Carcinogenesis edited by, R. Freudenthal and P. Jones, pp 139-141, Raven Press, New York.

20. Kouri, R.E., Salerno, R.A., and Whitmore, C.E. (1973): J. Natl. Cancer Inst., 50:363-368.

21. Kouri, R.E., Ratrie, H., and Whitmore, C.E. (1973): J. Natl. Cancer Inst., 51:197-200.

22. Kouri, R.E., Rude, T.H., Joglekar, R., Dansette, P.M., Jerina, D.M. Atlas, S.A., Owens, I.A., and Nebert, D.W. (1978): Cancer Res., 38: 2777-2783.

23. Nebert, D.W., Boobis, A.R., Yagi, H., Jerina, D.M., and Kouri, R.E. (1977): In: Biologically Reactive Intermediates edited by, D.J. Jollow, J.J. Kocsis, R. Snyder, and H. Vainio, pp. 125-145, Plenum Press, New York.

24. Thomas, P.E., Kouri, R.E., and Hutton, J.J. (1972): Biochem. Genet., 6:157-168.

25. Nebert, D.W., Goujon, F.M., and Gielen, J.E. (1972): Nature 236:107-110.

26. Nebert, D.W., Benedict, W.F., Gielen, J.E., Oesch, F., and Daly, J.W. (1972): Molec. Pharmacol., 8:374-379.

27. Benedict, W.G., Considine, N., and Nebert, D.W. (1973): Molec. Pharmacol. 9:266-277.

28. Burki, K., Liebelt, A.G., and Bresnick, E. (1973): J. Natl. Cancer Inst., 50:369-380.

29. DiGiovanni, J., Slaga, T.J., and Juchau, M.R. (1979): Proc. Amer. Assoc. Cancer Res., 20:134.

30. DiGiovanni, J., Slaga, T.J., Boutwell, R.K. (1980): Carcinogenesis, 1:381-389.

31. Brookes, P., and Lawley, P.D. (1964): Nature 202:781-784.

32. Phillips, D.H., Grover, P.L., and Sims, P. (1978): Int. J. Cancer, 22:487-494.

33. Phillips, D.H., Grover, P.L., and Sims, P. (1979): Int. J.

Cancer, 23:201-208.

34. Ashurst, S.W., and Cohen, G.M. (1981): Int. J. Cancer 27: 357-364.

35. Abbott, P., and Crew, F. (1981): Cancer Res., 41:4115-4120.

36. Abbott, P. (1983): Cancer Res., 43:2261-2266.

37. Pelkonen, O., Boobis, A.R., Levitt, R.C., Kouri, R.E., and Nebert, D.W. (1979): Pharmacology 18:281-293.

38. Colburn, N. (1986): In: Mechanisms of Environmental Carcinogenesis, Vol. 1, edited by J.C. Barrett, CRC Press, Inc., Boca Raton, FL., in press.

39. Sisskin, E.E., Gray, T., and Barrett, J.C. (1982): Carcinogenesis, 3:403-407.

40. Sisskin, E.E., and Barrett, J.C. (1981): Cancer Res., 41: 346-350.

41. Stenback, F., Garcia, H., and Shubik, P. (1974): In: The Physiopathology of Cancer, Vol. 1, Biology and Biochemistry, pp. 155-225, Karger, Basel.

42. Lewis, J.G., and Adams, D.O. (1986): Proc. Amer. Assoc. Cancer Res., 27:77.

43. Lewis, J.G., and Adams, D.O. (1986): Proc. Amer. Assoc. Cancer Res., 27:146.

44. Diamond, L. (1985): Pharmac. Ther. 26:89-145. .

45. Blumberg, P.M., Dunn, J.A., Jaken, S., Jeng, A.Y., Keach, K.L., Sharkey, N.A., and Yeh, E. (1984): In: Mechanisms of Tumor Promotion, Vol. 3, Tumor Promotion and Carcinogenesis In Vitro, edited by T.J. Slaga, p. 185, CRC Press, Inc., Boca Raton, FL.

46. Fujiki, H., and Sugimura, T. (1983): Cancer Surveys, 2:539.

47. Slaga, T.J., Solanki, V., and Logani, M. (1983): In: Radioprotectors and Anticarcinogens edited by O.F. Nygaard and M.G. Simic, pp. 471-485, Academic Press, New York.

48. Slaga, T.J., Jecker, L., Bracken, W.M., and Weeks, C. (1979): Cancer Lett., 7:51-59.

49. Scribner, N.K., and Scribner, J.D. (1980): Carcinogenesis 1:97-100.

50. Segal, A., Katz, C., and Van Duuren, B.L. (1971): J. Med. Chem. 14:1152-1154.

51. DiGiovanni, J., Decina, P.C., Prichett, W.P., Cantor, J., Aalfs, K.K., and Coombs, M.M. (1985): Cancer Res., 45:2584-2589.

52. Bock, F.G., and Burns, R. (1963): J. Natl. Cancer Inst., 30:393-398.

53. Scribner, J.D., Scribner, N.K., McKnight, B., and Mottel, N.K. (1983): Cancer Res., 43:2034-2041.

54. Strickland, P.T. (1982): Carcinogenesis, 3:1487-1489.

55. Poland, A., Palen, D., and Glover, E. (1982): Nature 300: 271-273.

56. Poland, A., Knutson, J., Glover, E., and Kende, A. (1983): In: Genes and Proteins in Oncogenesis edited by, I.B. Weinstein and H.J. Vogel, pp. 143-161, Academic Press,

New York.

57. Hennings, H., and Boutwell, R.K. (1970): Cancer Res., 30: 312-320.
58. Slaga, T.J., Fischer, S.M., Nelson, K., and Gleason, G.L. (1980): Proc. Natl. Acad. Sci. U.S.A., 77:3659-3663.
59. Furstenberger, G., Berry, D.L., Sorg, B., and Marks, F. (1981): Proc. Natl. Acad. Sci. U.S.A., 78:7722-7726.
60. Fischer, S.M., Hardin, L., Klein-Szanto, A., and Slaga, T.J. (1985): Cancer Lett., 27:323-327.
61. Furstenberger, G., and Marks, F. (1983). J. Invest. Dermatol., 81: 157s-161s.
62. Hennings, H., and Yuspa, S.H. (1985): J. Natl. Cancer Inst., 74: 735-740.
63. Wheldrake, J.F., Marshall, J., Ramli, J., and Murrary, A.W. (1982): Carcinogenesis, 3:805-807.
64. Blumberg, P.M., Delclos, K.B., and Jaken, S. (1983): In: Organ and Species Specificity in Chemical Carcinogenesis, edited by R. Langenbach, S. Nesnow, and J.M. Rice, pp. 201-220, Plenum Press, New York.
65. Garte, S.J., Edinger, F., and Mufson, R.A. (1985): Cancer Lett., 29:215-221.
66. Malkinson, A.M., Conway, K., Bartlett, S., Butley, M.S., and Conray, C. (1984): Biochem. Biophys. Res. Commun., 122:492-498.
67. Kreibich, G., Suss, R., Kinzel, V. (1974): Z. Krebsforsch., 81: 135-149.
68. Berry, D.L., Bracken, W.M., Fischer, S.M., Viaje, A., and Slaga, T.J. (1978): Cancer Res., 38:2301-2306.
69. Barrett, J.C., Brown, M.T., and Sisskin, E.E. (1982): Cancer Res., 42:3098-3101.
70. Shoyab, M., Warren, T.C., and Todaro, G.J. (1982): Nature, 295: 152-153.
71. Scribner, J.D., and Suss, R. (1978). Int. Rev. Pathol. 18:137-198.
72. Cerutti, P.A. (1985): Science, 227:375-381.
73. Fischer, S.M., Baldwin, J.K., and Adams, L.M. (1986): Carcinogenesis, 7:915-918.

Tumor Promoters: Biological Approaches for Mechanistic Studies and Assay Systems, edited by Robert Langenbach et al. Raven Press, New York © 1988.

LIVER TUMOR PROMOTION: MECHANISMS REVEALED BY OROTIC ACID

E. Laconi, S. Vasudevan, P.M. Rao, S. Rajalakshmi and D.S.R. Sarma

Department of Pathology, Medical Sciences Building, University of Toronto, Toronto, Ontario M5S 1A8 CANADA

PROMOTERS AND CARCINOGENESIS

Since the multistep nature of carcinogenesis was first established in the mouse skin model (3,6) a major area of research in the field deals with the role of tumor promoters in the sequence leading from an initiated cell to the overt appearance of cancer. Promoters are defined by their ability to selectively favour the growth of initiated cells over the surrounding tissue. Their contribution to the carcinogenic process could in this way be merely quantitative, in that they allow a differential expansion of the initiated cell population and the expanded population could then in turn be more likely to undergo the subsequent steps of progression. However, a more direct role of tumor promoters in the qualitative changes which undoubtedly take place during in vivo carcinogenesis cannot be ruled out at present.

From a mechanistic point of view the analysis of tumor promotion must take into account the differential effect observed on initiated cells as compared to the surrounding population. Based on the fact that the growth of focal areas is the key phenomenon during tumor promotion one line of investigation has focussed on the ability of promoters to act as mitogens for their respective target organs. Accordingly, TPA for the mouse skin (4) and a variety of promoters such as phenobarbital (16,18,19), α-hexachlorocyclohexane, nafenopin, cyproterone acetate (28), polychlorinated biphenyls (10,15) dichlorodiphenyltrichloroethane (17), 2,3,7,8-tetrachlorodibenzo-p-dioxin (20) and choline deficient diet (29) for the rat liver (1,7,28) have been shown to induce various degrees of cell proliferation in their target organs. Although in all these models one needs to explain how the mitogenic effect results in the selective growth of initiated cells as compared to the rest of the population, they have favoured the assumption that such a property is essential for a regimen to act as a promoter (27). This in turn has led to consider the possibility of introducing short term assays in which the promoting potential of an agent is tested based on its ability to induce either cell proliferation or cell cycle related enzymes such as ornithine decarboxylase.

THE OROTIC ACID MODEL

Some contribution to the understanding of these questions comes from the orotic acid (OA) model of rat liver tumor promotion (5,13,23). OA, a precursor for pyrimidine nucleotides, when given in diet to initiated rats increases the incidence of both precancerous lesions and hepatocellular carcinoma in these animals (Table 1) (5,13,23).

TABLE 1:   Promoting effect of orotic acid on
            rat liver carcinogenesis

Treatment	Incidence of	
	HCC	Metastasis
DENA + 1% orotic acid; 1 year	100%	33%
DENA + basal diet; 1 year	8%	0%

Male Fischer rats weighing 130–150 g were given diethylnitrosamine (DENA; 200 mg/kg, i.p.). After a one week recovery period on a semi–synthetic basal diet (diet No. 101, Dyets Inc. Bethlehem, PA) the rats were exposed to either the same basal diet or the basal diet containing 1% OA. At the end of one year the rats were killed. Liver, lungs and other organs that looked abnormal were excised and processed for histological and cytochemical examination. There were 12 rats in control group and 12 rats in OA exposed group at the time of killing. HCC, hepatocellular carcinoma.

In studies aimed to investigate the mechanism(s) of promotion, it was found that OA is not an inducer of cell proliferation either in the normal rat liver (23) or in γ-glutamyl transferase (γ-GT) positive foci (12). OA treatment was also unable to induce ornithine decarboxylase (ODC) activity in the liver. In normal liver the ODC activity was 2.1 ± 0.9 while in the livers of rats fed 1% OA for 2 wks it was 2.7 ± 0.7 nmoles CO_2/hr/g liver. Taken together these results suggest that the mitogenic potential is not a necessary requisite for tumor promoters and short term tests using this parameter as the end point therefore may not be appropriate. These results also point to the existence of other mechanisms by which promotion can be achieved. The resistant-hepatocyte (RH) model in the rat liver offers an example of how the selective growth of focal cells can be caused by a differential inhibition of the surrounding population (30). In this case initiated cells are resistant to the mitoinhibitory effect of 2-acetylaminofluorene and grow in the presence of a prolif-erative stimulus (30). This mechanism of promotion may not be unique to the RH model. There is evidence that chronic feeding of phenobarbital (PB) for several weeks exerts a mitoinhibitory effect on liver regeneration (2,18) despite the fact that PB is a liver mitogen upon acute administration (28). It is important to note that the promoting ability of PB correlates with chronic feeding, while acute exposure is ineffective (8). OA is not a strong inhibitor of liver cell proliferation (23). However, in a recent study we observed a slight decrease in the response of OA treated animals to partial hepatectomy compared to control (unpublished observation). If one considers that long exposure to OA is necessary for OA to be effective as a promoter, then even the observed slight difference may become important as a contributory factor for promotion. This point however needs further investigation.

NUCLEOTIDE POOLS IN PROMOTION

A second but not necessarily alternative hypothesis postulates that OA may exert its promoting effect by creating an imbalance in the cellular nucleotide pools. The rationale for this hypothesis stems from the observation that inhibition of the metabolism of orotic acid to form uridine nucleotides inhibited the promoting efficiency of orotic acid (25). The attractive feature of this hypothesis lies in the fact that an imbalance in nucleotide pools can exert a two pronged attack on DNA and membranes (24). Being precursors of nucleic acids, an imbalance in nucleotide pools can create pertur-bations in DNA (11,24). Like wise, since sugars are trans-ferred in the cell as nucleotide sugars, an imbalance in nucleotide pools can influence the glycosylation of the proteins and lipids of the membranes. Perhaps of greater significance is the prospect that, since nucleotide pools are normal cellular constituents, creation of an imbalance in nucleotide pools may be one common mechanism of tumor promotion in many organs. Recent evidence indicates that orotic acid, a liver tumor promoter also promotes duodenal carcinogenesis in rats initiated with azoxymethane (22).

These findings could also have clinical relevance. Porto-caval shunt which results in increased synthesis of orotic acid

(31) has been shown to exert a promoting effect in the rat (21). It would be of interest to determine whether conditions with liver dysfunction such as for example, livers with cirrhosis and with hepatitis B virus which exhibit an increased risk for liver cell cancer also result in increased levels of orotic acid.

At the nucleotide level the obvious question is how an imbalance in nucleotide pools promotes carcinogenesis, is it by creating perturbations in DNA and/or by causing changes in membranes especially in the glycosylation patterns of lipids and proteins of membranes. Once again one must explain the differential effect on initiated cells compared to the sur-rounding tissue. Liver nodules not exposed to orotic acid show increased levels of uridine and decreased levels of adenosine nucleotides compared to the surrounding tissue, a situation similar to that seen by feeding OA in the normal liver. However the magnitude of this change is less compared to what one observes in normal liver following exposure to OA (Table 2).

TABLE 2:   Nucleotide pools in rat liver nodules
             with and without exposure to orotic acid

Treatment	Tissue	Uridine (U) (mg/g tissue)	Inosine (I)+ Adenosine (A) (mg/g tissue)	Ratio of (I+A)/U
Basal diet	Nodules	0.7±0.03	1.2±0.03	1.7±0.04
	Surrounding liver	0.4±0.02	1.5±0.02	3.5±0.10
1% OA diet	Nodules	0.7±0.05	1.4±0.06	2.0±0.11
	Surrounding liver	1.2±0.08	1.2±0.06	1.0±0.12

Male Fischer 344 rats were initiated with a single dose of diethylnitrosamine and given either basal diet (BD) or BD with 1% OA. Animals were sacrificed at different times after initiation. Nodules (2-10 mm in diameter) and surrounding tissue were processed for nucleotides extraction. Ribo-nucleosides were determined by HPLC by methods as described (26). Data are mean ± S.E. of 6-8 samples

This type of pattern is also found during liver regeneration after partial hepatectomy (9) and seems therefore relatable to cell proliferation. Is it possible that a small increase in uridine nucleotides and a small decrease in adenosine nucleotides as seen in the nodules or in hepatocytes following PH offer an advantage for the liver cell to proliferate while a change of much greater magnitude as induced by OA may not offer such an advantage for the liver cell to proliferate. Interestingly, the nodules are relatively resistant to the nucleotide changes induced by orotic acid feeding (Table 2), and they show decreased incorporation of radiolabelled orotic acid in both the acid soluble and acid precipitable fractions of the homogenates. Similar resistance of hepatic nodules to OA was also observed by Lea et al. (14). The molecular basis for this resistance remains to be established, and whether this differential could be relevant for the nodular growth during orotic acid feeding needs to be explored.

In summary, the experimental data derived from the orotic acid model point to the fact that promoters are not necessarily inducers of cell proliferation. Moreover, there is increasing evidence that a mitoinhibitory environment created by either short term or chronic exposure to promoting regimens (2, 18,30) may be a more dominant pattern during promotion. Preliminary results obtained by us suggest that long term orotic acid feeding may also have inhibitory influence on liver cell proliferation. The induction of an imbalance in the cellular nucleotide pools by orotic acid seems to be a key factor in its promoting effect.

ACKNOWLEDGEMENTS

We wish to thank Lori Cutler for her excellent secretarial help. The study was supported in part by U.S. PHS grants CA 37077 and CA 23958 from the National Cancer Institute and from the National Cancer Institute, Canada. E.L. was supported by Associazione Italiana per la Ricerca sul Cancro.

REFERENCES

1.   Abanobi, S.E., Lombardi, B., and Shinozuka, H. (1982): Cancer Res., 42:412-415.
2.   Barbason, H., Rassenfosse, C., and Betz, E.H. (1983): Br. J. Cancer, 47:517-525.
3.   Berenblum, I., and Shubik, P. (1947): Br. J. Cancer, 1:379-382.
4.   Boutwell, R.K. (1974): CRC Crit. Rev. Toxicol., 2:419-443.
5.   Columbano, A., Ledda, G.M., Rao, P.M., Rajalakshmi, S., and Sarma, D.S.R. (1982): Cancer Lett., 16:191-196.
6.   Friedevald, W.F., and Rous, P. (1944): J. Exp. Med., 8:101-106.

7. Ghoshal, A., and Farber, E. (1983): Carcinogenesis, 4:801–804.
8. Goldsworthy, T., Moran, S., Weeks, J., Campbell, H.A., and Pitot, H.C. (1981): Proc. Am. Assoc. Cancer Res., 22:130.
9. Jackson, R.C., Lui, M.S., Bortizki, T.J., Morris, H.P., and Weber, G. (1980): Cancer Res., 40:1286–1291.
10. Kimura, N.T., Kanematsu, T., and Baba, T. (1976): Zeitschrift fur Krebsförschüng, 87:257–266.
11. Kunz, B.A. (1982): Environ. Mutagen., 4:695–725.
12. Laconi, E., Vasudevan, S., Rao, P.M., Rajalakshmi, S., and Sarma, D.S.R. (1987): in Non-genotoxic Mechanisms in Carcinogenesis". Banbury Reports, Cold Spring Harbor Laboratory, New York, in press.
13. Laurier, C., Tatematsu, M., Rao, P.M., Rajalakshmi, S., and Sarma, D.S.R. (1984): Cancer Res., 44:2186–2191.
14. Lea, M.A., Oliphant, V., and Tesoriero, J.V. (1986): Proc. Am. Assoc. Cancer Res. 27:18.
15. Nishizumi, M. (1979): Gann, 70:835–837.
16. Peraino, C., Fry, R.J.M., and Staffeldt, E. (1971): Cancer Res., 31:1506–1512.
17. Peraino, C., Fry, R.J.M., Staffeldt, E., and Christopher, J.P. (1975): Cancer Res., 35:2884–2890.
18. Peraino, C., Richards, W.L., and Stevens, F.J. (1983): in Mechanisms of Tumor Promotion: Tumor Promotion in Internal Organs, edited by T.J. Slaga, pp. 1–53, CRC Press, Inc., Boca Raton.
19. Pitot, H., Barsness, L., Goldworthy, T., and Kitagawa, T. (1978): Nature, 271:456–458.
20. Pitot, H.C., Goldworthy, T., Campbell, H.M., and Poland, A. (1980): Cancer Res., 40:3616–3620.
21. Preat, V., Pector, J.C., Taper, H., Lans, M., de Gerlache, J., and Roberfroid, M. (1984): Carcinogenesis, 5:1151–1154.
22. Rao, P.M., Laconi, E., Rajalakshmi, S., and Sarma, D.S.R. (1986): Proc. Am. Assoc. Cancer Res., 27:142.
23. Rao, P.M., Nagamine, K., Ho, R.K., Roomi, M.W., Laurier, C., Rajalakshmi, S., and Sarma, D.S.R. (1983): Carcinogenesis, 4:1541–1545.
24. Rao, P.M., Nagamine, Y., Roomi, M.W., Rajalakshmi, S. and Sarma, D.S.R. (1984): Toxicol. Pathol., 12:173–178.
25. Rao, P.M., Rajalakshmi, S., and Sarma, D.S.R. (1985): Proc. Am. Assoc. Cancer Res., 26:119.
26. Rao, P.M., Vasudevan, S., Laconi, E., Rajalakshmi, S., and Sarma, D.S.R. (1986): in Nutritional Diseases: Research Directions in Comparative Pathology, edited by D.G. Scarpelli and G. Migaki. pp. 411–421. Alan R. Liss Inc., N.Y.
27. Schulte-Hermann, R. (1985): Arch. Toxicol., 57:147–158.

28. Schulte-Hermann, R., Ohde, G., Schuppler, J., and Timmermann-Trosiener, I. (1981): Cancer Res. 41:2556–2562.
29. Sells, M.A., Katyal, S.L., Sell, S., Shinozuka, H., and Lombardi, B. (1979): Br. J. Cancer, 20:274–283.
30. Solt, D.B., and Farber, E. (1976): Nature (London) 263:702–703.
31. Steele, R.D. (1984): J. Nutr., 114:210–216.

Tumor Promoters: Biological Approaches for Mechanistic Studies and Assay Systems,
edited by Robert Langenbach et al.
Raven Press, New York © 1988.

QUANTITATIVE STUDIES ON MULTISTAGE

HEPATOCARCINOGENESIS IN THE RAT

Henry C. Pitot and Harold A. Campbell

McArdle Laboratory for Cancer Research
Departments of Oncology and Pathology
The Medical School
University of Wisconsin
Madison, Wisconsin 53706

In experimental rodent systems chemical carcinogenesis, defined as the natural history of neoplastic disease induced by chemicals, occurs in two or more sequential stages in a number of histogenetic systems both in vivo (51,65) and in vitro (5,40,79). This symposium has emphasized the stage of tumor promotion, but it has been possible to distinguish at least three stages in the development of malignant disease resulting from the treatment of rodents with chemicals or mixtures of chemicals. Furthermore, some chemicals may exert their predominant effects primarily at one specific stage of carcinogenesis as distinct from chemicals that exert effects at all stages of carcinogenesis. This discussion is concerned with the quantitation of the effects of chemicals at the various stages of carcinogenesis by use of a specific model histogenetic system: multistage hepatocarcinogenesis in the rat.

CHARACTERISTICS OF THE STAGES OF HEPATOCARCINOGENESIS IN THE RAT

In most of the models of multistage hepatocarcinogenesis in the rat, at least three different stages can be distinguished on the basis of their morphologic and biologic characteristics. These stages and a number of their features are noted in Table 1.

Initiation

The first stage, initiation, is irreversible as judged by an extended separation between the point of initiation and that of the beginning of the second stage, promotion (43,46).

TABLE 1. <u>Initiators, promoters, and early lesions in various organ systems in experimental animals</u>[a]

Tissue	Initiating Agent	Early Lesions	Promoting Agent
Dog bladder	2-Naphthylamine	Alkaline phosphatase-deficient foci	D,L-Tryptophan
Rat bladder	Methylnitrosourea		Saccharin
Rat bladder	N-[4]-(5-nitro-2-furyl)2-thiazolylformamide		Allopurinol
Rat colon	N-Methyl-N'-nitro-N-nitroso-guanosine	Proliferative foci	Lithocholic acid
Rat colon	1,2-Dimethylhydrazine		Na barbiturate
Rat bone marrow (leukemia)	N'N'-2,7-Fluorenylbis-acetamide		Blood loss
Mouse embryo fibroblasts (in culture)	3-Methylcholanthrene		Tetradecanoylphorbol acetate (TPA)
	Ultraviolet radiation		TPA
	Ionizing radiation		TPA
Mouse forestomach	3-Methylcholanthrene, benzo[a]pyrene, dimethylbenzo[a]-anthracene		Croton oil or lime oil
Rat liver	2-Acetylaminofluorene, diethylnitrosamine, azo dyes	Hyperplastic nodules; enzyme-altered foci	Phenobarbital, DDT, PCB's, butylated hydroxytoluene (BHT), estrogens, 2,3,7,8-tetrachloro-dibenzo-p-dioxin (TCDD)
Mouse lung	Urethan		BHT
Mouse lung	4-Nitroquinoline-l-oxide		Glycerol[b]

TABLE 1. (continued)

Rat mammary gland	7,12-Dimethylbenz[a]-anthracene	Ductular hyperplasia; hyperplastic alveolar nodule	Phorbol, prolactin
Rat pancreas	Azaserine	Adenomas	Unsaturated fat
Rat stomach, glandular	N-Methyl-N'-nitro-N-nitroso-guanidine		Croton oil
Rat trachea	7,12-Dimethylbenzanthracene	Metaplasia-dysplasia	TPA
Rat kidney	N-Ethyl-N-hydroxyethyl-nitrosamine Diethylnitrosamine	Dysplastic foci	$KBrO_3$[c] Na_3 nitrilo-acetate[d] Nicotinamide[e]
Rat thyroid	N-Bis(2-hydroxypropyl)-nitrosamine	Adenoma	Phenobarbital[f]

[a] Adapted from Pitot, H. C. J. Urol., 23 (suppl.): 9–17, 1984.

[b] Inayama, Y. Jpn. J. Cancer Res. (Gann) 77: 345–350, 1986.

[c] Kurokawa, Y., Aoki, S., Imazawa, T., Hayashi, Y., Matsushima, Y., and Takamura, N. Jpn. J. Cancer Res. (Gann) 76: 583–589, 1985.

[d] Hiasa, Y., Kitahori, Y., Konishi, N., and Shimoyama, T. Carcinogenesis 6: 907–910, 1985.

[e] Rosenberg, M. R., Novicki, D. L., Jirtle, R. L., Novotny, A., and Michalopoulos, G. Cancer Res. 45: 809–814, 1985.

[f] Hiasa, Y., Kitahori, Y., Ohshima, M., Fujita, T., Yuasa, T., Konishi, N., and Miyashiro, A. Carcinogenesis 3: 1187–1190, 1982.

However, for initiation to be effective, the process must occur within a relatively short time of hepatocyte replicative DNA synthesis and cell division (32,77). Such concepts of irreversibility and "fixation" of initiation by cell division have been reported in several other systems in vivo and in vitro (8,74).

As yet, single initiated hepatocytes cannot be unequivocally identified by known methodologies. The presumptive early clonal progeny of an initiated cell after as few as four rounds of cell division has been identified (17). However, such clones must be considered as resultants of the second stage of hepatocarcinogenesis, promotion. Much more significant is the question of "spontaneous" or "fortuitous" initiated cells whose presence has been identified in rodent liver by their immediate progeny (42,52,64). In the absence of exogenous promotion, the number of identifiable clones derived from spontaneously initiated cells, as well as the total volume (cell number) occupied by such alterations in the liver, increases with the age of the animal (42,64). However, when exogenous promoting agents are administered, the number of such foci increases during the first 2 months of life but remains unchanged thereafter (50). This latter finding has been interpreted to indicate that spontaneous initiation in the liver is dependent on the fixation of cell division, which occurs early in the life of the animal but is relatively rare thereafter.

The sensitivity of the stage of initiation during hepatocarcinogenesis to modulation by exogenous factors is well known. Williams (76) has reviewed a number of examples of the inhibition of hepatocarcinogenesis during the stage of initiation by the administration of a variety of chemicals, many exhibiting promoting activity during multistage hepatocarcinogenesis. 5-Azacytidine (14) and inhibitors of poly(ADP) ribosylation (69) enhance the process of initiation during multistage hepatocarcinogenesis in the rat. The process of initiation in multistage hepatocarcinogenesis in the rat is a linear, dose-related phenomenon, which does not exhibit a readily measurable threshold. This fact was first demonstrated by Scherer and Emmelot (58), who reported a linear dose response of the appearance of enzyme-altered foci following a single dose of diethylnitrosamine to rats subjected to a 70% partial hepatectomy. An analogous experiment may be seen in Fig. 1, where the diethylnitrosamine was replaced by dimethylbenzanthracene (DMBA). In this instance some groups of animals were given phenobarbital (PB) in the diet as a promoting agent (vide infra). With or without the promoting agent, the number of enzyme-altered foci increased almost linearly with the dose of DMBA. Furthermore, only those animals given the promoting agent developed tumors; a background level of enzyme-altered foci that can be promoted with phenobarbital is shown at the zero dose. As expected, some of these animals developed tumors within the time period of the experiment.

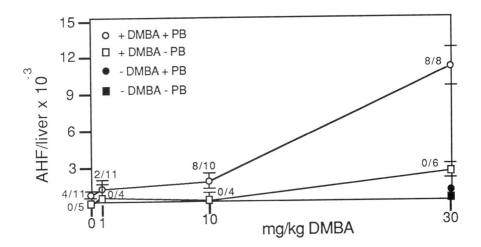

FIG. 1.   Dose-response relationship between the number of
enzyme altered foci induced and the dose of dimethylbenzanthracene (DMBA) administered. A single dose of DMBA was given to
Fisher 344 female rats, 200 g body weight, 24 hr following a
70% partial hepatectomy (27), and 2 wk later those groups
designated "+ phenobarbital" (upper curve) were placed on 0.05%
phenobarbital (PB) in the diet. All groups were fed an NIH-07
diet for 6 months and sacrificed. Foci quantitation was carried out by the method of Campbell et al. (12). The brackets
indicate the standard error of the mean of 6-10 animals. The
points in the lower right hand corner indicate the number of
foci in animals given DMBA but with no partial hepatectomy.
The fractional values at each point indicate the number of
animals with hepatic tumors/total number of animals analyzed.

Promotion

   The major characteristic of the stage of tumor promotion in
multistage hepatocarcinogenesis that distinguishes it from the
stages of initiation and progression is that of its reversibility. In essentially all model systems of multistage hepatocarcinogenesis in the rat, this feature has been characteristic
of the stage of promotion (24,41,68,70). Thus, on removal of
the promoting stimulus, whether promotion be in the form of a
selection of altered cells (67) or the continued administration
of a promoting agent for extended periods following initiation
(48), many of the promoted cell populations (clones)--i.e.,
enzyme-altered foci or islands--disappear by one or more mechanisms (2). Farber and his associates (70) presented evidence
that the "disappearance" of enzyme-altered foci following
initiation and "selection-promotion" is the result of "remodel-
ing" of hepatocytes from their altered appearance within

enzyme-altered foci to normal-appearing hepatocytes. On the other hand, Schulte-Herrmann and his associates (9) and others (13) have indicated that the disappearance of such focal lesions is due to the process of apoptosis, or individual cell death, of such altered cells. Hanigan and Pitot (29) have presented evidence that cells derived from enzyme-altered foci during the stage of promotion in multistage hepatocarcinogenesis in the rat can be transplanted into syngeneic hosts, with their subsequent development only if such hosts are treated continuously with a promoting agent, phenobarbital. This study indicates that the existence of altered hepatocytes within enzyme-altered foci is dependent on the continuing presence of the promoting agent. Such a phenomenon is very analogous to the "dependent" neoplasms of endocrine tissues described by Furth many years ago (22).

If such focal lesions, which are the clonal progeny of initiated cells (55,60), are dependent on the continued administration of the promoting agent during the stage of promotion and disappear upon its removal, do the "stem cells" or original initiated cells also disappear, or do they remain on withdrawal of the promoting agent? Recent studies from this laboratory (26) have demonstrated that the extended feeding (6 months) of a crude grain-based diet in the absence of phenobarbital after initiation and promotion for 4-6 months results in no significant change in the population of foci. More recent studies have demonstrated that under more controlled conditions removal of the promoting agent, phenobarbital, results in a rapid loss of enzyme-altered foci, whose number can then be recovered by refeeding the promoting agent to the animals even after 30 or more days without the promoting agent (Fig. 2). These studies argue strongly that the initiated cell population remains inherent in the liver, even though its clonal progeny is dependent on the presence of the promoting agent for its existence.

The morphology of enzyme-altered foci has been extensively investigated, and various nomenclatures have arisen. Bannasch (1) has identified three types of focal lesions as seen under the light microscope with routine staining procedures: clear and acidophilic, mixed, and basophilic focal lesions. More recently, he and his associates (3) have added another type, the tigroid cell focus, to this classification. Both Bannasch and his coworkers (3), as well as Ward (72), have used similar descriptions for more advanced, grossly nodular lesions in the liver and have indicated that the histologic appearance of the larger lesions is similar to, if not identical with that of the smaller lesions. Schulte-Hermann and his associates (63) have demonstrated that the administration of several different promoting agents stimulates DNA synthesis in the altered hepatocytes of both foci and nodules to a greater degree than in non-focal and non-nodular hepatocytes within the same liver. More recently, however, Ward and Ohshima (73) presented evi-

A

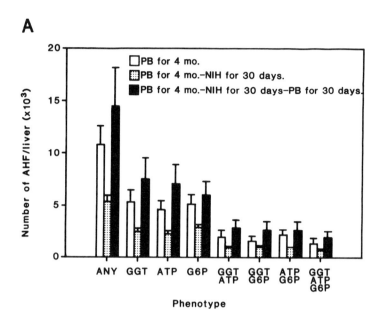

FIG. 2. Effects of withdrawal and readministration of phenobarbital (PB) on the number of enzyme-altered foci (labeled
AHF, altered hepatic foci) in livers of animals initiated with
DEN/partial hepatectomy. The format for initiation and promotion was that described by Pitot et al. (48). The open bars
represent the number of AHF in livers of animals promoted with
0.05% phenobarbital (PB) for 4 months on a laboratory chow
diet. The dotted bars indicate the number of AHF in livers of
animals subjected to the same period of promotion but removed
from the promoting agent for a period of 30 days and then
sacrificed. The black bars indicate the number of foci in
livers of animals promoted for 4 months followed by an absence
of phenobarbital for 30 days and then readministration of 0.05%
PB in the diet for the subsequent 30 days, at which time they
were sacrificed. The calculations were performed according to
Campbell et al. (12). The designation ANY denotes the total
number of foci with any histochemical alteration. GGT = gamma-
glutamyltranspeptidase-positive foci; ATP = canalicular ATPase-
deficient foci; G6P = glucose-6-phosphatase-deficient foci.
Quantitation of foci exhibiting the seven possible phenotypes
are noted in the figure (Hendrich, S., Glauert, H. P., and
Pitot, H. C., Carcinogenesis, in press).

dence that phenobarbital did not have this effect on the basophilic lesions. Numerous investigations (10,21,28,37,44,61)
have demonstrated the varied histochemical staining of the
altered foci and nodules. Pitot and his coworkers have emphasized the diversity of such "phenotypes" as determined by
quantitative stereologic techniques (48), while Farber and his
colleagues (18) have proposed that altered xenobiotic metabolism is common to essentially all such focal and nodular alterations. Since both phenotypic diversity and altered xenobiotic
metabolism are characteristic of hepatocellular carcinomas, it
is reasonable to suggest that the latter develops from the
former, although only occasionally (48). On the other hand,
Pugh and Goldfarb (54) demonstrated that focal lesions exhibiting the most deviant phenotype based on histochemical alterations exhibited the most rapid rate of DNA synthesis. Similar
results have been described by Peraino et al. (44) and
Estadella et al. (19). Peraino and his associates (44) have
also demonstrated that tumors resulting from promotion by
phenobarbital exhibit predominantly the most deviant phenotypes. Thus, these correlative studies on the morphologic and
histochemical characteristics of lesions during the stage of
promotion further argue that the latter are derived from the
former.

Finally, the dose of the promoting agent required to stimulate the formation of foci exhibits a measurable threshold or
no-effect level for its action on the initiated cells (25).
This would be expected on the basis of the reversible nature
of tumor promotion. Furthermore, the action of phenobarbital
demonstrates a "maximal effect" in promoting a finite number
of cells initiated by a finite dose of initiating agent (25).

Progression

The stage of progression during hepatocarcinogenesis in the
rat has not yet been clearly defined; however, on the basis of
the action of promoting agents and analogous to the studies of
multistage carcinogenesis in other tissues, in this stage
irreversible benign and/or malignant neoplasms are character-
istically seen (62). Progression has been defined (47) as
that stage of carcinogenesis exhibiting measurable (by
recombinant DNA technology or similar methods) and/or morphologically discernible (karyotypic) changes in the activity or
structure of the cell genome. Environmental alterations during
progression may produce effects on the growth rate of the cells
during this stage. Agents that act only during this stage,
especially to advance a cell from promotion to progression,
have not been definitively characterized in multistage hepatocarcinogenesis in the rat. Theoretically such agents should
be capable of inducing the genetic changes defined above
for the entrance of a cell into the stage of progression.

Perhaps the best morphologic evidence for the existence of
a transition between the stages of promotion and progression
during multistage hepatocarcinogenesis in the rat is the induction of "foci-within-foci" as described by Scherer et al. (59)
and by others (20,31). However, Scherer has extended the
morphologic findings to suggest that the cells undergoing such
"second" alterations, induced by the administration of a second
initiating agent during the stage of promotion, are probably
the direct precursors of malignant neoplasms (57). The initi-
ation-promotion-initiation format was previously discussed by
Potter (53) and experimentally demonstrated in the mouse epidermis by Hennings et al. (30), who found that when the usual
initiation-promotion format for this tissue was followed by
the application of a second complete carcinogen, a rapid high
incidence of carcinoma resulted, in contrast to the original
initiation-promotion format, which gave primarily benign neoplasms during the time span of the experiment. Yokoyama and
Lombardi have presented evidence for a similar format in rat
liver, with a choline-devoid diet as the promoting agent (78).
The occurrence of foci-within-foci in the usual initiation-
promotion protocol, such as that described by Pitot et al.
(48) in rat liver, is quite infrequent. However, one would
expect this if this alteration actually represents the earliest
demonstrable lesion at the interface of promotion and progression, since this model system results in very few malignant
neoplasms compared with the large number of enzyme-altered
foci seen during neoplastic development. Since the morphology
of many of the focal lesions developing within enzyme-altered
foci established during promotion is identical with that of
hepatocellular carcinomas, this finding is further evidence
for the origin of malignant neoplasms from such focal and/or
nodular lesions.

From these characteristics and previous definitions of the
three stages of neoplastic development in multistage hepatocarcinogenesis, it can be noted that two stages, initiation
and progression, probably involve changes in the structure of
the genome of the cell. Such changes are clearly demonstrable
during progression, and there is overwhelming evidence that
initiation results in alterations in the genetic material of
the cell (39). In this concept of the natural history of the
development of hepatic neoplasia, there is an analogy between
the two genetic alterations of initiation and progression and
the two-hit theory of Knudson (34) developed from studies of
neoplasms in the human that exhibit a clear Mendelian pattern
of inheritance.

THE QUANTITATION OF THE EFFECTS OF CHEMICALS ON INDIVIDUAL
STAGES OF MULTISTAGE HEPATOCARCINOGENESIS IN THE RAT

As noted earlier in this discussion, carcinogenic chemicals
may act at one, two, or all three of the stages of multistage

carcinogenesis. Table 2 gives a classification of agents with respect to their action on the stages of carcinogenesis. A complete carcinogen is an agent exhibiting action at all three stages of carcinogenesis and thus by itself is capable of inducing cancer. On the other hand, an incomplete carcinogen--an agent exhibiting initiating activity only--is in itself unable to induce cancer, although it may initiate cells. As shown in Fig. 1, DMBA is an incomplete carcinogen for the liver, but is a well-known complete carcinogen for a variety of other tissues (39). A true incomplete carcinogen may be difficult to demonstrate in view of the presence of numerous promoting agents in our environment and even in that of the laboratory animal (6). Studies from this laboratory have indicated that proflavin may be a weak incomplete carcinogen for the liver, although it is not known to be carcinogenic for other tissues (27).

TABLE 2. Classification of chemical carcinogens by their
effect on individual stages of carcinogenesis

	Initiation	Promotion	Progression
Complete carcinogen	+	+	+
Incomplete carcinogen (initiating agent)	+	-	-
Promoting agent	-	+	±
Progressor agent	-	-	+

Similarly, promoting agents do not exhibit initiating activity and act primarily during the reversible stage of promotion. However, some promoting agents such as tetradecanoyl phorbol acetate (TPA) may have some of the characteristics of progressor agents (vide supra) in that they are capable of indirect effects on DNA, especially producing clastogenic effects (15). On the other hand, the hepatic promoting agents--phenobarbital (65), dioxin (35), and peroxisome proliferators (56)--have all been shown to induce hepatocellular carcinomas on long-term, chronic feeding but do not exhibit appreciable initiating action as judged from studies in vivo (23,26,49) or in vitro (38,56,75). The formation of malignant neoplasms after the chronic administration of promoting agents in all likelihood results from the promotion of spontaneous or fortuitously initiated cells (64). In support of this hypothesis is the usual finding that the incidence of neoplasms resulting from the chronic administration of promoting agents occurs only after prolonged administration of the agent and then not always in 100% of the animals.

Progressor agents are largely a theoretical consideration at the present time, although, as progression is defined, such agents should exist and in all likelihood will be found to induce grossly discernible alterations in the cellular genome such as aneuploidy, nondisjunction of chromosomes, and chromosome breakage. The best example of such an agent, benzoyl peroxide (66), has been described as active in multistage epidermal carcinogenesis in the mouse. That such agents do not exhibit appreciable promoting action may be presumed from their characteristic irreversible effects on the structure of the genome. However, until more such agents can be identified and characterized in different systems, progressor agents will remain largely in the theoretical realm.

Relative Efficiences of the Action of Chemical Agents on Individual Stages of Hepatocarcinogenesis in the Rat

In several model systems of hepatocarcinogenesis in the rat, it has been possible to estimate the relative efficiency or potency of a chemical's action at one or more stages of carcinogenesis. Ito and his associates (33) have classified a number of chemicals on the basis of their activity in promoting enzyme-altered foci and nodules following initiation with DEN, using the number/cm^2 and area/cm^2 of focal lesions as the endpoint. Using a system devised in our laboratory, we have been able to quantitate both the number and volume occupied by enzyme-altered foci within the liver. The techniques and instrumentation for this were described previously (12). Basically the methods of quantitative stereology are utilized to determine on a statistical basis the number of focal lesions that occur within the entire liver. Such a three-dimensional calculation is critical, since it takes into account the differing sizes of the lesions that occur in most model systems (11). On the other hand, the volume occupied by the focal lesions, calculated from the areas noted on the slides that are analyzed, is a direct function of the area, and thus either area or volume may be utilized for this parameter. Such a parameter is critical, since it reflects the actual number of cells within the sum of the focal lesions.

We have thus far developed techniques for determining the relative efficiency (potency) of a chemical as an initiating agent and/or promoting agent. Both parameters may be calculated for any single agent. The following relationships describe these two parameters:

Initiation Index = log [no. foci · liver^{-1} · mmole^{-1}]

Promotion Index = V_f/V_c · mmole^{-1} · wk^{-1}

where V_f is the total volume occupied by enzyme-altered foci in the liver of animals treated with the test agent and V_C is the total volume of enzyme-altered foci in the control animals, which have only been initiated. Since volume is directly related to cell number, the measurement of effectiveness of a promoting agent is related to its ability to stimulate and/or allow the replication of the promoter-dependent progeny of initiated cells. The initiation index is determined after promotion for at least 6 months in order to demonstrate the progeny of all initiated cells. The promotion index is usually determined after 6 months' treatment with the promoting agent, but other time intervals could be used as well.

Some representative initiation and promotion indices can be seen in Table 3. The initiating and promoting potencies vary with the dose of the same compound, possibly because of a lesser "toxicity" at the lower levels, where the compounds are more efficient in their action.

It is also of interest that the initiation and promotion potencies of a single compound may be quite different. DEN is a potent initiator but a relatively poor promoting agent. 1'-Hydroxysafrole is a poor initiating agent but is much more effective as a promoter (7). Both of these agents are recognized as complete carcinogens on the basis of their effects in vivo. However, the peroxisomal próliferating agent Wy-14,643, like 2,3,7,8-tetrachlorodibenzo-p-dioxin (TCDD), is not muta-

TABLE 3. Initiating and promoting potencies of several agents as hepatocarcinogens in the rat

	Initiating Index[a]	Promoting Index[b]
Diethylnitrosamine	6.6	0.7[c]
Dimethylbenzanthracene	6.6	---
L-Ethionine	2.5	---
Phenobarbital	0.0	324
2,3,7,8-Tetrachloro-dibenzo-p-dioxin	0.0	8.7×10^6
WY-14,643[d]	---	29
1'-Hydroxysafrole[e]	2.5	680

[a] Log (foci/liver/mmole).

[b] V_f/V_c/mmole/wk. See text for further explanation.

[c] Calculated from Kunz et al. (36).

[d] In female Fisher-344 rats. All others in Sprague-Dawley female rats.

[e] Calculated from data of Boberg (Ph.D. dissertation, Univ. Wisconsin-Madison, 1986, ref. 7).

genic or DNA-damaging (56,75), but is carcinogenic. These agents, like phenobarbital, are effective promoting agents.

As discussed previously (see above), dioxin is a very potent promoting agent, perhaps the most potent yet reported, but lacks measurable initiating action. Conversely, butylated hydroxyanisole is a weak promoting agent by comparison with phenobarbital (27). Although the number of compounds subjected to this analysis is not as yet great, the results to date demonstrate that it is possible to estimate with reasonable quantitative data the relative potency of a chemical as an initiating and/or promoting agent. Unfortunately, it is not yet possible to quantitate the relative efficiency of a chemical as a progressor agent. We anticipate that this can be done by quantitating the number of "foci-in-foci" (57), which are the most likely initial lesions seen in the stage of progression in multistage hepatocarcinogenesis. If this can be accomplished, it will be possible in the future to quantitate the potency of complete carcinogens at any of the three stages of carcinogenesis, as well as to quantitate the relative efficiency of chemicals that fall into the other three classifications.

CONCLUSIONS

The multistage nature of hepatocarcinogenesis in the rat is rapidly becoming well characterized. Although all of the features of the stages of carcinogenesis described in this paper are not completely characterized in this model system, it is unlikely that carcinogenesis in the rat liver proceeds by pathways other than those described herein. Furthermore, there is now ample evidence for a similar multistage process of hepatocarcinogenesis in the mouse (71) and in the human (4,16). Many features of multistage hepatocarcinogenesis are extremely analogous to multistage epidermal carcinogenesis in the rat. As we learn more of the characteristics of multistage carcinogenesis in other histogenetic systems, it is quite likely that quantitative analysis of the action of chemicals during the various stages in hepatocarcinogenesis can be accomplished as well.

At the present time the determination of the carcinogenic activity of a chemical is a qualitative analysis. No attempt is made to distinguish the action of chemical agents at the various stages of carcinogenesis; rather, all agents are assumed to be complete carcinogens (45). Since it is now apparent that such an assumption is false, it behooves the regulatory agencies to begin to take account of the action of chemicals at the various stages of carcinogenesis and to relate such actions to the risk involved in exposure of the human population to such agents. Such risk estimations always involve quantitative parameters, and it is to be expected that quantitation of the relative efficiencies of chemicals in animal systems will aid in quantitative risk estimations in the future.

REFERENCES

1. Bannasch, P. (1984): J. Cancer Res. Clin. Oncol., 108:11-22.
2. Bannasch, P. (1986): Carcinogenesis, 7:689-695.
3. Bannasch, P., Benner, U., Enzmann, H., and Hacker, H. J. (1985): Carcinogenesis, 6:1641-1648.
4. Bannasch, P., and Klinge, O. (1971): Virchows Arch. Abt. A Pathol. Anat., 352:157-164.
5. Barrett, J. C. (1980): Cancer Res., 40:91.
6. Berenblum, I. (1985): Cancer Res., 45:1917-1921.
7. Boberg, E. (1986): Ph.D. Dissertation. University of Wisconsin-Madison.
8. Borek, C., and Sachs, L. (1968): Proc. Natl. Acad. Sci., 59:83-85.
9. Bursch, W., Lauer, B., Timmermann-Trosiener, I., Barthel, G., Schuppler, J., and Schulte-Hermann, R. (1984): Carcinogenesis, 5:453-458.
10. Cameron, R., Kellen, J., Kolin, A., Malkin, A., and Farber, E. (1978): Cancer Res., 38:823-829.
11. Campbell, H. A., Pitot, H. C., Potter, V. R., and Laishes, B. A. (1982): Cancer Res., 42:465-472.
12. Campbell, H. A., Xu, Y.-D., Hanigan, M. H., and Pitot, H. C. (1986): J. Natl. Cancer Inst., 76:751-767.
13. Columbano, A., Ledda-Columbano, G. M., Rao, P. M., Rajalakshmi, S., and Sarma, D. S. R. (1984): Amer. J. Pathol., 116:441-446.
14. Denda, A., Rao, P. M., Rajalakshmi, S., and Sarma, D. S. R. (1986): Carcinogenesis (in press).
15. Dzarlieva-Petrusevska, R. T., and Fusenig, N. E. (1985): Carcinogenesis, 6:1447-1456.
16. Edmondson, H. A., Reynolds, T. B., Henderson, B., and Benton, B. (1977): Ann. Int. Med., 86:180-182.
17. Emmelot, P., and Scherer, E. (1980): Biochim. Biophys. Acta, 605:247-304.
18. Eriksson, L., Ahluwalia, M., Spiewak, J., Lee, G., Sarma, D. S. R., Roomi, M. J., and Farber, E. (1983): Environ. Health Perspect., 49:171-174.
19. Estadella, M. D., Pujol, M. J., and Domingo, J. (1984): Oncology, 41:276-279.
20. Farber, E. (1973): Methods Cancer Res., 7:345-375.
21. Fischer, G., Ullrich, D., and Bock, K. W. (1985): Carcinogenesis, 6:605-609.
22. Furth, J. (1968): Hormones and Neoplasia: Thule International Symposia on Cancer and Aging, pp. 131-151. Nordiska Bokhandelns Förlag, Stockholm.

23. Glauert, H. P., Beer, D., Rao, M. S., Schwarz, M., Xu,
    Y.-D., Goldsworthy, T. L., Coloma, J., and Pitot, H. C.
    (1986): Cancer Res., 46: (in press).
24. Glauert, H. P., Schwarz, M., and Pitot, H. C. (1986):
    Carcinogenesis, 7:117-121.
25. Goldsworthy, T., Campbell, H. A., and Pitot, H. C. (1984):
    Carcinogenesis, 5:67-71.
26. Goldsworthy, T. L., and Pitot, H. C. (1985): Carcinogene-
    sis, 6:1261-1269.
27. Goldsworthy, T. L., and Pitot, H. C. (1985): J. Toxicol.
    Environ. Health, 16:389-402.
28. Hacker, H. J., Moore, M. A., Mayer, D., and Bannasch, P.
    (1982): Carcinogenesis, 3:1265-1272.
29. Hanigan, M., and Pitot, H. C. (1985): Cancer Res.,
    45:6063-6067.
30. Hennings, H., Shores, R., Mitchell, P., Spangler, E. F.,
    and Yuspa, S. H. (1985): Carcinogenesis, 6:1607-1610.
31. Hirota, N., and Yokoyama, T. (1985): Acta Pathol. Jpn.,
    35(5):1163-1179.
32. Ishikawa, T., Takayama, S., and Kitagawa, T. (1980):
    Cancer Res., 40:4261-4264.
33. Ito, N., Tatematsu, M., Nakanishi, K., Hasegawa, R.,
    Takano, T., Imaida, K., and Ogiso, T. (1980): Gann,
    71:832.
34. Knudson, A. G., Jr. (1985): Cancer Res., 45:1437-1443.
35. Kociba, R. J., Keyes, D. G., Beyer, J. E., Carreon, R. M.,
    Wade, C. E., Dittenber, D. A., Kalnins, R. P., Frauson,
    L. E., Park, C. N., Barnard, S. D., Hummel, R. A., and
    Humiston, C. G. (1978): Toxicol. Appl. Pharm. 46:279.
36. Kunz, H. W., Tennekes, H. A., Port, R. E., Schwartz, M.,
    Lorke, D., and Schaude, G. (1983): Environ. Health
    Persp., 50:113.
37. Lindahl, R., Clark, R., and Evces, S. (1983): Cancer
    Res., 43:5972-5977.
38. McCann, J., Choi, E., Yamasaki, E., and Ames, B. N.
    (1975): Proc. Natl. Acad. Sci. U.S.A., 72:5135-5139.
39. Miller, E. C. (1978): Cancer Res., 38:1479-1496.
40. Mondal, S., Brankow, D. W., and Heidelberger, C. (1976):
    Cancer Res., 36:2254-2260.
41. Moore, M. A., Hacker, H.-J., and Bannasch, P. (1983):
    Carcinogenesis, 4:595-603.
42. Ogawa, K., Onoe, T., and Takeuchi, M. (1981): J. Natl.
    Cancer Inst., 67:407-412.
43. Peraino, C., Fry, R. J. M., and Staffeldt, E. (1977):
    Cancer Res., 37:3623.
44. Peraino, C., Staffeldt, E. F., Carnes, B. A., Ludeman,
    V. A., Blomquist, J. A., and Vesselinovitch, S. D. (1984):
    Cancer Res., 44:3340-3347.
45. Perera, F. P. (1984): Environ. Res., 34:175-191.
46. Pitot, H. C. (1978): The Induction of Drug Metabolism
    Symposium, Ashford Castle, Ireland, edited by R. W.

Estabrook and E. Lindenlaub, p. 471. F. K. Schattauer Verlag, Stuttgart, New York.

47. Pitot, H. C. (1986): Fundamentals of Oncology, 3rd edition, Marcel Dekker, Inc., New York.
48. Pitot, H. C., Barsness, L., Goldsworthy, T., and Kitagawa, T. (1978): Nature, 271:456-457.
49. Pitot, H. C., Goldsworthy, T., Campbell, H. A., and Poland, A. (1980): Cancer Res., 40:3616-3620.
50. Pitot, H. C., Grosso, L. E., and Goldsworthy, T. (1985): Carcinogenesis, 10:65-79.
51. Pitot, H. C., and Sirica, A. E. (1980): Biochim. Biophys. Acta, 605:191-215.
52. Popp, J. A., Scortichini, B. H., and Garvey, L. K. (1985): Fund. Appl. Toxicol., 5:314-319.
53. Potter, V. R. (1981): Carcinogenesis, 2:1375-1379.
54. Pugh, T. D., and Goldfarb, S. (1978): Cancer Res., 38:4450-4457.
55. Rabes, H. M., Bücher, Th., Hartmann, A., Linke, I., and Dünnwald, M. (1982): Cancer Res., 42:3220-3227.
56. Reddy, J. K., Scarpelli, D. G., Subbarao, V., and Lalwani, N. D. (1983): Tox. Path., 11:0192.
57. Scherer, E. (1984): Biochim. Biophys. Acta, 738:219-236.
58. Scherer, E., and Emmelot, P. (1975): Europ. J. Cancer, 11:689-696.
59. Scherer, E., Feringa, A. W., and Emmelot, P. (1984): Models, Mech. Etiol. Tumor Prom., 56:57.
60. Scherer, E., and Hoffmann, M. (1971): Europ. J. Cancer, 7:369-371.
61. Schor, N. A. (1978): Cancer Lett., 5:167-171.
62. Schulte-Hermann, R. (1985): Arch. Toxicol., 57:147-158.
63. Schulte-Hermann, R., Ohde, G., Schuppler, J., and Timmermann-Trosiener, I. (1981): Cancer Res., 41:2556-2562.
64. Schulte-Hermann, R., Timmermann-Trosiener, I., and Schuppler, J. (1983): Cancer Res., 43:839-844.
65. Scribner, J. D., and Süss, R. (1978): Intl. Rev. Exp. Path., 18:137.
66. Slaga, T. J., Klein-Szanto, A. J. P., Triplett, L. L., and Yorn, L. P. (1981): Science, 213:1023-1025.
67. Solt, D. B., Medline, A., and Farber, E. (1977): Amer. J. Pathol., 88:595-618.
68. Takahashi, S., Lombardi, B., and Shinozuka, H. (1982): Int. J. Cancer, 29:445-450.
69. Takahashi, S., Nakae, D., Yokose, Y., Emi, Y., Denda, A., Mikami, S., Ohnishi, T., and Konishi, Y. (1984): Carcinogenesis, 5:901-906.
70. Tatematsu, M., Nagamine, Y., and Farber, E. (1983): Cancer Res., 43:5049-5058.
71. Uchida, E., and Hirono, I. (1979): Gann, 70:639-644.
72. Ward, J. M. (1981): Virchows Arch. [Pathol. Anat.], 390:339-345.

73. Ward, J. M., and Ohshima, M. (1985): <u>Carcinogenesis</u>, 6:1255-1259.
74. Warwick, G. P. (1971): <u>Fed. Proc.</u>, 30:1760-1765.
75. Wassom, J. S., Huff, J. E., and Loprieno, N. (1977/1978): <u>Mutat. Res</u>. 47:141-160.
76. Williams, G. M., and Furuya, K. (1984): <u>Carcinogenesis</u>, 5:171-174.
77. Ying, T. S., Enomoto, K., Sarma, D. S. R., and Farber, E. (1982): <u>Cancer Res</u>., 42:876-880.
78. Yokoyama, S., and Lombardi, B. (1985): <u>Cancer Lett</u>., 25:171-176.
79. Yuspa, S. H., Hennings, H., and Lichte, U. (1981): <u>J. Supramol. Struct. Cell. Biochem</u>., 17:245.

Tumor Promoters: Biological Approaches for
Mechanistic Studies and Assay Systems,
edited by Robert Langenbach et al.
Raven Press, New York © 1988.

CHEMICAL AND ONCOGENE MODULATION OF
GAP JUNCTIONAL INTERCELLULAR COMMUNICATION

J.E. Trosko and C.C. Chang

Center for Environmental Toxicology
Department of Pediatrics and Human Development
College of Human Medicine
Michigan State University
East Lansing, Michigan 48824

CRISIS IN TOXICOLOGY: INADEQUACY OF THE
CONCEPT OF GENOTOXICITY

Obviously, exposure to chemicals can lead to both benefi-
cial/adaptive and harmful/maladaptive responses at the whole
organism level. At the cell level, the chemical could (a)
alter the genetic information [mutagenicity]; (b) induce cell
death by a wide variety of mechanisms (e.g., lethal mutations, enzyme inhibition, membrane destruction) [cytotox-
icity]; and/or (c) modulate gene expression [epigenetic
modulation] (97). Depending on a wide variety of factors,
such as the stage of development (early embryonic versus
adult stage); how many cells have been affected; concentration of the chemical; genetic defense mechanisms of the
organism; synergisms or antagonisms with other endogenous or
exogenous chemicals; how many and which genes might be affected; whether the affected cell is clonally amplified or
not, etc.], the biological consequences of this mutagenic,
cytotoxic or epigenetic change could vary from the undetect-
able, to acute toxic reactions and death, to various chronic
diseases (91,92).

In recent years, one of the most powerful paradigms to
study chemical toxicity has been the introduction of the
concept of "genotoxicity" (14). Clearly, since the fidelity
of the genetic information in both germ and somatic cells are
needed for maintenance of all levels of the biological
hierarchy in multi-cellular organisms, induction of gene and
chromosomal mutations are known or suspected to be associated
with a wide spectrum of genetic and somatic diseases
(2,3,52,57,69,95). Therefore, to study mutagenesis and to
detect environmental mutagens have been, and will continue to
be, an important elements of toxicology.

Unfortunately, this paradigm, as important as it is, has
blinded us to other mechanisms by which chemicals could be
toxic to organisms. In other words, while it is true and

clear that mutagens can be harmful, not all harmful chemicals are mutagenic!(89). In this report, we will present another paradigm, namely chemical modulation of gap junctional intercellular communication as a cellular mechanism of chemical toxicity which could lead to a wide variety of harmful endpoints. Specifically, we and others have postulated that chemical modulation of gap junctional communication can lead to teratogenesis (49,94,108), promote initiated cells during carcinogenesis (93), cause neurotoxic effects (99), bring about reproductive dysfunction and other dysfunctional physiological states (90).

GAP JUNCTIONAL INTERCELLULAR COMMUNICATION
IN MULTI-CELLULAR ORGANISMS

Distribution, structure and role of Gap Junctions

Gap junctions are communicating membrane channels between neighboring cells that allow passive transport of ions and small molecules up to approximately 1500 D (51). They have been found in every phyla of multicellular organisms and in most cells in the body except circulating blood cells and skeletal muscle cells (27). Although the molecular/biochemical structure of the gap junction has not yet been unequivocally delineated, it appears to consist of one non-glycosylated protein, with possible post translational modifications in certain tissues within and between species (74).

The fact that gap junctions are found in all multi-cellular animals implies they play a very fundamental role in these organisms. Using the adage of Theodosius Dobzhansky, "Nothing in biology makes sense except in the light of evolution", this observation of the presence of gap junctions in multi-cellular organisms, but not in single celled, undifferentiated organisms, together with their suspected functional roles in multicellular organisms, implies the appearance of the genes coding for the structure and regulatory components of the gap junction might well have been the main evolutionary change behind the ability to form adaptive differentiated tissue in the multi-cellular organisms.

In general, gap junctional intercellular communication has been correlated with growth control and differentiation [by ionic and chemical metabolic coupling] in unexcitable, proliferatable cells, (50), with controlling organ function, such as synchronizing heart (75) or uterine muscle fibers (20), with ionic and nutrient dependence of non-proliferating, excitable brain cells (3,10), and with the embryonic (48) and wound-healing or regenerative process (112).

Modulation of Gap Junctions

One of the important points to understand when one considers gap junctional intercellular communication is that the process must involve at least four functional operations:

(a) the adhension or "docking" of the potentially communicating cells. Cell adhension molecules [CAM'S] (22), different from the gap junction proteins, are needed (73); (b) gap junction subunits (connexons) of the communicating cells must unite and be functionally open; (c) the existence and transfer of signaling ions and critical small regulatory molecules needed to establish normal physiological homeostasis must occur; and (d) normal reaction to the transferred ions and molecules must happen. If all four steps are accomplished, intercellular communication can be considered to have occurred. Any one or more of these steps, if inhibited, would interfer with the gap-junctional mediated intercellular communication process.

It is becoming increasingly clear that these gap junctions are not "cast in concrete" in the membranes of cells. As Larsen and Risinger (45) have characterized, the gap junction has a "dynamic life history." Indeed, there is ample evidence that early embryonic cells do not seem to have gap junction function (i.e., they are under developmental genomic control) (48). In addition, many endogenous factors appear to modulate their appearance or disappearance (i.e., hormones) (45). More recently, exogenous chemicals, such as drugs [i.e., phenobarbital (43)], food additives [i.e., saccharin (96)], environmental pollutants [i.e., polybrominated biphenyls(100)], natural plant and animal toxins [i.e., phorbol esters (68,113)], and many natural dietary chemicals (i.e., unsaturated fatty acids (7)], and many solvents and metabolites (18,60), have been shown to modulate their regulation. Increased intracellular Ca^{++}, H^+, as well as voltage changes, has been correlated with channel occlusion (75). On the other hand, increased C-AMP levels appears to be correlated in some cell systems with increased gap junction function (21,28,56,62,82,101).

One speculation to explain how a wide number of genomic or external factors could modulate gap junctions, and therefore, their physiological functions, would be that all these factors could modulate the ubiquitous, but critical, cellular signals of Ca^{++}, pH and C-AMP. For example, if a pollutant (i.e., DDT) increases intracellular Ca^{++} by inhibiting the efflux of Ca^{++} (59), the gap junction function would diminish (81). On the other hand, if a hormone or differentiation factor increased C-AMP in the target cell, increased communication might occur, blocking cell proliferation and inducing differentiation.

Many diverse, structurally unrelated chemicals products have been shown to modulate gap junctional structure/function both in vivo and in vitro (45,53,61,75). Indeed, more recently, several oncogene products appear to be able to modulate gap junction function (6,8,17). By logical implication, if gap junctional communication serves as a critical function to regulate growth and differentiation of proliferatable cells, homeostatic control of cells within tissues, and compartmentalization of functions in non-proliferatable cells, the unscheduled modulation of gap junction function could lead to many developmental, physiological dysfunctions (see below).

Possible Mechanisms Modulating Gap Junctional Communication

By examining this diverse set of gap-junctional modulating factors, it seems, at first glance, that a unifying or simple mechanism for regulating gap junction function could not exist. Although little is known of the biophysical/biochemical mechanism(s) regulating gap junction function, several cellular factors seem to be correlated with gap junction intercellular communication, and since many of these factors are known to cause homeostatic disruption of either intracellular Ca^{++}, pH and/or C-AMP, and since Ca^{++}, pH and C-AMP have been shown to be related to the modulation of gap junction function, it is reasonable to speculate a unifying mechanism to explain chemical modulation of gap junctions. In addition to chemical modulation of gap junctional communication, it is conceivable that temperature might affect gap junctions (4). Elevated temperature of a fever associated with infections might be the result of the biological toxin-inhibition of intercellular communication which, then, might lead to additional inhibition of cell communication. The implication of disrupted body functions, dependent on gap junctional communication, at either elevated or depressed body temperatures, will have to be examined.

Possible Role of Protein kinases and Oxygen Radicals
in the Modulation of Gap Junction Function

One might ask how chemicals, such as the phorbol esters, DDT or saccharin, might inhibit gap junctional intercellular communication by creating disruptions of homeostatic regulation by Ca^{++}, pH, C-AMP or voltage. Although there are several ways to approach this problem, it seems reasonable to ask what seems to be one of the major cellular functions of gap junctional communication and the major cellular consequences of disrupting this normal function.

Normal potentially proliferatable cells "contact-inhibit" to stop growth. Gap junctional intercellular communication is associated with these stationary phase cells. Cell death, cell removal and exposure to mitogenic chemicals presumably release these cells from contact-inhibition (by operational definition), and therefore, by implication, inhibit gap junctional communication to allow intracellular built up of critical molecules needed for cell division (90).

In addition, tumor promoting chemicals or conditions (i.e., partial hepatectomy), which reduce gap junction function, are, by definition, mitogenic for the initiated cell, in that they bring about the clonal amplification of the initiated cell clone. In other words, promoting chemicals are mitogens, not mutagens (97).

In trying to understand this complex mitogenic process, calcium has been long implicated as a "second" messenger for regulating mitogenesis or differentiation in proliferatable stem or precursor cells (11). Cellular pH, the other modulator of gap junctions, has also been linked to a mitogenic signal (34,39,63,78,103). There also might be other mechanisms causing the alteration of gap junction function.

Recently, two major hypotheses have been offered to explain how TPA-like tumor promoters might be acting to cause clonal expansion of initiated cells. First, the activation of protein kinase C is thought to be the primary action of the tumor promoter (71). The calcium dependent-phospholipid kinase (PK-C), once activated, then sets off a chain reaction to phosphorylate a series of cellular structures and proteins. PK-C has also been implicated in the inhibition of intercellular communication, since chemicals such as TPA and teleocidin (15,32), as well as the endogenous activation of PK-C, diacyglycerol (24,33), do inhibit gap junctional communication. Whether all tumor promoters, not binding to PK-C (i.e., DDT, saccharin), work through this mechanism is not yet known. However, the possible role these non-PK-C binding promoters might be doing is causing homeostatic disruption of intracellular free calcium, thereby making it possible to activate PK-C. The observation of synergistic effects of TPA and calcium ionophores (70,106), and some of our own preliminary observations on TPA and DDT [unpublished data], suggest a role of PK-C and gap junctional regulation. At this stage, it is not known whether the effect of PK-C is direct (i.e., phosphorylation of the gap junction protein) or indirect (i.e., phosphorylation of other enzymes/proteins, which, then, inactivates the gap junction).

The activation of a C-AMP-dependent protein kinase and the phosphorylation of gap junctional protein by chemicals which increase gap junctional communication (42,109) suggest a potential phosphorylation/dephosphorylation model of regulation of this critical structure/function (54).

A competing model of the mechanism of TPA-like tumor promoters is that of the induction of the "pro-oxidative" state by tumor promoters (16). While there seems to be strong evidence for the production of oxygen-radical species by many chemical tumor promoters, the critical point is, "What is the cellular molecular target for these reactive species?". Some have argued that DNA is the target; ergo, chemicals, such as TPA, PBB's, phenobarbital etc., by damaging DNA, could act as tumor promoters.

We, and others, have argued that if tumor promoters damaged DNA, via oxygen radicals, "What would be the mechanistic difference between initiators and promoters?" and "How could "mutagens" be "mitogens"?". While some experimental evidence has been interpreted as indicating the production of DNA damage by tumor promoters (i.e., alkaline elution, UDS,

sister chromatid and Ames assay data), it has been argued
that these valid observations have been misinterpreted due to
ignoring the known artifacts or limitations linked to these
assays (89,93). Several in vivo initiation/promotion studies
have indicated no mutagenic potential related to the promotion process, per se, (31,37,79,80,84).

It must be stressed, however, if promotion is operationally the process to amplify the initiated or mutated cell in
order to enhance the probability of additional genetic "hits"
in the cell (93), those additional mutations occur during DNA
replication of the mitogenic or promotion process. In other
words, promotion, although not a mutagenic process, does
facilitate production of gene mutations and other genomic
changes (i.e., gene amplification, non-disjunction, etc.)
which can only occur during mitogenesis.

Therefore, since oxygen radicals can be produced by promoters and since radical savangers have been shown to negate
the tumor promoting effects of some chemicals (55), what
might be alternative cellular/molecular targets other than
DNA. One speculation would be the membrane. This is supported by the observation that benzoyl peroxide has been shown
to be a tumor promoter and to inhibit gap junctional communication (46,87). If oxygen radicals could either damage
membrane molecules, thereby affecting membrane function
(i.e., Ca^{++}-ions regulation, gap junctional integrity/func-
tion, activation of protein kinase C by increases of intracellular Ca^{++} through "leaking" damaged membranes, etc.), one
might be able to integrate the two hypotheses together.

There is a possibility that the PK-C and pro-oxidative
hypotheses, and the known involvement of Ca^{++} as a mitogenic/
differentiation signal, as well as a factor involved in cell
killing (25), could help explain (a) the known mitogenic/
differentiation effects of tumor promoters; (b) how both non-
cytotoxic, mitogenic chemicals, as well as cytotoxic, non-
genotoxic chemicals [i.e. alcohol] or conditions, can be mitogenic and promoting stimuli; (c) how tumor promoters which
are membrane-interacting chemicals modulate both enzyme acti-
vation/deactivation, as well as enzyme and gene induction
(65).

The potential role of the tumor promoter-induced oxygen
radicals in the activation of the ADP-ribosyl transferase and
the ADP-ribosylation of proteins to inactive enzymes and
genes (16), and of the promoter-activated PK-C, by activating
proteins, enzymes and genes (71), could, in principle, provide a complementary regulation system to convert a quiescent
cell to a mitogenic cell.

The Functional Consequence of Chemical Inhibition
of Gap Junctional Communication

Assuming gap junctional communication does play a critical
function (a) during embryogenesis and development; (b) regeneration and wound-healing of tissue; (c) regulation of mito-

sis in proliferatable cells; and (d) maintenance of homeostatic function within specialized cells, both proliferatable and differentiated, of a given organ; and (e) control of adaptive responses in terminally differentiated cells, together with the fact that endogenous and exogenous factors can modulate (enhance or decrease) gap junctional communication, it seems reasonable to speculate that chemicals, which alter gap junctions at critical stages (in early embryogenesis) or for chronic periods of time (in initiated liver) or in specific organs (gonads, brain), might induce non-adaptive disruptions, such as teratogenesis, tumor promotion, reproductive dysfunction or neurotoxicity, respectively.

In addition, if one further assumes that gap junction regulation is ostensibly the same in all cells of all tissues, and that most cells have gap junctions that can be modulated, it would be predicted that a given chemical, depending on pharmacokinetics/metabolism, would affect many organ-specific, gap junction-dependent functions. Interestingly, there seems to be several observations which are consistent with that prediction. Chemicals, such as the retinoic acid analogues, which are modulators of cell differentiation in certain cell lines (13), also modulate gap junctional communication in the target cells (23,76,85,111), ameliorate TPA-inhibition of cell-cell communication (111), as well as act as teratogens (58), anti-tumor promoters against TPA-promotion of skin tumorigenesis (12,102), and tumor-promoters under certain conditions (30,38,107).

In other words, if, by increasing gap junctions in cells during the critical stages of embryogenesis, certain cells have altered communication patterns, differentiation and normal development is altered. In the initiated skin, TPA seems to reduce gap junctional communication (53), induces hyperplasia and alters differentiation (5), and brings the clonal expansion of initiated cells (i.e., promotes tumors). Retinoic acid can, possibly by reversing the TPA reduction of gap junctions, stop the hyperplasia and induce differentiation of initiated cells, thereby acting as an "anti-tumor promoter."

Finally, as a note of speculation, to explain how a single chemical can lead to so many different kinds of toxicological/pharmacological responses in the same organism, one need only recognize the many different functions gap junctions normally fulfill during the development, homeostatic maturation and adaptive phases of an organism's existence.

Phenobarbital, alcohol, diazepam, DDT, dieldrin and aldrin, while being able to modulate brain function, are also tumor promoting chemicals, and in certain cases, structural or behavior teratogens (99). It should also be noted that there is little, if any, evidence any of these chemicals are genotoxic (99).

Major questions as to why any of these and other similar chemicals seem to show species, organ, tissue and/or cell type specificity, in terms of toxic responses, have to be understood. For example, phenobarbital, which is a liver tumor promoter in the mouse and rat, has not yet been shown to be correlated with tumor promotion in human beings, nor does it seem to be a skin tumor promoter in the mouse. Saccharin, a bladder tumor promoter in rats (19), can modulate gap junction function, in vitro, in Chinese hamster V79 cells (96), but not in normal human fibroblasts (64).

In the brain, where gap junctions might play an important role as supplier of nutrients and possible coupler of ionic signals between terminally differentiated excitable neurons and potentially proliferatable glial and astrocytic cells, inhibition of communication for critical periods might not only be non-adaptive in terms of complex brain-dependent behaviors, but might lead to permanent brain damage. One could envisage certain neuron regions of the brain atrophying by the inhibiting the gap junction transfer of critical ions and molecules needed for survival.

In the heart or uterus, where gap junctional communication is needed for ionic and metabolic coupling, respectively (20,75), inhibition of this form of communication could lead to major organ dysfunction.

In summary, although we still need to know much about the actual function of gap junctions in all organs during the development and adaptive life-time of all multi-cellular organisms, and that we need to understand the basic biochemical regulatory function of gap junctions in each organ, it seems that gap junctions do have many important functions in excitable and non-excitable cells, which are potentially proliferatable or are terminally differentiated. Modulation of these gap junctions is part of the adaptive function of these gap junctions. On the other hand, conditions for increasing or decreasing gap junction function, depending on circumstances, can be maladaptive.

POSSIBLE ROLE OF ONCOGENES ON INTERCELLULAR COMMUNICATION AND THE REGULATION AND PROLIFERATION AND DIFFERENTIATION

By definition, oncogenes are sequences of DNA information with a proven cancer association that appear to function primarily in the regulation of cellular proliferation and differentiation (44). Recently, with the explosion of knowledge in the field of oncogene research, Hunter (92) has pointed out that, the understanding of the cellular basis of cancer means being able to describe the biochemistry of the regulated pathways between cell surface and nucleus that control cell growth. However, while this perspective is necessary, it is incomplete, in that, as Potter has stressed, "The cancer problem is not merely a cell problem, it is a problem of cell interaction, not only within tissues, but with distant cells in other tissues" (77).

While our understanding of the number and roles of the oncogenes is far from complete, it does seem clear that these
gene products seem to function as growth factors, growth factor receptors, and regulators of macromolecular synthesis
(105). The expression of several oncogenes have been correlated with dramatic changes taking place in cells during
proliferation and differentiation (1,9,26,29,35,41,66,67,72,
83,88,104,114).

Starting with the assumptions that (a) gap junctions are
critical structures needed for the regulation of proliferation and differentiation (50); (b) chemical tumor promoters,
which are known to modulate proliferation and differentiation
(110), inhibit gap junctional communication and cause clonal
expansion of initiated cells (68,113); and (c) growth factors
and their receptors must trigger events which overcome "contact inhibition" or gap junction-mediated suppression of cell
proliferation, a role of oncogene products in the regulation
of gap junctional communication, at any of its component
steps (98), seems reasonable.

In the last several years, several oncogenes have been
implicated in normal development and differentiation, and in
the differentiation of cells (1,9,26,29,35,41,66,67,83,88,104
114). The fact that several oncogenes [i.e., erb B and sis]
seem to code for growth factors or growth factor receptors
indicates that these oncogenes might play a role in the regulation of gap junction function (98). We (17) and others (6,
8) have demonstrated that several oncogenes (i.e., src, mos,
ras] seem to interfere with gap-junctional communication.

Although growth factors have not yet been tested as tumor
promoters, Lipton et al (47) have shown that platelet-derived
growth factor, coded by c-sis gene, similar to v-sis oncogene, causes the enhancement of growth of HSF-2 transformed
HDF cells in the cheek pouch of hamsters, whereas no tumor
growth was observed in the appropriate control.

Finally, the possible involvement of mutation and clonal
expansion of a mutated oncogene in the initiation/promotion
process of skin tumorigenesis (79) and of the modulation of
oncogenes by the phorbol ester tumor promoter (86) provides a
basis for testing the possible role of oncogenes in the
intercellular regulation of the cancer process.

SUMMARY

Gap junctional communication appears to be an important
biological process involved in the regulation of proliferation, differentiation and adaptive responses of differentiated cells. The process of gap junctional-intercellular is
operationally dependent on a cell's ability to recognize and
"dock" with another cell, to organize the gap junction subunits into functional channels, to transfer regulatory ions
and small molecules and to have appropriate subcellular com-

ponents to respond to these regulatory signals. The biophysical/biochemical chemical nature of the gap junction structure, while not yet unequivocally delineated, seems to be modulated by several important factors, including Ca^{++}, pH, C-AMP, voltage changes, and temperature. Endogenous and exogenous chemicals have been shown to affect gap junction structure/function. Many chemicals which affect gap junctional communication have been shown to stimulate the activity of either protein kinase C or the C-AMP–dependent protein kinase, or to generate oxygen radicals, as well as to modulate intracellular homeostatic control of Ca^{++}, pH or C-AMP.

The biological consequences of modulating gap junction function can be either adaptive or maladaptive, depending on many circumstances, including the time of modulation, the duration of modulation, and the tissue or organ of modulation. The species and organs specificity of chemical modulation is still unknown. Finally, implications for the development of universal in vitro assays to detect chemical modulators of gap junctional communication seems unlikely due to species, organ and cell-type specificity to chemical modulation of gap junction function.

ACKNOWLEDGMENT

The authors wish to express our appreciation to Mr. Mohamed El-Fouly, Dr. B.V. Madhukar, Dr. Toshio Mori, Dr. Saw Yin Oh and Ms. Mary McCrae for discussions pertaining to the manuscript and to Mrs. Darla Conley for the typing of the manuscript. Research, on which this manuscript was based, was supported by the National Cancer Institute (CA21104), the Air Force Office of Scientific Research (AFOSR-86-0084). The U.S. Government is authorized to reproduce and distribute reprints for Government purposes notwithstanding any copyright notion thereon.

REFERENCES

1. Alemia, S., Casalbone, P., Agostin, E., and Tato, F. (1985): Nature 316:557-559.
2. Ames, B.N. (1979): Science 204:587-593.
3. Andrew, R.D., MacVicar, B.A., Dudek, F.E., and Hatton, G.I. (1981): Science 211:1187-1189.
4. Arancia, G., Malorni, W., Mariutti, G., and Trovalusci, P. (1986): Rad. Res. 106:47-55.
5. Argyris, T.S. (1985): CRC Critical Rev. Toxicol. 14: 211-258.
6. Atkinson, M., and Sheridan, J. (1986): J. Membr. Biol. 91:53-64.
7. Aylsworth, C.F., Jone, C., Trosko, J.E. and Chang, C.C. (1984): J. Natl. Cancer Instit. 72:637-645.

8. Azarnia, R., and Loewenstein, W.R. (1984): J. Membr. Biol. 82:191–205.
9. Bar-Sagi, D., and Feramisco, J.R. (1985): Cell 42:841–848.
10. Bennett, M.V.L., and Goodenough, D.A. (1978): Neurosci. Res. Bull. 16:373–486.
11. Berridge, M.J. (1975): J. Cyclic Nucleot. Res. 1:305–320.
12. Boutwell, R.K., and Verma, A.K. (1979): Pure and Appl. Chem. 51:857–866.
13. Breitman, T.R., Selonick, S.E., and Collins, S.J. (1980): Proc. Natl. Acad. Sci. USA 77:2936–2940.
14. Brooks, P., Druckrey, H., Lagerlof, B., Litwin, J., and Williams, G. (1973): In: Ambio. Special Report: Evaluation of Genetic Risks of Environmental Chemicals, edited by C. Ramel, pp. 15–16. Univ. of Stockholm Press, Stockholm.
15. Castagna, M., Takai, Y., Kaibuchi, K., Sano, K., Kikkawa, U., and Nishizuka, Y. (1982): J. Biol. Chem. 257:7847–7851.
16. Cerutti, P.A. (1985): Science 227:375–381.
17. Chang, C.C., Trosko, J.E., Kung, H.J., Bombick, D., and Matsumura, F. (1985): Proc. Natl. Acad. Sci. USA 82:5360–5364.
18. Chen, T.H., Kavanagh, T.J., Chang, C.C., and Trosko, J.E. (1984): Cell Biol. Toxicol. 1:155–171.
19. Cohen, S.M., Murasaki, G., Ellwein, L.B., and Greenfield, R.E. (1983): In: Mechanisms of Tumor Promotion, Vol. 1, edited by T.J. Slaga, pp. 131–150. CRC Press, Baco Raton, Florida.
20. Cole, W.C., Garfield, R.E., and Kirkuldy, J.S. (1985): Am. J. Physiol. 249:C20–C31.
21. DeMaziere, A.M.G.L., and Scheuermann, D.W. (1985): Cell Tiss. Res. 239:651–655.
22. Edelman, G.M. (1983): Science 219:450–457.
23. Elias, P.M., Grayson, S., Caldwell, T.M., and McNutt, N.S. (1980): Lab. Invest. 42:469–474.
24. Enomoto, T., and Yamasaki, H. (1985): Cancer Res. 45:3706–3710.
25. Farber, J.L. (1981): Life Sciences 29:1289–1295.
26. Filmus, J., and Buick, R.N. (1985): Cancer Res. 45:822–825.
27. Finbow, M.E., and Yancey, S.B. (1981): In: Biochemistry of Cellular Regulation, Vol. IV, edited by M.J. Clemens, pp. 215–249. CRC Press, Boca Raton, Florida.
28. Flagg-Newton, J.L., Dahl, G., and Loewenstein, W.R. (1981): J. Membr. Biol. 63:105–121.
29. Foldes, I., and Minarovits, J. (1984): Acta Microbiol. Hung. 31:325–334.

30. Forbes, P.D., Urbach, F., and Davies, R.E. (1979): Cancer Letts. 7:85-90.

31. Fry, R.J.M, Rey, R.D., Grube, D., and Staffeldt, E. (1982): In: Carcinogenesis, Vol. 7, edited by H. Hecker, N.E. Fusenig, W. Kunz, F. Marks, and H.W. Thielmann, pp. 155-165. Raven Press, New York.

32. Fujiki, M., Tanaka, Y., Miyake, R., Kikkawa, U., Nishizuka, Y., and Sugimura, T. (1984): Biochem. Biophys. Res. Commun. 120:339-343.

33. Gainer, H.C., and Murray, A.W. (1985): Biochim. Res. Commun. 126:1109-1113.

34. Gerson, D.F., Kiefer, H., and Eufe, W. (1982): Science 216:1009-1010.

35. Grosso, L.E., and Pitot, H.C. (1985): Cancer Res. 45:847-850.

36. Hartman, P.E. (1983): Environ. Mut. 5:139-152.

37. Hennings, H., Shores, R., Wenk, M.L., Spangler, E.F., Tarone, R., and Yuspa, S.H. (1983): Nature 304: 67-69.

38. Hennings, H., Wenk, M.L., and Donahoe, R. (1982): Cancer Lett. 16:1-5.

39. Hesketh, T.R., Moore, J.P., Morris, J.D.H., Taylor, M.V., Rogers, J., Smith, G.A., and Metcalfe, J.C. (1985): 313:481-484.

40. Hunter, T. (1986): Nature 322:14-16.

41. Jakobovits, A., Schwab, M., Bishop, J.M., and Martain, G.R. (1985): Nature 318:188-190.

42. Johnson, K.R., Panter, S.S., and Johnson, R.G. (1985): Biochim. Biophys. Acta 844:367-376.

43. Jone, C., Erickson, L.M., Trosko, J.E., Netzloff, M.L., and Chang, C.C. (1985): Teratog. Carcinogen. Res. 5:379-391.

44. Lacey, S.W. (1986): Amer. J. Med. Sci. 29:39-46.

45. Larsen, W.J., and Risinger, M.A. (1985): Modern Cell Biol. 4:151-216.

46. Lawrence, N.J., Parkinson, E.J., and Emmerson, A. (1984): Carcinogenesis 5:419-421.

47. Lipton, A., Kepner, N., Rogers, C., Witkoski, E., and Leitzel, K. (1982): In: Interaction of Platelets and Tumor Cells, edited by G.A. Jamieson, pp. 233-248. Alan R. Liss, Inc., New York.

48. Lo, C.W., and Gilula, W.B. (1979): Cell 18:411-422.

49. Loch-Caruso, R., and Trosko, J.E. (1985): CRC Critical Rev. Toxicol. 16:157-183.

50. Loewenstein, W.R. (1979): Biochim. Biophys. Acta 560: 1-65.

51. Loewenstein, W.R. (1981): Physiol. Rev. 61:829-913.

52. Lower, G.M., and Kanarek, M.S. (1982): J. Epidemiol. 115:803-817.

53. Kalimi, G., and Sirsat, S.M. (1984): Carcinogenesis 5:1671-1677.

54. Kanno, Y. (1985): Japan. J. Physiol. 35:693-707.
55. Kensler, T.W., Bush, D.M., and Kozumbo, W.J. (1983): Science. 221:75-77.
56. Kanno, Y., Enomoto, T., Shiba, Y., and Yamasaki, H. (1983): Exp. Cell Res. 152:31-37.
57. Knudson, A.G., Jr. (1979): Am. J. Genet. 31:401-413.
58. Maden, M. (1982): Nature 295:672-675.
59. Madhukar, B.V., Yoneyama, M., Matsumura, F., Trosko, J.E., and G. Tsushimoto (1983): Cancer Lett. 18:251-259.
60. Malcolm, A.R., Mills, L.J., and McKenna, E.J. (1985): Cell Biol. Toxicol. 1:269-283.
61. Malcolm, A.R., Mills, L.J., and Trosko, J.E. (1985): In: Carcinogenesis, edited by M.J. Mass, pp. 305-318. Raven Press, New York.
62. Mehta, P.P., Bertman, J.S., and Loewenstein, W.R. (1986): Cell 44:187-196.
63. Moolenaar, W.H., Tertoolen, L.G.J., and de Laat, S.W. (1984): Nature 312:371-374.
64. Mosser, D.D., and Bols, N.C. (1983): Carcinogenesis 4:991-995.
65. Mueller, G.C., and Wertz, P.W. (1982): In: Carcinogenesis, Vol. 7, edited by E. Hecker, N.E. Fusenig, W. Kunz, F. Marks, and H.W. Thielmann, pp. 499-511. Raven Press, New York.
66. Muller, R., Curran, T., Muller, D., and Guilbert, L. (1985): Nature 314: 546-548.
67. Muller, R., and Wagner, E.F. (1984): Nature 311:438-442.
68. Murray, A.W., and Fitzgerald, D.J. (1979): Biochem. Biophys. Res. Commun. 91:395-401.
69. Neel, J.V. (1978): Canad. J. Genet. Cytol. 20:295-306.
70. Nishizuka, Y. (1984): Nature 308:693-698.
71. Nishizuka, Y. (1986): Science 233:305-312.
72. Noda, M., Ko,M., Ogura, A., Liu, D., Amano, T., Takuno, T., and Ikawa, Y. (1985): Nature 318:73-75.
73. Obrink, B. (1986): Exp. Cell Res. 163:1-21.
74. Paul, D.L. (1986): J. Cell Biol. 103:123-134.
75. Peracchia, C., and Girsch, S.J. (1985): Am. J. Physiol. 248:H765-H782.
76. Pitts, J.D., Hamilton, A.E., Kam, E., Burk, R.R., and Murphy, J.P. (1986): Carcinogenesis 7:1003-1010.
77. Potter, V.R. (1973): In: Cancer Medicine, edited by J. Holland and E. Frei, pp. 178-192. Lea and Febiger, Philadelphia.
78. Pouyssegur, J., Franchi, A., L'Allemain, G., and Paris, S. (1985): FEBS 190:115-119.
79. Quintanilla, M., Brown, K., Ramsden, M., and Balmain, A. (1986); Nature 322:78-80.
80. Reddy, A.L., and Fialkow, P.J. (1983): Nature 304:69-71.

81.   Rose, B., Simpson, I., and Loewenstein, W.R. (1977): Nature 265:625–627.
82.   Saez, J.C., Spray, D.C., Nairn, A.C., Hertzberg, E., Greengard, P., and Bennett, M.V.L. (1986): Proc. Natl. Acad. Sci. USA 83:2473–2477.
83.   Schartl, M., and Barnekow, A. (1984): Devel. Biol. 105:415–422.
84.   Scherer, E., Feringa, A.W., and Emmelot, P. (1984): In: Models, Mechanisms and Etiology of Tumor Promotion, edited by M. Borzonyi, N.E. Day, K. Lupis, and H. Yamasaki, pp. 57-66. IARC Scientific Publ., Lyon, France.
85.   Shuin, T., Nishimura, R., Noda, K., Umeda, M., and Ono, T. (1983): Gann 74:100–105.
86.   Skouv, J., Christensen, B., Skibshj, I., and Autrup, H. (1986): Carcinogenesis 7:331-333.
87.   Slaga, T.J., Klein-Szanto, A.J.P., Triplett, L.L., Yotti, L.P., and Trosko, J.E. (1981): Science 213:1023–1025.
88.   Thiele, C.J., Reynolds, C.P., and Israel, M.A. (1985): Nature 313:404–406.
89.   Trosko, J.E. (1984): Environ, Mut. 6:767–769.
90.   Trosko, J.E., and Chang, C.C. (1983): Pharmacol. Rev. 36:137–144.
91.   Trosko, J.E., and Chang, C.C. (1985): In: Methods for Estimating Risk of Chemical Injury: Human and Non-Human Biota and Ecosystems, edited by V.B. Vouk, G.C. Butler, D.G. Hoel, and D.B. Peakall, pp. 181-200. J. Wiley & Sons, Chichester.
92.   Trosko, J.E., and Chang, C.C. (1986): In: Antimutagenesis and Anticarcinogenesis: Mechanism, edited by D.M. Shankel, P.E. Hartman, T. Kada, and A. Hollaender. Plenum Press, New York.
93.   Trosko, J.E., Chang, C.C., and Medcalf, A. (1983): Cancer Invest. 1:511-526.
94.   Trosko, J.E., Chang, C.C., and Netzloff, M. (1982): Terat. Carcinog. Mutag. 2:31-45.
95.   Trosko, J.E., Chang, C.C., and Wade, M.H. (1984): In: Genetics: New Frontier, edited by V.L. Chopra, B.C. Joshi, R.P. Sharma, and H.C. Bansal, Vol. 1, pp. 352-346. Oxford and IBH Publ., New York.
96.   Trosko, J.E., Dawson, B., Yotti, L.P., and Chang, C.C. (1980): Nature 284:109–110.
97.   Trosko, J.E., Jone, C., and Chang, C.C. (1983): In: Cellular Systems for Toxicity Testing, edited by G.M. Williams, V.C. Dunkel, and V.A. Ray, pp. 316-327. New York Acad. Sciences, New York.

98. Trosko, J.E., Jone, C., and Chang, C.C. (1984): Cellular Interactions by Environmental Tumor Promoters, edited by H. Fujiki, E. Hecker, R.E. Moore, T. Sugimura, and I.B. Weinstein, pp. 101-113. Japan Scientific Soc. Press, Tokyo.

99. Trosko, J.E., Jone, C., and Chang, C.C. (1986): Mol. Toxicol., in press.

100. Tsushimoto, G., Trosko, J.E., Chang, C.C., and Aust, S.F. (1983): Carcinogenesis 3:181-185.

101. In't Veld, P., Schuit, F., and Pipeleers, D. (1985): J. Cell Biol. 36:269-276.

102. Verma, A.K., Conrad, E.A., and Boutwell, R.K. (1982): Cancer Res. 42:3519-3525.

103. Vicentini, L.M., and Villereal, M.L. (1986): Life Sci. 38:2269-2276.

104. Watanabe, T., Sariban, E., Mitchell, T., and Kufe, D. (1985): Biochem. Biophys. Res. Commun. 126:999-1005.

105. Weinberg, R.A. (1985): Science 230:770-776.

106. Weissmann, G., Azaroff, L., Davidson, S., and Dunham, P. (1986): Proc. Natl. Acad. Sci. USA 83:2914-2918.

107. Welsch, C.W., Goodrich-Smith, M., Brown, C.K., and Crowe, N. (1981): J. Natl. Cancer Instit. 67:935-938.

108. Welsch, F., and Stedman, D.B. (1984): Teratog. Carcinog. Mutag. 4:285-301.

109. Wiener, E.C., and Loewenstein, W.R. (1983): Nature 305:433-435.

110. Yamasaki, H. (984): In: Mechanisms of Tumor Promotion, Vol. IV, edited by T.J. Slaga, pp. 1-26. CRC Press, Baco Raton, Florida.

111. Yamasaki, H., Enomoto, T., Hamel, H., and Kanno, Y. (1984): In: Cellular Interactions by Environmental Tumor Promoters, edited by H. Fujiki, E. Hecker, R.E. Moore, T. Sugimura, and I.B. Weinstein, pp. 221-233. Japan Scientific Soc. Press, Tokyo.

112. Yancey, S.B., Easter, D., and Revel, J.P. (1979): J. Ultrast. Res. 67:229-249.

113. Yotti, L.P., Chang, C.C., and Trosko, J.E. (1979): Science 206:1089-1091.

114. Zimmerman, K.A., Yancopoulos, G.D., Collum, R.G., Smith, R.K., Kohl, N.E., Denis, K.A., Nau, M.M., Witte, O.N., Toran-Allerand, D., Gee, C.E., Minna, J.D., and Alt, F.W. (1986): Nature 319:780-783.

Tumor Promoters: Biological Approaches for
Mechanistic Studies and Assay Systems,
edited by Robert Langenbach et al.
Raven Press, New York © 1988.

DISRUPTION OF CELL-CELL CHANNELS AS AN EVENT COMMON TO THE

POTENTIAL MECHANISM OF ACTION OF SOME CHEMICALS WITH

TERATOGENIC AND CARCINOGENIC ACTIVITY

F. Welsch

Department of Cell Biology
Chemical Industry Institute of Toxicology
Research Triangle Park, North Carolina 27709

BACKGROUND

Based on in vitro studies regarding disruption of gap junction-mediated intercellular communication by tumor promoting chemicals and on certain commonalities between carcinogenesis and teratogenesis, Trosko and his associates postulated that disruption of cell-cell communication may also be a mechanism by which some chemical teratogens act (24,37). The common feature in both cases is that normal cell differentiation is disrupted. The complexity of normal embryogenesis and the lack of understanding of its controlling factors have hindered studies on the induction of abnormal development. There is agreement that teratogens are likely to act through a multitude of mechanisms, and alteration of membrane functions is one among them. This may result in failure of proper cell-cell interactions (30,44). Morphogenetic communication in embryos has been studied for quite some time, and the phenomenon is described in the literature as "morphogenetic tissue interactions" or "inductive tissue interactions". Although many observations suggest that the cell membrane is a target site, very little specific data exist with respect to alteration of membrane function caused by chemical teratogens.

Cell-Cell Channels in Embryogenesis

Among several modes of cell-cell communication (synonymous with intercellular communication) is one specific way how cells in close proximity can communicate with one another through a low resistance pathway. Hydrophilic cell-to-cell channel traverse apposing cell membranes and form aggregates known as gap junctions. Such pathways were first postulated based on functional studies and their existence was then confirmed by ultrastructural analysis (25,31). Considerable progress has been made as regards the structure, distribution, permeability and biochemical make-up of these junctions (8,10,27,31,32). Knowledge about the physiological role of the junctions has advanced comparatively modestly, yet the term "junctional (or gap junctional) communication" is readily accepted in the literature.

It is believed that during embryogenesis gap junctions are involved in the regulation of cell growth, pattern formation and differentiation by allowing the cell-to-cell transmission of as yet unidentified molecular signals (1,15,23,25,26,45). Lower vertebrate embryos have been studied most intensely because they have large, identifiable cells with gap junctions. The cell size makes them suitable for multiple simultaneous micropipet impalements which are desirable for ion coupling studies (9,32,39). In mammalian development cell-cell communication has been measured by electrocoupling and fluorescent dye coupling in pre- and postimplantation mouse embryos (23). In reviewing the accumulated data, Lo (23) observed that "in order to discern the role of cell-cell communication in embryogenesis, it would be necessary to be able to specifically inhibit gap junctional communication and study the subsequent effects on development." Indeed, a major obstacle in testing the numerous hypotheses about the role of gap junctions has been lack of a specific and reversible probe to interfere with junctional permeability (23,24).

More recently the effect of antibodies against highly purified gap junction protein was studied and the results strongly suggest an association between cell-cell channel function and progressive development. An indentified, single cell of xenopus embryos was injected with antibodies, and within minutes dye and electrical coupling to adjacent cells were disrupted. The effect was long-lasting, and in many instances grossly malformed embryos developed (39,40). While this example has particular relevance to the role of gap junctional communication in embryogenesis, antibodies have also been shown to affect gap junctional conductance in other tissues (9). Antibodies have been used to demonstrate by indirect immunofluorescence the presence of gap junctions in tissues rich in junctions such as mouse or rat liver (3,7).

The abundance of gap junctions throughout embryonal development and their appearance or disappearance coincident with specific developmental events supports the idea that cell-to-cell channels provide a pathway for intercellular signals of a transient nature. They may also facilitate the build-up of chemical gradients during development (24,25,45). Gap junctional communication can be measured with methods requiring very different levels of technical sophistication. Although several laboratories are pursuing quantification of gap junction proteins with techniques of immunology and molecular biology (7,10,27), there is to date no method more readily available than morphometry to correlate functional measurements of cell coupling with the structural existence and extent of gap junction plaques (22). This relationship is of particular interest when pharmacological agents are applied that alter gap junctional communication.

Disruption of Gap Junctions by Teratogens

In our laboratory gap junctional communication has been studied with three different methods involving cell culture. The first observations were made in V79 Chinese hamster cells using the metabolic cooperation assay (36) and showed that some well established chemical teratogens apparently inhibited gap junctional communication (41). However, the long chemical exposure time of 3 days in this assay seemed incompatible with the speed of events in embryogenesis. Therefore we adopted a much more sensitive autoradiographic method and applied it a cell line derived from the palate region of a human embryo. This allowed to assess communication competence after only 3 hr exposure to an embryotoxin (42). We selected 12-O-tetradecanoylphorbol-13-acetate (TPA) for a more detailed analysis that involved correlation of gap junction function and quantitative morphometry. TPA is quite potent in whole embryo culture where it interferes with yolk sac function of cultured rat embryos (11,12), and *in vivo* TPA induces kidney malformations in mouse offspring (13). Common features between carcinogenesis and embryogenesis are suggested by some of the biological effects that TPA exerts on the epidermis of adult mice. The drug causes the skin to assume several biochemical characteristics of embryonal skin as evidenced by a decrease in histidase activity, an increase in protease and ornithine decarboxylase activities, the appearance of two embryonal proteins and the induction of stem cells with resemblance to embryonal cells (13).

More recently all-trans-retinoic acid (RA) has been studied in cultures of mouse limb bud mesenchyme cells which undergo morphological and biochemical differentiation. This compound and structurally related congeners called retinoids have been investigated very actively in carcinogenesis. Only quite recently have retinoids attracted considerable attention in teratology because 13-cis-retinoic acid (ACCUTANE) was approved by the FDA for the therapy of severe human skin diseases. By now numerous cases of malformations in human babies are recorded resulting from inadvertent exposure to the drug *in utero* (5). These effects were not unanticipated since it has been known for about 20 years that RA is a potent animal teratogen in several species with multiple target sites including the limbs (18). Thus two compounds which because of their profound biologic activities have been investigated much more intensely in tumorigenesis where they are known to affect cell differentiation profoundly were used in our studies. The common denominator is that the mechanism of action of TPA and RA in carcinogenesis and teratogenesis may ultimately affect gap junction permeability. Available evidence indicates that a receptor-mediated biochemical cascade is involved whose complexity increases all the time as new data are generated. Our observations suggest that the teratogens disrupted the function of cell-to-cell channels and affected gap junctions at the time when intercellular communication was impaired.

MATERIALS AND METHODS

1) Intercellular communication experiments with human embryonal palate mesenchyme (HEPM) cells: Transfer of ^{3}H-uridine labeled nucleotides was measured with methods described in detail (28,42), and the inhibitory effects of TPA were correlated with ultrastructural analysis of the incidence of gap junctions.

2) Intercellular communication between mouse embryo limb bud mesenchyme cells: Male and female Crl:CD-1 ICR BR (CD-1) mice were obtained from Charles River Breeding Laboratories, Inc. (Kingston, N.Y.). Upon arrival the animals were quarantined for 2 weeks, housed in polycarbonate cages in a mass air displacement room (Bioclean, Hazleton Systems Inc., Vienna, Va.) and provided NIH-07 open formula diet (Zeigler Brothers, Gardner, Pa.) and water <u>ad</u> <u>libitum</u>. Males were housed individually, while females were kept in groups of 5/cage. The animal room was maintained at 22 ± 1.5°C with a relative humidity of 50 ± 10% and was illuminated from 1000 to 2200 hr daily. Nulliparous females of about 25-35 g body weight were paired in the home cage of the males for the last 1.5 hr of the dark cycle. Females with copulation plugs were presumed to be pregnant. These animals were weighed, and the next 24 hr period was designated as gestation day (gd) 0.

On gd 11 (about 40-44 somites) dams were killed by cervical dislocation, and the uterine horns were removed aseptically. Embryos were obtained, and forelimb buds were excised. Pooled limb buds were dissociated into single cells with 0.25% trypsin-containing, calcium and magnesium-free, saline solution for 20 min at 37°C. The resultant cell suspension was filtered through a 20 μm Nitex microfilament screen to remove any remaining large cell clumps. The cell suspension was then centrifuged for 10 min at 600x g and the supernatant was removed. Complete culture medium consisting of CMRL-1066 (Gibco, Grand Island, NY) containing 10% fetal bovine serum, 2 mM L-glutamine and gentamicin was added to result in a final cell concentration of 1×10^7 cells/ml. For routine cultures 20 μl aliquots (~200,000 cells) were seeded in 35 mm culture dishes. After a 2 hr incubation to allow cell attachment the resultant spot cultures were fed with 2 ml of complete medium, and incubation was continued at 37°C in a humidified atmosphere of 95% air and 5% CO_2. These conditions at high density ("micromass cultures") are conducive to cartilaginous differentiation of limb mesenchymal cells and to the production of chondrogenic matrix (17,26,47). Cartilage nodules are clearly recognizable after about 48 hr in culture. At this time all-trans retinoic acid (RA; Sigma Chemicals, St. Louis, MO) in concentrations ranging from 0.01 μg to 10.0 μg/ml culture medium (0.033-33 μM) dissolved in ethanol (volume not exceeding 0.5% of the culture volume) was added to the medium.

In dishes destined to undergo chondrogenic differentiation the culture medium was changed 24 hr later, i.e. 3 days after initiation. Fresh medium containing RA was added for 3 more days. On day 6 the cultures were stained for 2 hr with Alcian Blue (0.5% Alcian Blue in 3% glacial acetic acid, pH adjusted to 1.0 with HCl). Unbound dye was removed by washing 3 times with 3% acetic acid (pH 1.0). The dye bound to the extracellular matrix was extracted overnight with 1.0 ml of 4 M guanidine HCl, an aliquot of which was transferred to a 96 well microtiter plate. The absorbance of Alcian Blue was determined at 600 nm with a Titertek multiskan spectrophotometer.

In dishes designated for dye coupling, measurements were performed with the equipment described elsewhere (35). Briefly, about 48 hr after seeding the cells and within less than 1 hr after their first exposure to RA, pneumatic microinjections of picoliter volumes of Lucifer Yellow CH (Sigma Chemical) were delivered from the Picospritzer 2 (General Valve Corporation, Fairfield, N.J.). Dye was injected into cells associated with chondrogenic foci which were clearly recognizable at 200 fold magnification. Dye spread into cells in direct and indirect contact with an injected cell was recorded 5 min later when maximal fluorescence labeling had occurred by counting the number of cells containing Lucifer Yellow. In later experiments, the exposure time to RA was as short as 2 min before the first dye injections were made. The reversibility of RA-induced inhibition of dye coupling following 1 hr of drug exposure was studied after washing the cultures 3 times with phosphate buffered saline which contained 10% bovine serum albumin.

Cells were grown in preparation for ultrastructural analysis of gap junctions. In order to obtain enough cells, multiple spots of dissociated limb bud cells were plated in 150 cm^2 culture flasks, keeping the cell density/ml medium corresponding to the one used in dye coupling studies. Following exposure to ethanol vehicle or to 0.1 and 1.0 μg RA/ml for 1 hr as in most of the dye coupling experiments, cells were detached from the substratum with a rubber policeman and pelleted by mild centrifugation. Cells were then fixed by resuspending the pellet in 2% glutaraldehyde/2% paraformaldehyde in 0.1 M phosphate buffer, pH 7.2. Further preparation for freeze-fracture and electron microscopic examination of replicas followed the procedure described elsewhere (42).

RESULTS AND DISCUSSION

In HEPM cells, ^{3}H-uridine labeled nucleotides were transferred from pulse-labelled potential donor cells to potential recipient cells during 3 hr coculture. This process met all established specificity criteria (28) and was therefore assumed to be occurring through gap junctions. Various concentrations of TPA or of 4α-phorbol-12,13-di-decanoate (4α-PDD, which lacks skin tumor promoting capacity) were added during the coculture phase. Only TPA inhibited the transfer of radioactive nucleotides to potential recipient cells in a concentration-related manner. Ultrastructural analysis revealed that HEPM cells had gap junctions, and quantitative morphometry showed that TPA caused a significant reduction in the number of gap junctions (Table 1).

Table 1. <u>Incidence of gap junctions in HEPM cells</u>[+]

	Control	TPA exposed
No. of cells examined at x20,000	119	111
Total area examined (μm^2)	1096.73	1149.42
μm^2/field ± SD	9.22±3.24	10.35±2.91
No. of cells with gap junctions	25	11
Total no. of gap junctions	48	14

Cells were exposed to 4.0 ng TPA/ml for 3 hr.
[+]Reprinted from ref. 42, with permission.

This effect is similar to the one in V79 cells after much longer TPA exposure (46). A disadvantage of (the otherwise very sensitive) autoradiographic method to measure gap junctional communication quantitatively is that several hours of coculture are required so that enough labeled nucleotides are transferred to produce sufficient grain counts on autoradiograms. During this time the cells are continuously exposed to the teratogen. Although the method was a vast improvement over the 3 days of chemical teratogen presence in our V79 cell studies, the 3 hr exposure time is still quite long considering the rapidity of biochemical reactions in living cells and the speed of onset of inhibitory effects of TPA which we observed in later experiments with dye coupling (35). Nevertheless, the results further supported the hypothesis that gap junctions might be affected by some chemical teratogens.

For the next phase of the investigations two considerations entered into the experimental design. One was to use a method that would allow more rapid assessment of gap junctional communication and the second was to use a biological system that undergoes progressive development as cells in embryos do. The first objective was accomplished by adopting the dye coupling technique. Its advantage for detecting intercellular communication is that dye distribution from a single injected cell into neighboring cells with direct membrane apposition can be observed within seconds and that final distribution is reached within minutes. The other goal was met by the selection of primary cultures of mouse embryo limb bud mesenchyme cells which undergo chondrogenic differentiation. Cell-cell interactions between cells of limb buds in situ and in vitro are believed to be critical for normal limb development (14,15,33,34). There is persuasive evidence derived from transmission electron microscopic (TEM) studies that the appearance of gap junctions in high density cultures precedes in time chondrogenic differentiation and is a prerequisite for initiation of this process (26). Although the exact nature of the interactions and the chemical messengers which are potentially involved are unknown, 3',5'-cyclic adenosine monophosphate (cAMP) has emerged as an agent that enhances chondrogenic differentiation of cultured limb mesenchyme cells (4,20,21,34). Another attractive feature was that mouse embryo limb buds exposed to RA in utero are highly susceptible to RA-induced malformations (18,19) and that RA and other retinoids interfere with chondrogenic differentiation in high density cultures (6,16,17,47). Dye coupling was studied under control conditions and after exposure to RA or dibutyryl cAMP (dbcAMP). Data on cell coupling were correlated with the synthesis of Alcian Blue stained extracellular cartilaginous matrix. Exposure to RA inhibited the differentiation of mesenchyme cells to chondrocytes and the synthesis of cartilaginous matrix in a concentration-dependent manner (Figure 1; Table 2).

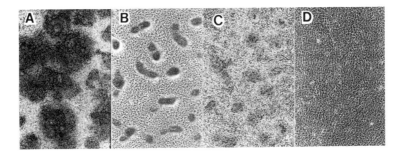

FIG. 1. Chondrogenic differentiation of limb bud cells. Culture conditions as in Table 2. All-trans retinoic (RA) acid was added 48 hr later and remained present for 4 days. The photomicrographs demonstrate the extent of the chondrogenic foci which consist of chondrocytes (not visible at this enlargement) and Alcian Blue stained cartilage extracelluar matrix. Panel A is a control culture, while the others illustrate the RA concentration-dependent inhibition of matrix synthesis : 0.1 (B), 1.0 (C) and 10.0 (D) $\mu g/ml$. More and more of the culture dish surface is occupied by cells which do not undergo chondrogenic differentiation. Magnification 25 x.

Table 2. Inhibition of chondrogenesis

Retinoids	0.01 μg/ml	0.1 μg/ml	1.0 μg/ml	10 μg/ml
All-trans-retinoic acid (RA)	67	18	10	4
13-Cis-RA	57	45	24	8

Values are % of control (Alcian Blue stain)
Limb bud mesenchyme cells were explanted in high density micromass culture on gestation day 11, and 48 hr later retinoids were added. The cultures were terminated after 6 days, fixed and stained with Alcian Blue, which was extracted and quantitated by spectrophotometry. All values are expressed in percent of control.

When Lucifer Yellow was injected 48 hr after explantation into cells undergoing chondrogenic differentiation, dye spread into neighboring cells was rapid and maximal judged by labeling intensity within a few minutes (Figure 2, A and B). Routinely the number of fluorescent cells was counted 5 min after injection. A disadvantage of the dye coupling method in the multilayer high density cultures was that its applicability is limited to the periphery of chondrogenic nodules where not too many layers grow on top of one another. Otherwise it is impossible to count the number of fluorescent cells into which the dye has spread reliably.

Within 1 hr or less RA affected dye coupling depending on the concentration (Figure 2, panel B; Table 3). When the potencies of RA and 13-cis-RA are compared, it is difficult to decide whether the concentration differences at which they interfered

Table 3. Inhibition of dye coupling

Retinoids (μg/ml)	Control	0.01	0.1	1.0	10
All-trans-retinoic acid (RA)[a]	12.14 ±0.89	9.95 ±0.76	6.27[b] ±0.37	3.33[b] ±0.54	0.067[b] ±0.057
13-Cis-RA[a]	9.43 ±1.12	ND	11.2 ±1.19	9.20 ±0.85	0.00[b] ±0.0

ND - not determined; [a]Values are means ± SE of at least 20 injected cells; [b]p<0.001
Culture conditions as in Table 2. About 48 hr later cultures were exposed to the retinoids, and dye coupling was quantitated within 1 hr. Numbers show the number of recipient cells 5 min after microinjections of Lucifer Yellow into a single donor cell and are the mean ± S.E. of at least 20 injected cells.

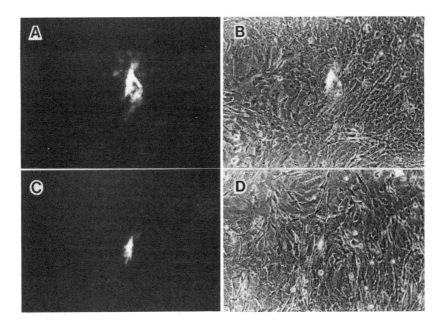

FIG. 2.   Dye coupling during chondrogenic differentiation.
Culture conditions as in Table 2. About 48 hr later Lucifer
Yellow was microinjected into single cells. Panel A and B:
Control culture in fluorescent (A) and brightfield (B)
illumination dye spread recorded 5 min after injection into the
bright glowing cell has occurred into many neighboring cells
(A). Panel C and D: Inhibition of dye coupling after exposure
to 1.0 μg RA/ml for 1 hr (C). Even in the brightfield picture
the injected cell is recognizable (D). Magnification 50 x.

with dye coupling reflect the in vivo observations.   At
equimolal doses RA is a more potent teratogen than 13-cis-RA is
(18), and it appears as if the in vivo differences can be
explained on pharmacokinetic grounds (19).   When formation of
cartilaginous matrix was used as the assay endpoint, there was
no remarkable difference between RA and 13-cis-RA in vitro.
Using the same endpoint, Kistler found correlations with the in
vivo teratogenicity among retinoids with free carboxyl end-
groups (17).
    Additional support for the contention that a relationship
exists between cell coupling, chondrogenic differentiation and
cartilaginous matrix formation derives from the effects of
dbcAMP. While we have not performed a systematic analysis of the
chronology, an enhancement of dye coupling was first detectable
5 hr after the addition of 1 mM to cells which were explanted
about 48 hr earlier. In parallel dishes chondrogenesis was more
than doubled (Table 4). These findings agree with those first

Table 4.   <u>Effects of dibutyryl-3',5'-cyclic AMP on dye coupling</u>
           <u>and on chondrogenic differentiation</u>

Treatment	Dye coupling	Alcian Blue absorption
Control	16.00 ± 7.95	0.124 (=100%)
dbcAMP (1 mM)	31.93 ± 8.14	0.301 (241%)

Culture conditions as in Table 2.   About 48 hr later cultures
were exposed to dbcAMP. Dye coupling was assessed 24 hr later,
and the data show the   number   of fluorescent recipient cells ±
S.D. resulting from injections   into   at   least 20 cells. Alcian
Blue was quantitated 6 days after initiating culture.

described by Loewenstein and   associates, who demonstrated that
cAMP enhanced   cell   coupling   and   the   number of cell-to-cell
channels (25).   Our   observations   confirm those made by several
investigators   who   reported   that   during   chondrogenic
differentiation of mouse limb bud cells <u>in vitro</u>, cAMP or other
molecular   signals   that   elevate   its intracellular levels
stimulate the synthesis of cartilaginous matrix (4,20,21,34).
    Judged by inhibition of dye spread both 0.1 and 1.0 μg RA/ml
disrupted cell-cell channel function.   Our observations agree
with those   reporting   inhibitory   effects   of   RA on metabolic
cooperation between rat liver cells   after 6.5 to 24 hr exposure
(38)   and   alterations   of   the   gap junctional conductance
characteristics (32).   More   detailed measurements regarding the
onset of inhibitory effects on dye coupling were performed with
RA because it was recently   reported   that in BRL rat epithelial
cells RA at the   high   concentration   of 100 μM blocked dye
coupling almost completely within 2 min (29).   We examined 1 μg
RA/ml (3.3 μM) and 10 μg/ml (33 μM) and observed that at 1.0 μg
the onset of inhibitory effects   on dye coupling was gradual and
significant after 30   min   (Table   5).   At   the   higher
concentration, the onset of dye coupling blockade was so rapid
that after the technically   unavoidable   delay (~ 2 min) between
adding microliter amounts of   RA, mixing, repositioning the dish
on the microscope stage   and   impaling cells for dye injection,
there   was   already   complete   blockade   of gap junctional
communication (Table 5).
    Recent results obtained in cells   growing in monolayer have
suggested that the inhibitory effect of   10 μM (2) or 100 μM RA
(29) on gap junctional   communication   was readily reversible
after washing. With respect   to our limb mesenchyme cell system
such concentrations   of   RA are   extremely high.   Significant
effects on chondrogenic differentiation as judged by Alcian Blue
extracted after 6   days   are   observed   following treatment with
0.01 μg RA/ml (Table 2). Unfortunately, Alcian Blue staining to
quantitate the   amount   of cartilaginous extracellular matrix is
too insensitive to allow synchronization of the endpoints of

Table 5.   Onset of inhibitory effects of retinoic acid on
dye coupling

	2 min	5 min	Drug Exposure Time 10 min	30 min	1 hr	2 hr
1 μg/ml (3.3 μM)	ND	11.46 ±3.96	7.00 ±3.10	2.00 ±2.76	0	0
10 μg/ml (33 μM)	0	0	0	ND	ND	ND

Control was 14.33 ± 3.73 in this experimental series

ND-not determined.
Culture conditions as in Table 2.   About 48 hr later cells were
exposed to all-trans-retinoic acid.   Numbers shown indicate the
number of recipient cells   labelled   5 min after microinjections
of Lucifer Yellow into a single donor cell.   Values are the mean
± S.E. of at least 20 injected cells.

inhibited   dye   coupling   and   reduced   matrix   synthesis.   The
concentration-effect relationship as   regards   dye coupling also
revealed significant inhibition by 0.1   μg within 1 hr after the
cells were first exposed (Figure 3).
    When micromass cultures of limb   bud   cells exposed to 1.0 or
10 μg RA/ml for 1 hr   were   washed as .described in Methods, the
return of   communication   competence was   much   slower   than in
fibroblasts (2) or BRL cells (29)   growing in monolayer.   In our
chondrocyte cultures dye coupling returned to the control levels
only after   about   2 hr (Table 6).   The   differences may be
attributable to the fact   that   RA   is quite lipophilic and that
washing removes the drug   much   less efficiently from multilayer
chondrocyte cultures than it   does   from the monolayers examined
in the other studies.
    The results by quantitative   morphometry were correlated with
those   obtained   in   dye   coupling   and   cartilaginous   matrix
determinations, both of which were used as functional indicators
of cell-cell interactions.   One hr   after exposure to 0.1 or 1.0
μg RA/ ml, when inhibition of dye coupling was well established
or   complete,   respectively,   cells   were   prepared   for freeze-
fracture analysis in a double blind fashion.   The codes were not
broken until all numbers were   assembled.   The data reveal that
after examining   a   comparable   number   of   cells   and total PF-
membrane surface area, the   incidence   of gap junctions appeared
to be higher in cells   exposed   to   0.1 g RA/ml than in controls
(Table 7).   However, individual gap junctions were smaller after
treatment with this drug   concentration.   Although the average
size of the   remaining   individual   gap   junctions was unchanged
compared to control after   treatment   with   1.0   μg RA/ml, the
number of junctions was apparently decreased.   This is reflected

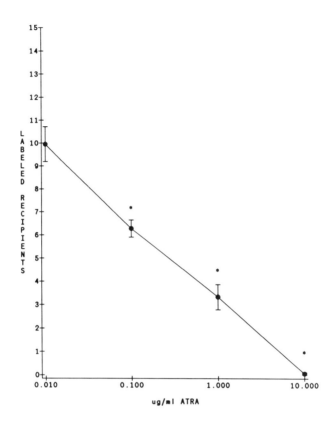

FIG. 3.   Retinoic acid (RA) concentration effects on dye
coupling. Cultures conditions as in Table 2. About one hour
after exposure to the RA concentrations indicated on a
logarithmic scale in the abscissa, cells were injected with
Lucifer Yellow. The number of labeled cells shown on the
ordinate was counted 5 min later. Each point is the mean ± SE
of at least 20 injected cells. The control value in this series
was 12.14 ± 0.89, and values marked with an asterisk differ
significantly (p < 0.01) from that control.

in the trend towards a decline of total gap junctional area when
the size of all individual junctions is summed. The apparent
action of RA to reduce gap junction incidence is also reflected
by the reduction of the fractional cell surface area occupied by
gap junctions in relationship to the total protoplasmic membrane
area of the cells (Table 7).   Analysis of the differences
between treatment-specific means after a log 10 transformation
with an unpaired t-test (pooled variance) did not quite reach
significance at p <0.05.   The ultrastructural data show that
limb mesenchyme cells undergoing chondrogenic differentiation

Table 6. <u>Effect of washing on retinoic acid-induced inhibition of dye coupling</u>

| | Time after completing wash procedure | | | | | |
	2 min	5 min	10 min	30 min	1 hr	2 hr
1.0 μg/ml	ND	ND	0	1.08	4.36	10.71
(3.3 μM)				$\pm$1.44	$\pm$2.20	3.34
10 μg/ml	ND	0	0	4.59	3.27	11.92
(33 μM)				$\pm$3.66	$\pm$3.66	$\pm$ 4.32

Control was 12.63 $\pm$ 4.11 in this experimental series

ND-not determined.
Culture conditions as in Table 2. About 48 hr later cells were treated for 1 hr with all-trans-retinoic acid. Values shown are mean $\pm$ S.E. of at least 20 injected cells.

Table 7. <u>Incidence of gap junctions (gj) in differentiating mouse embryo limb bud cells</u>

| | | All-trans retinoic acid | |
	Control	0.1 μg/ml	1.0 μg/ml
No. of fields examined at x2000	104	115	99
Total area examined (μm^2)	791	676	733
Total no. of gj	22	30	15
Gj/ 100 μm^2	2.78	4.44	2.04
Area of individual gj	11.88	6.47	13.49
(nm^2, mean $\pm$ S.E.)	$\pm$ 3.38	$\pm$ 1.21	$\pm$ 4.39
Total gj area (μm^2)	0.2614	0.1942	0.2023
Gj area as % of total area	3.30x10^{-4}	2.87x10^{-4}	2.76x10^{-4}

Culture conditions as in Table 2. About 48 hr later cultures were exposed to all-trans retinoic acid for 1 hr and then fixed and prepared for freeze-fracture and quantitative morphometry of gj.

have few and small gap junctions (Figure 4). This is reflected by the low number of junctions and the small fractional area that they occupy compared to the total cell surface area. Other cells, for example in the liver or membrana granulosa cells in the ovary, have much more favorable relationships with single junctions as large as 40 μm^2 and fractional total gap junctional area occupying 20% of the surface of a single cell. Mathematical analysis of our data projects that in order to raise the power of the statistical test, the sample size would need to be increased to about 100 gap junctions per treatment condition. Quantitative morphometry of gap junctions is time consuming. Therefore considerable effort would be required to

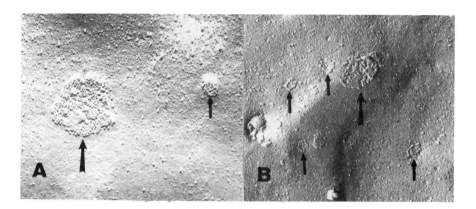

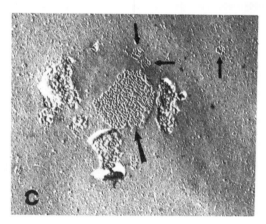

FIG. 4. Gap junctions (gj) of differentiating cells. Culture
conditions as in Table 2. One hour after all-trans retinoic acid
(RA) exposure cells were fixed and prepared for freeze-fracture.
Arrows point to gj on the protoplasmic face (PF) of the
fractured membrane where they apppear as aggregates of
particles, each constituting one cell-to-cell channel. A:
Control with one relatively large and one small gj; B: several
small and one larger gj from cells exposed to 0.1 μg RA/ml; C:
one large and several small gj from cells exposed to 1.0 μg
RA/ml. Regardless of RA treatment other PF membrane-associated
particles appear to be randomly distributed over the membrane
surface. Magnification 60000 x.

scrutinize more cells. The incidence of gap junctions in
mesenchymal cells of the limb bud is much lower than it is in
ectodermal cells of the apical ectodermal ridge (14). This

structure is intimately associated with morphogenetic cell-cell interactions with the underlying mesenchyme during limb development (14,15). It appears more worthy to invest the time into examining cells form this source after RA treatment to facilitate the procurement of substantive quantitative morphometric data than to pursue the limb chondrocyte cells.

The effects of RA on gap junctions have been discussed elsewhere in greater detail (43), and only selected references will be cited here to studies in which the exposure conditions are somewhat similar to those applied in our chondrocyte cultures. An increase in the number of gap junctions seems incompatible with the reduction of dye coupling observed after 1 hr exposure to 0.1 μg RA/ml (compare Figure 2 and 3 with Table 7). At the same time, however, a decline in average size was apparent. Both phenomena in chondrocyte culture resemble those described by Larsen (22). He found that cumulus and membrana granulosa cells of the rat ovary responded to hormonal stimulation by the rapid disappearance of larger gap junctions from the surface and that loss was reflected in a significant increase in the appearance of smaller gap junction plaques. The results were interpreted to indicate that some small junctions may be leftover fragments of larger gap junctions in the process of breaking up and that such smaller junctions are indicative of terminal surface membrane aggregates rather than newly formed aggregates. These findings raise questions about the functional identity of all junctions within a given population (22). It is also relevant to mention that the reduction in the number of gap junctions following 1.0 μg RA/ml is reconcilable with observations made in high density mouse limb bud cultures (47). In that case, limb bud cells were also explanted on gd 11 and retinoid effects on cells examined by TEM. No clear-cut gap junctions were found after 3 days continuous retinoid exposure to concentrations identical to those used in our study. This observation appears compatible with the inhibition of dye coupling and with the reduced incidence of gap junctions caused by 1.0 μg RA/ml in the present experiments.

The experimental results described here have provided additional evidence in support of the hypothesis that some chemical teratogens may act by disrupting intercellular communication. Future studies in our laboratory will examine the relationship between gap junction number, size of individual plaques and fractional gap junction area compared to total cell surface area before and after retinoid exposure in epithelial cells of the limb bud apical ectodermal ridge. The direction that this work will take is built on the extensive morphometric analyses with respect to gap junction dynamics and cell function performed by Larsen and his associates (22).

ACKNOWLEDGMENTS

I am indebted to Dr. Thomas Starr for his advice regarding the statistical analysis of the morphometric gap junction data.

Expert technical assistance was provided by Mr. Donald B. Stedman.

REFERENCES

1. Caveney, S. (1985): Annu. Rev. Physiol. 47:319-335.

2. Davidson, J.S., Baumgarten, I.M. and Harley, E.H. (1985): Carcinogenesis 6: 645-650.

3. Dermietzel, R., Leibstein, A., Frixen, U., Janssen-Timmen, U., Traub, O. and Willecke, K. (1984): EMBO J. 3:2262-2270.

4. Elmer, W.A., Smith, M.A. and Ede, D. (1981): Teratology 24:215-223.

5. Hall, J.G. (1984): J. Pediat. 105:583-584.

6. Hein, R., Krieg, T., Mueller, P.K. and Braun-Falco, O. (1984): Biochem. Pharmacol. 33:3263-3267.

7. Hertzberg, E.L. and Skibbens, R.V. (1984): Cell 39:61-69.

8. Hertzberg, E.L. (1985): Annu. Rev. Physiol. 47:305-318.

9. Hertzberg, E.L., Spray, D.C. and Bennett, M.V.L. (1985): Proc. Natl. Acad. Sci. USA 82:2412-2416.

10. Heynkes, R., Kozjek, G., Traub, O. and Willecke, K. (1986): FEBS Letters, in press.

11. Huber, B.E. and Brown, N.A. (1983a): Cancer Res. 43:5541-5551.

12. Huber, B.E. and Brown, N.A. (1983b): Cancer Res. 43:5552-5559.

13. Huber, B.E. and Brown, N.A. (1985): Res. Comm. Chem. Pathol. Pharmacol. 49:17-34.

14. Kelley, R.O. and Fallon, J.F. (1983): In: Limb Development and Regeneration, Part A, edited by J.F. Fallon and A.I. Caplan, pp. 119-130. Alan Liss, New York.

15. Kelley, R.O., Fallon, J.F, and Kelly, R.E., Jr. (1984): In: Issuues and Reviews in Teratology, Vol. 2, edited by H. Kalter, pp. 219-265. Plenum Press, New York.

16. Kistler, A. and Hummler, H. (1985): Arch. Toxicol. 58:50-56.

17. Kistler, A. (1985): In: Concepts in Toxicology, Vol. 3, edited by F. Homburger, pp. 86-100. Karger, Basel.

18. Kochhar, D.M., Penner, J.D. and Tellone, C.I. (1984): Teratog. Carcinog. Mutag. 4:377-387.

19. Kochhar, D.M. (1987): In: Approaches to Elucidate Mechanisms in Teratogenesis, edited by F. Welsch, (in press). Hemisphere Publishers, Washington.

20. Kosher, R.A. (1983): In: Limb Development and Regeneration, Part A, edited by J.F. Fallon and A.I. Caplan, pp. 279-288. Alan Liss, New York.

21. Kosher, R.A. and Gay, S.W. (1985): Cell Differ. 17:159-167.

22. Larsen, W.J. (1985): In: Gap Junctions, edited by M.V.L. Bennett and D.C. Spray, pp. 289-306. Cold Spring Harbor Laboratory.

23. Lo, C.W. (1980): In: Development of Mammals, Vol. 4, edited by M.H. Johnson, pp. 39-80. Elsevier, New York.

24. Loch-Caruso, R. and Trosko, J.E. (1985): Crit. Rev. Toxicol. 16:157-183.

25. Loewenstein, W.R. (1981): Annu. Rev. Physiol. 61:829-913.

26. Merker, H.-J., Zimmermann, B. and Barrach, H.-J. (1984): Acta Biol. Hung. 35:195-203.

27. Paul, D.L. (1986): J. Cell Biol. 103:123-134.

28. Pitts, J.D. and Simms (1977): Exp. Cell Res. 104:153-163.

29. Pitts, J.D., Hamilton, A.E., Kam, E., Burk, R.R. and Murphy, J.P.(1986): Carcinogenesis 7:1003-1010.

30. Saxen, L. (1977): In: Handbook of Teratology, Vol. 2, edited by J.G. Wilson and F.C. Fraser, pp. 171-197. Plenum Press, New York.

31. Sheridan, J.D. and Atkinson, M.M. (1985): Annu. Rev. Physiol. 47:337-353.

32. Spray, D.G. and Bennett, M.V.L. (1985): Annu. Rev. Physiol. 47:281-303.

33. Solursh, M., Reiter, R.S., Ahrens, P.B. and Vertel, B.M. (1981): Dev. Biol. 83:9-19.

34. Solursh, M. (1983): In: Cartilage, Vol. 2, edited by B.K. Hall, pp. 121-141. Academic Press, New York.

35. Stedman, D.B. and Welsch, F. (1985): Carcinogenesis 6:1599-1605.

36. Trosko, J.E., Yotti, L.P., Dawson, B., and C.C. Chang (1981): In: Short Term Tests for Chemical Carcinogens, edited by H.F. Stich and R.H.C. San, pp. 420-427. Springer, New York.

37. Trosko, J.E., Chang, C.C. and Netzloff, M. (1982): Teratog. Carcinog. Mutag. 2:31-45.

38. Wälder, L. and Lützelschwab, R. (1984): Exp. Cell Res. 152:66-76.

39. Warner, A.E., Guthrie, S.C. and Gilula, N.B. (1984): Nature 311:127-131.

40. Warner, A.E. (1985): In: Gap Junctions, edited by M.V.L. Bennett and D.G. Spray, pp. 275-288. Cold Spring Harbor Laboratories.

41. Welsch, F. and Stedman, D.B. (1984): Teratog. Carcinog. Mutag. 4:285-301.

42. Welsch, F., Stedman, D.B. and Carson, J.L. (1985): Exp. Cell Res. 159:91-102.

43. Welsch, F., Stedman, D.B. and Carson, J.L. (1987): In: Approaches to Elucidate Mechanisms in Teratogenesis, edited by F. Welsch, (in press). Hemisphere Publishers, Washington.

44. Wilson, J.G. (1977): In: Handbook of Teratology, Vol. 1, edited by J.G. Wilson and F.C. Fraser, pp. 47-74. Plenum Press, New York.

45. Wolpert. L. (1978): In: Intercellular Junctions and Synapses, edited by J. Feldman, N.B. Gilula and J.D. Pitts, pp. 83-94. Chapman & Hall, London.

46. Yancey, S.B., Edens, J.E., Trosko, J.E., Chang, C.C. and Revel, J.P. (1982): Exp. Cell Res. 139:329-340.

47. Zimmermann, B. and Tsambaos, D. (1985): Arch. Dermatol. Res. 277:98-104.

Tumor Promoters: Biological Approaches for
Mechanistic Studies and Assay Systems,
edited by Robert Langenbach et al.
Raven Press, New York © 1988.

THE ROLE OF SELECTIVE JUNCTIONAL COMMUNICATION IN

CELL TRANSFORMATION

H. Yamasaki, and D. J. Fitzgerald

Division of Environmental Carcinogenesis
International Agency for Research on Cancer
150 cours Albert-Thomas, 69372 LYON cedex 08, France

INTRODUCTION

Functional and morphological behaviour of cells in a given tissue is rigidly controlled through various forms of inter-cellular communication. Since tumor cells behave independently from surrounding normal cells, it is considered that tumor cells participate in local or humoral intercellular communication in a manner different from normal counterparts. The idea is then extended to ask, in regard to such communication, whether (and if so, when) a potential cancerous cell deviates from normal cells during the process of carcinogenesis.

In late 1979, simultaneous and independent reports appeared from the laboratories of Andrew Murray (62) and James Trosko (89) demonstrating that phorbol ester tumor promoters can inhibit membrane-mediated (probably gap-junctional) cell-cell communication. On the basis of their observations, these investigators suggested that such a property of tumor promoters may explain how, in the initiation-promotion scheme of carcino-genesis, an initiated cell could evade the imposition of junction-mediated local tissue discipline and proliferate to form a neoplasm. These observations were confirmed and extended by many other research groups, including ours. In this article, we will review the progress made in this field of study, with a special emphasis on the role of selective intercellular communi-cation in cell transformation and in the maintenance of the transformed phenotype.

GAP JUNCTIONAL CELL-CELL COMMUNICATION

Among various forms of intercellular communication, it is believed that gap-junctional communication plays an essential role in the maintenance of homeostasis in a given tissue (48, 49, 53). Control of cellular functions is also regulated by other forms of communication such as are mediated by receptors (e.g., growth factors, hormones) or cell-cell recognition factors (cell adhesion molecules, glycolipids). Although it is conceivable that all these avenues of communication play important roles during carcinogenesis, much attention has been drawn to the study of gap-junctional intercellular communication, since this is the only form of communication in which intracellular factors are directly exchanged between cells.

It is generally considered that the gap junction is the membrane-residing conduit traversing apposed cells of most metazoan tissues and through which various ions and metabolites (less than 1 000 daltons) can be directly exchanged (49). In this fashion, gap junctions may function in dissemination of molecular information and co-ordination of the responses of tissues and organs to varied stimuli. During embryogenesis, cells arise with selective communication capacity (8, 33, 68) and may play a major role in the creation of morphogenetic fields, compartmentalization and resulting differentiation pathways. Recently, Warner and colleagues (77) demonstrated that microinjection of gap junction antibody into one cell of early Xenopus embryos resulted in various developmental defects in the stage 36 animals.

Numerous studies have focussed on how gap-junctional communication may function in control of cell proliferation, particularly as it relates to cancerous growth. Using measurements of ionic coupling, Loewenstein and Kanno (50) first demonstrated that cells of normal rat liver were electrically coupled, i.e. were communication-competent, while cells within carcinogen- induced or transplanted liver tumors were communication-incompetent (a recent study using gap junction antibody reveals that rat hepatocarcinomas have a reduced complement of gap junctions (38)). The same phenomenon was soonafter observed in normal and cancerous human stomach (41). From these and some ensuing investigations emerged the tentative conclusion that neoplastic growth is characterized by loss of gap junctions and/or communication capacity from the constituent cells of a neoplasm. However, in the intervening years since these reports, a series of related studies of various cancer cells in vivo and in vitro have not entirely given credence to this conclusion (23, 59, 66, 78). It is possible though that qualitative changes in communication profile, such as alterations in selectivity of communication (23, 37), may be important along with quantitative changes. Nonetheless, these studies used already-tumorigenic cells and, in attempting to define whether or not these events are causally related to the neoplastic process, it is clear that different approaches are required. One procedure has been to examine the effects on cell-cell communication of tumor promoters, the agents of the two-stage model of carcinogenesis responsible for eliciting a tumor response (5).

TUMOR PROMOTER EFFECTS ON CELL-CELL COMMUNICATION

Since the original demonstration that cell-cell communication, as measured in metabolic cooperation assays, was inhibited by phorbol esters which are known in vivo tumor promoters, numerous investigators have corroborated and extended these findings employing a broad range of communication assay techniques and cell types including human cells. Table 1 provides a collation of these different techniques and some of the cell types utilized.   In addition to the in vivo promoting stimuli shown in this table, various other known or suspected in vivo tumor promoters have been tested as positive in cell-cell communication assays (34, 46, 56, 75).   Some of these assays are being rigorously studied in order to determine their validity as short-term tests to detect tumor promoting activity of chemicals (16, 90). Furthermore, in view of the proposed role of gap junctional communication in embryogenesis, these assays may also predict teratogenic potential of xenobiotics (47, 80).

In the light of the ability of phorbol ester tumor promoters to inhibit cell-cell communication, some earlier observations from experiments employing phorbol esters may be explained by this action of these compounds. For example, Sivak and van Duuren (70), treating mixed populations of mouse 3T3 cells (excess) and SV40-transformed 3T3 cells with a tumor promoting phorbol ester-containing purified resin fraction of Croton tiglium L., observed a significant increase in the number of transformed clones.   In addition, Hsaio et al. (13) reported that the tumor promoters 12-0-tetradecanoylphorbol-13- acetate (TPA) and teleocidin enhance transformation of mouse C3H 10T1/2 fibroblasts after transfection with a cloned human bladder cancer H-ras oncogene. Similarly, Connan et al. (36) reported that after introducing c-myc, v-myc, or polyoma plt oncogenes into secondary rat embryo fibroblasts or established FR3T3 rat fibroblasts, exposure to TPA elicited marked focus formation. In these cited instances, it is possible that nascent transformed cells were permitted to clonally expand if their initial suppression by virtue of intercellular communication with nontransformed cells was abolished by the tumor promoters.

The exact mechanism of phorbol ester inhibition of junctional communication is presently unknown.   However, it appears to involve specific binding of phorbol esters to membrane receptors (21, 35). These receptors, identified as protein kinase C (63), bind also the supposed endogenous analogue of TPA, i.e. diacylglycerol (69), which in turn can rapidly inhibit communication as shown in BALB/c 3T3 cells (20) and mouse epidermal cells

TABLE 1.   Inhibition of gap junctional intercellular communication by tumor promoting stimuli

Method of junctional communication measurement	Promoting stimulus	Target cells or tissue	Reference
Metabolic cooperation			
3H-uridine metabolites transfer	Phorbol esters	Mouse epidermal cell line /Swiss 3T3 cells	62
HGPRT$^+$/HGPRT$^-$[a]	Phorbol esters and many other tumor promoting agents	Chinese hamster V79	89
		Human fibroblasts	61
		Rat hepatocytes/rat liver epithelial cells	81
ASS$^-$/ASL$^-$[b]	Phorbol esters	Human fibroblasts/V79	14
AK$^+$/AK$^-$[c]	Phorbol esters	Chinese hamster V79	32
Electrical coupling	Phorbol esters	Human amniotic membrane epithelial cells	22
	Phorbol esters	BALB/c 3T3 cells	86
	Skin wounding[d]	Urodele skin	51
Dye transfer			
Microinjection	Phorbol esters and certain other tumor promoting agents	Human colon epithelial cells	27
		Mouse epidermal cell line, rat myoblasts	25
		BALB/c 3T3 cells	21
		Chinese hamster V79	90
	Partial hepatectomy	Rat liver	60

TABLE 1. Cont'd

Method of junctional communication measurement	Promoting stimulus	Target cells or tissue	Reference
Photobleaching	TPA, dieldrin	Human teratocarcinoma cells	76
Scrape loading	TPA, dieldrin and other tumor promoting agents	Chinese hamster V79, rat glial and glioma cells, rat liver cells, human teratocarcinoma cells, human fibroblasts	17
Gap junction structure analysis			
Electron microscope	Phorbol esters	Chinese hamster V79	88
	Phorbol esters	Mouse skin in vivo	40
	Phenobarbital, DDT	Rat liver in vivo	73
Gel electrophoresis analysis	Phorbol esters	Chinese hamster V79	24
Analysis with gap junction antibody	Partial hepatectomy	Rat liver in vivo	74

(a) HGPRT, hypoxanthine guanine phosphoribosyltransferase
(b) ASS⁻, argininosuccinate synthetase-deficient; ASL⁻, argininosuccinate lyase-deficient
(c) AK, adenosine kinase
(d) Mouse skin wounding promotes tumorigenesis (12).

(29); diacylglycol also mimics a variety of other TPA effects (31, and refs. therein).

Knowledge of the events linking protein kinase C activation to gap junction perturbations is currently sparse. Elevation of endogenous cyclic AMP levels in mouse epidermal cells can abrogate TPA or diacylglycerol effects on communication (30); likewise, a protective effect of cyclic AMP was observed in BALB/c 3T3 (21) and human FL cells (42). This is reminiscent of the positive modulation of junctional communication by cyclic AMP (upregulation) as reported previously (26). Perhaps, then, protein kinase C activation results in decreased cyclic AMP levels, leading to gap junction downregulation. This explanation may be naive since an anti-TPA effect of cyclic AMP was not observed for TPA-inhibited communication in rat liver epithelial cells (59). Another candidate to interpose protein kinase C activation and gap junction modulation is Ca^{++} (65). In the human fibroblast/V79 cooperation assay of Davidson et al. (14), the effectiveness of TPA to inhibit communication was diminished in the absence of Ca^{++}, while in V79 cells, TPA and DDT increased cellular Ca^{++} uptake and inhibited cell-cell communication (54, 90). It is clear that further studies are required to fully elucidate the biochemical mechanism of promoter-inhibited communication.

The inhibition of junctional intercellular communication by phorbol esters is associated with a decreased number of gap junctions in treated Chinese hamster V79 cells in culture (88). On the other hand, when phorbol esters are removed from the culture medium of mouse epidermal cells and human FL cells, the cells resume their communication even in the presence of RNA or protein synthesis inhibitors (25, 85), thus indicating that phorbol ester-treated cells are able to re-establish functional gap junctions in the absence of de novo RNA or protein synthesis. From these experimental results, it is reasonable to assume that phorbol esters decrease or eliminate gap junctions by dispersing component subunits into the plasma membrane milieu, rather than by completely destroying gap junction proteins.

CORRELATION OF CELL TRANSFORMATION WITH DIMINISHED INTERCELLULAR COMMUNICATION

Currently, there exists considerable experimental data which suggest that diminished intercellular communication is involved in the clonal expansion of initiated cells, i.e., the process of tumor promotion. For example, when phorbol esters were utilized in the in vitro two-stage transformation of BALB/c 3T3 cells, there was a good correlation between the extent of inhibition of intercellular communication and enhancement of cell transformation (19, 84). However, in a different in vitro transformation system, namely that employing C3H 10T1/2 cells, no such correlation was found (15).

Rivedal et al. (67) have studied the effect of TPA on inter-cellular communication and enhancement of transformation using various Syrian hamster embryo (SHE) cell lines. TPA inhibited communication only in a cell line in which it enhanced cell transformation, and had no effect in a TPA-resistant line, suggesting a correlation between inhibition of communication and enhancement of cell transformation. However, it should be emphasized that this transformation system uses colony formation as its endpoint, whereas the BALB/c 3T3 and C3H10T1/2 systems are focus assays. In the SHE cell system, TPA induces morpho-logical transformation of colonies within a day, while four to five weeks are required for the expansion and appearance of transformed colonies in the other two systems. Therefore, it is likely that in BALB/c 3T3 and C3H10T1/2 cells, TPA enhances the process of cell transformation while in SHE cells, TPA enhances the expression of morphological transformation. Regardless, these results intimate that diminished junctional communication may be involved both in the process and expression of cell transformation.

Use of BALB/c 3T3 cell variants has provided another line of evidence for the involvement of blocked intercellular communi-cation in cell transformation. When a variant that is sensitive (clone A31-1-13) was compared to one that is resistant (clone A31-1-8) to induction of transformation by UV radiation or chemical carcinogens, no difference was seen in the ability to metabolize carcinogens, to bind these metabolites to DNA, to repair DNA damage or in the susceptibility to induction of mutation (39, 52). However, there was a drastic difference in the intercellular communication capacity of the two variants: although this capacity was similar at the logarithmic phase, transformation- sensitive but not transformation-resistant cells became virtually communication-incompetent at confluency (86). We interpret these results to indicate that these transforma-tion-sensitive cells have an intrinsic ability to express a TPA-like effect (inhibited communication) at confluence, leading to enhanced transformation in this cell line.

An involvement of aberrant junctional communication in cell transformation is further implied from recent studies of viral and oncogene actions in tissue culture. Atkinson and co-workers (1) first showed that cell-cell dye transfer in normal rat kid-ney cells was rapidly and markedly reduced upon incubation with a temperature-sensitive mutant of avian sarcoma virus at the viral permissive temperature. Similar findings have been reported by Azarnia and Loewenstein (2, 4) who studied the effect on various cell types of mutants of Rous sarcoma virus and simian virus 40. Recently, it was shown by Chang et al. (11) that transfection of NIH/3T3 cells with a plasmid bearing the v-src oncogene resulted in transformed clones which com-prised cells of reduced communication competence. Thus, it has been proposed that $pp60^{src}$, the src gene product, may be involved in perturbing cell-cell communication which in turn may be causally linked to subsequent uncontrolled growth of cells. From a mechanistic consideration, pp60^{src} and its tyrosine-phosphorylated substrate(s) localize on the plasma membrane (55, 82) where conceivably they may directly or indirectly alter gap junction fidelity. Such an alteration may be independent of transformation-associated changes to the cytoskeleton (3).

As discussed so far, there are several lines of evidence from in vitro studies that inherent or induced deficiency of cell-cell communication capacity may be involved in the loss of growth control (see Table 2 for a summary of the evidence which speaks for and against the proposed causal link of disturbed communication to cell transformation). In the tumor promotion concept of multi-stage carcinogenesis (5) where the loss of growth control is evidenced by the appearance of a benign or malignant neoplasm, one central unanswered question is how does a cell, having been initiated by a carcinogen, escape the orderly and disciplinary confines of the surrounding cells and clonally expand to form a neoplasm ? Assuming that various tumor promoters may function by blocking cell-cell communication, two further questions arise from this. Firstly, are there in fact growth-controlling substances that are transmitted between cells by junctional communication ? In the literature, there are some reports from in vitro studies that normal or non-neoplastic cells in contact with neoplastic cells can prohibit the growth of the latter (7, 10, 72, 79). In perhaps not a dissimilar mechanistic manner, tumorigenic cells lose their tumorigenicity when hybridized with non-tumorigenic cells (44, 71). Perhaps then, negative growth modulators originating within the normal cells could directly pass to the neoplastic cells. In a recent report this notion is given considerable credence. Using co-cultures of transformed and non-transformed C3H10T1/2 cells and assaying cell-cell communication with dye transfer, Mehta and colleagues (57) demonstrated that non-transformed cells inhibited the growth of contacting, transformed cells only when such contact included heterologous cell-cell communication; otherwise, no growth inhibition occurred. The identification of these growth modulatory substances will definitely represent a major advance.

Secondly, could blockage of cell-cell communication and "isolation" of an initiated or preneoplastic cell from contiguous normal cells be solely responsible for eliciting a tumor promoter response ? Probably not. For example, the incomplete but second-stage mouse skin tumor promoter, phorbol 12-retinoate 13-acetate (PRA) (28), can inhibit cell-cell communication (84); if communication inhibition was the sole mechanism of tumor promotion, then PRA should act as a complete promoter. It is likely, however, that during the hyperplasia that accompanies tumor promotion, both initiated and non-initiated cells proliferate but clearly there arises an unequal expansion of the preneoplastic clone over surrounding normal tissue. This is a highly

TABLE 2. Evidence for and against the involvement of blocked cell-cell communication in cell transformation

Cell transformation system	Observation	Reference
	Affirmative evidence	
BALB/c 3T3	Transformation enhanced by agents that block communication but not by agents which do not block communication.	19, 20, 84
BALB/c 3T3	Transformation-sensitive cells lose communication ability at confluence; not so for transformation-resistant cells.	86
BALB/c 3T3	Agents that abrogate selective communication also inhibit transformation.	43
SHE	TPA inhibits communication in a cell line that is sensitive to TPA-induced transformation but does not inhibit communication in a cell line that resists TPA-induced transformation.	67
NRK & various other cells	Certain oncogenic viruses rapidly inhibit cell-cell communication at the viral permissive-temperature.	1, 2, 4
NIH/3T3	v-src-transformed cells have reduced communication competence.	11
C3H10T1/2	Correlation of growth inhibition of transformed cells by normal cells to the degree of heterologous communication.	57
	Negative evidence	
C3H10T1/2	Lack of correlation of TPA dose response for inhibition of communication and transformation enhancement.	15
	TCCD promotes transformation but does not inhibit communication.	9
C3H10T1/2	Retinoic acid suppresses communication but does not enhance transformation.	6, 57
BALB/c 3T3	TGF-β enhances MCA-initiated cell transformation but does not inhibit communication.	*

*Unpublished observations

complex process and certainly is linked to the genetic lesions of initiated cells and probably to the ability of tumor promoters to alter and/or express patterns of differentiation (83). Inhibition of cell-cell communication may be one of the key factors in permitting this differential expansion. The recent development of molecular probes, such as cDNA clones (35, 45, 64) or monoclonal antibodies against gap junctions (38), makes available molecular approaches for the study of the relationship between cell-cell communication and carcinogenesis.

SELECTIVE INTERCELLULAR COMMUNICATION

In addition to promoter inhibition of cell-cell communication, we have observed a related but different phenomenon in BALB/c 3T3 cell transformation studies. Cells within carcinogen-induced transformed foci were microinjected with fluorescent dye and seen to communicate among themselves (18). There was, however, no apparent dye transfer to surrounding normal cells. The converse was also true, i.e., normal cells were found to communicate among themselves but not with contacting focus cells. Thus transformed cells displayed selective communication; this however was not the case for communication between normal cells and cells of non-transformed foci (Type I) where heterologous dye transfer did occur. Since, we have found that selective communication is a feature of BALB/c 3T3 transformed foci generated by a carcinogen (MCA), an oncogene (EJ-ras) and by MCA with TPA (87, unpublished results), and a feature also of tumorigenic rat liver epithelial cells in co-culture with non-tumorigenic counterparts (87, and see Figure 1). Furthermore, it later became apparent that agents which are anti-transforming in the BALB/c 3T3 cell transformation system can abolish this selective communication (43).

There exists therefore a way in which normal cell influence can be barred from an emerging population of transformed cells and where the constant presence of a transforming agent is not required. It seems then, at least in the described instance of the transformed BALB/c 3T3 foci, that the transforming agent was directly responsible for the lesion, resulting in lack of heterologous communication. Since transformed cells as well as surrounding non-transformed cells were capable of efficient dye transfer within their respective compartments, this is evidently no general effect on communication per se. Seemingly, the key aberration is at the normal cell/transformed cell interface where one can surmise that lack of cell-cell recognition prevents sufficient aligning of appropriate apposing membrane components to allow gap junction formation. Selective communication has been observed also with pairs of normal/abnormal C3H10T1/2 cells (57). However, in the C3H10T1/2 transformation focus assay, it was seen that focus cells displayed loss of homologous cell-cell communication capacity (Boreiko, in this

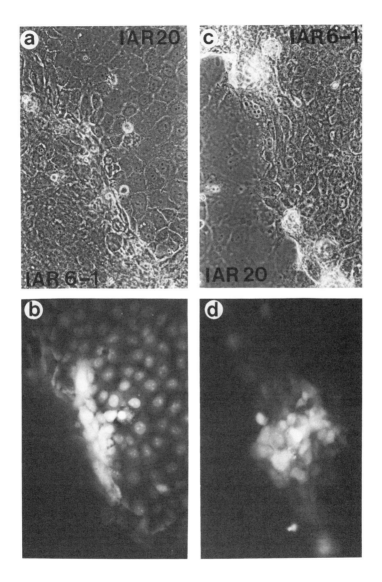

FIG. 1., Selective cell-cell communication between transformed and non-transformed rat liver epithelial cells in culture.
    Tumorigenic (IAR 6-1) and non-tumorigenic (IAR-20) cells were co-cultured and Lucifer Yellow dye was microinjected into IAR-20 cells (a, b) or into IAR 6-1 cells (c, d). Note that only dye transfer among homologous cells was observed. b, d, UV fluorescence photographs of, respectively, a, c.

volume). Nonetheless, these apparently different results still merge at a common point, i.e., transformed cells do not communicate with surrounding, non-transformed counterparts.

These findings led us to formulate some speculation. If lack of cell-cell recognition can explain selective communication, then perhaps it can also explain the mechanism by which tumor promoters inhibit junctional communication, i.e., loss of communication ability induced by promoters may occur secondarily and as a direct consequence of perturbed cell-cell recognition apparatus. Another query arises from this; namely, can the growth-controlling influences of normal cells vis-à-vis transformed cells be imparted by cell-cell contact-dependent means other than junctional communication ? Some recent work in our laboratory suggests, although indirectly, that they may. We have observed that primary rat hepatocytes alone in culture rapidly lose differentiative functions. These functions, however, are resumed when cells are co-cultured with biliary epithelial cells. This influence on hepatocyte gene expression was shown to be dependent on establishment of heterologous cell-cell contact and independent of heterologous junctional communication; contacting biliary cells and hepatocytes did not exchange micro-injected dye (58). This indicates the existence of an information transfer process, which requires cell-cell contact but not junctional communication, and which functions in alteration of gene expression. In the context of carcinogenesis, perhaps some of the suppressive influences of normal cells on transformed cell gene expression may operate via this process. Hence evasion of transformed cells from suppressive normal cells could be effected by agents that act to disrupt this process. Whether or not tumor promoters operate thus is a point for future study.

There is an interesting parallel that may be drawn between embryogenesis and the above reports on selective communication. As mentioned earlier, the establishment of morphogenetic fields and compartmentalization within the developing embryo may be closely linked to the appearance of communication domains which arise as certain cells exhibit selective communication. Perhaps, the selective communication in our transformed foci is akin to that in embryogenesis, heralding rapid growth and accompanied by major changes in differentiation. Hence, insight may be gained from studies aimed at understanding cell-cell recognition processes in developmental systems.

CONCLUSIONS

The notion that cancerous growth may be linked to disturbances in gap-junctional intercellular communication remains an attractive and much-studied hypothesis. Further interest has been generated in this area since various tumor promoters were demonstrated to inhibit cell-cell communication, and many

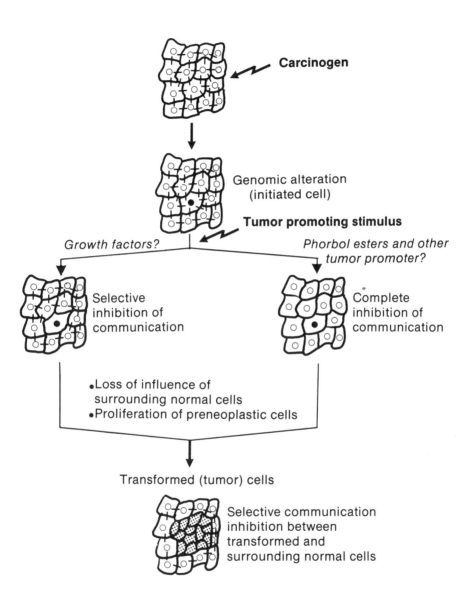

FIG. 2., Schematic representation of the hypothesized involvement of complete or selective inhibition of cell-cell communication in carcinogenesis. Interconnecting lines represent functional gap junctions.

studies are presently aimed at understanding the mechanism by which gap junctions are perturbed by these agents. In addition, we have observed a selective communication between transformed and non-transformed cells in the BALB/c 3T3 cell transformation system (18), and, as discussed, other examples of selective communication have been discovered suggesting that this may be a general phenomenon. It is possible that as a direct result of selective communication or promoter-inhibited cell-cell communication, preneoplastic cells are no longer influenced by growth regulatory molecules emanating from normal cells via gap junctions. Such a hypothesis is schematically presented in Figure 2. However, the _in vivo_ cell-cell communication characteristics of emerging neoplasms and surrounding normal tissue need to be elucidated. Also, further studies are required to examine the cell-cell recognition systems that are likely to be involved in the establishment of selective communication.

ACKNOWLEDGEMENTS

We thank Mr Marc Mesnil for his contribution and Ms C. Fuchez for her secretarial help. Part of this work was supported by NCI Grant No. R01 CA4053401.

REFERENCES

1. Atkinson, M.M., Menko, A.S., Johnson, R.G., Sheppard, J.R., and Sheridan, J.D. (1981): J. Cell Biol., 91: 573-578.
2. Azarnia, R., and Loewenstein, W.R. (1984): J. Membrane Biol., 82: 191-205.
3. Azarnia, R., and Loewenstein, W.R. (1984): J. Membrane Biol., 82: 207-212.
4. Azarnia, R., and Loewenstein, W.R. (1984): J. Membrane Biol., 82: 213-220.
5. Berenblum, I. (1982): In: Cancer, a Comprehensive Treatise, vol. 1 (2nd ed.), ed. F.F. Becker, pp. 451-484, Plenum Press, New York.
6. Bertram, J.S. (1980): Cancer Res., 40: 3141-3146.
7. Bertram, J.S., and Faletto, M.B. (1985): Cancer Res., 45: 1946-1952.
8. Blennerhasett, M.G., and Caveney, S. (1984): Nature, 309: 361-364.
9. Boreiko, C.J., Abernethy, D.J., Sanchez, J.H., and Dorman, B.H. (1986): Carcinogenesis, 7: 1095-1099.
10. Borek, C., and Sachs, L. (1966): Proc. Natl. Acad. Sci. USA, 56: 1705-1711.
11. Chang, C-C., Trosko, J.E., Kung, H-J., Bombick, D., and Matsumura, F. (1985): Proc. Natl. Acad. Sci. USA, 82: 5360-5364.

12. Clarke-Lewis, I., and Murray, A.W. (1978): Cancer Res., 38: 494-497.
13. Connan, G., Rassoulzadegan, M., and Cuzin, F. (1985): Nature, 314: 277-279.
14. Davidson, J.S., Baumgarten, I., and Harley, E.H. (1985): Cancer Res., 45: 515-519.
15. Dorman, B.H., Butterworth, B.E., and Boreiko, C.J. (1983): Carcinogenesis, 4: 1109-1115.
16. Elmore, E., Korytynski, E.A., and Smith, M.P. (1985): Progr. Mut. Res., 5: 597-612.
17. El-Fouly, M.H., Trosko, J.E., and Chang, C-C. (1986): Exp. Cell Res., in press.
18. Enomoto, T., and Yamasaki, H. (1984): Cancer Res., 44: 5200-5203.
19. Enomoto, T., and Yamasaki, H. (1985): Cancer Res., 45: 2681-2688.
20. Enomoto, T., and Yamasaki, H. (1985): Cancer Res., 45: 3706-3710.
21. Enomoto, T., Martel, N., Kanno, Y., and Yamasaki, H. (1984): J. Cell. Physiol., 121: 323-333.
22. Enomoto, T., Sasaki, Y., Shiba, Y., Kanno, Y., and Yamasaki, H. (1981): Proc. Natl. Acad. Sci. USA, 78: 5628-5632.
23. Fentiman, I.S., Hurst, J., Ceriani, R.L., and Taylor-Papadimitriou, J. (1979): Cancer Res., 39: 4739-4743.
24. Finbow, M.E., Shuttleworth, J., Hamilton, A.E., and Pitts, J.D. (1983): EMBO J., 2: 1479-1486.
25. Fitzgerald, D.J., Knowles, S.E., Ballard, F.J., and Murray, A.W. (1983): Cancer Res., 43: 3614-3618.
26. Flagg-Newton, J.L., Dahl, G., and Loewenstein, W.R. (1981): J. Membrane Biol., 63: 105-121.
27. Friedman, E.A., and Steinberg, M. (1982): Cancer Res., 42: 5096-5105.
28. Furstenberger, G., Berry, D.L., Sorg, B., and Marks, F. (1981): Proc. Natl. Acad. Sci. USA, 78: 7722-7726.
29. Gainer, H.St.C., and Murray, A.W. (1985): Biochem. Biophys. Res. Commun., 126: 1109-1113.
30. Gainer, H.St.C., and Murray, A.W. (1986): Exp. Cell Res., 166: 171-179.
31. Giroldi, L., Hamel, E., and Yamasaki, H. (1986): Carcinogenesis, 7: 1183-1186.
32. Gupta, R.S., Singh, B., and Stetsko, D.K. (1985): Carcinogenesis, 6: 1359-1366.
33. Guthrie, S.C. (1984): Nature, 311: 149-151.
34. Hartman, T.G., and Rosen, J.D. (1983): Proc. Natl. Acad. Sci. USA, 80: 5305-5309.
35. Heynkes, R., Kozjek, G., Traub, O., and Willecke, K. (1986): FEBS Lett., 205: 56-60.
36. Hsaio, W-L. W., Gattoni-Celli, S., and Weinstein, I.B. (1984): Science, 226: 552-554.
37. Hunter, G.K., and Pitts, J.D. (1981): J. Cell Sci., 49: 163-175.

38. Janssen-Timmen, U., Traub, O., Dermietzel, R., Robes, H.M., and Willecke, K. (1986): Carcinogenesis, 7: 1475-1482.
39. Kakunaga, T., and Crow, J.D. (1980): Science, 209: 505-507.
40. Kalimi, G.H., and Sirsat, S.M. (1984): Cancer Lett., 22: 343-350.
41. Kanno, Y., and Matsui, Y. (1968): Nature, 218: 775-776.
42. Kanno, Y., Enomoto, T., Shiba, Y., and Yamasaki, H. (1984): Exp. Cell Res., 152: 31-37.
43. Katoh, F., and Yamasaki, H. manuscript in preparation.
44. Koi, M., and Barrett, J.C. (1986): Proc. Natl. Acad. Sci. USA, 83: 5992-5996.
45. Kumar, N.M., and Gilula, N.B. (1986): J. Cell Biol., 103: 767-776.
46. Lawrence, N.J., Parkinson, E.K., and Emmerson, A. (1984): Carcinogenesis, 5: 419-421.
47. Loch-Caruso, R., and Trosko, J.E. (1986): CRC Crit. Rev. Toxiol., 16: 157-183.
48. Loewenstein, W.R. (1979): Biochim. Biophys. Acta, 560: 1-65.
49. Loewenstein, W.R. (1981): Physiol. Rev., 61: 829-913.
50. Loewenstein, W.R., and Kanno, Y. (1966): Nature, 209: 1248-1249.
51. Loewenstein, W.R., and Penn, R.D. (1967): J. Cell Biol., 33: 235-242.
52. Lo, K.Y., and Kakunaga, T. (1982): Cancer Res., 42: 2644-2650.
53. MacDonald, C. (1985): Essays in Biochem., 21: 86-118
54. Madhukar, B.V., Yoneyama, M., Matsumura, F., Trosko, J.E., and Tsushimoto, G. (1983): Cancer Lett., 18: 251-259.
55. Maher, P.A., Pasquale, E.B., Wang, J.Y.J., and Singer, S.J. (1985): Proc. Natl. Acad. Sci. USA, 82: 6576-6580.
56. Mazzoleni, G., Ragnotti, G., Enomoto, T., and Yamasaki, H. (1985): Carcinogenesis, 6: 1477-1482.
57. Mehta, P.P., Bertram, J.S., and Loewenstein, W.R. (1986): Cell, 44: 187-196.
58. Mesnil, M., Fraslin, J-M., Piccoli, C., Yamasaki, H., and Guguen-Guillouzo, C. Submitted for publication.
59. Mesnil, M., Montesano, R., and Yamasaki, H. (1986): Exp. Cell Res., 165: 391-402.
60. Meyer, D.J., Yancey, S.B., and Revel, J-P. (1981): J. Cell Biol., 91: 505-523.
61. Mosser, D.D., and Bols, N.C. (1982): Carcinogenesis, 3: 1207-1212.
62. Murray, A.W., and Fitzgerald, D.J. (1979): Biochem. Biophys. Res. Commun., 91: 395-401.
63. Niedel, J.E., Kuhn, L.J., and Vandenbark, G.R. (1983): Proc. Natl. Acad. Sci. USA, 80: 36-40.
64. Paul, D.L. (1986): J. Cell Biol., 103: 123-134.
65. Peracchia, C., and Peracchia, L.L. (1980): J. Cell Biol., 87: 708-718.
66. Pitelka, D.R., Hamamoto, S.T., and Taggart, B.N. (1980): Cancer Res., 40: 1588-1599.

67. Rivedal, E., Sanner, T., Enomoto, T., and Yamasaki, H. (1985): Carcinogenesis, 6: 899-902.
68. Schultz, R.M. (1985): Biol. Reprod., 32: 27-42.
69. Sharkey, N.A., Leack, K.L., and Blumberg, P.M. (1984): Proc. Natl. Acad. Sci. USA, 81: 607-610.
70. Sivak, A., and van Duuren, B.L. (1967): Science, 157: 1443-1444.
71. Stanbridge, E.J., Der, C.J., Doersen, C.J., Nishimi, R.Y., Peehl, D.M., Weissman, B.E., and Wilkinson, J.E. (1982): Science, 215: 252-259.
72. Stoker, M. (1964): Virology, 24: 165-174.
73. Sugie, S., Mori, H., and Takahashi, M. (1984): Int. Cell Biol., p. 316 (abstract).
74. Traub, O., Druge, P.M., and Willecke, K. (1983): Proc. Natl. Acad. Sci. USA, 82: 7330-7334.
75. Trosko, J.E., Yotti, L.P., Warren, S.T., Tsushimoto, G., and Chang, C-C. (1982): In: Carcinogenesis, vol. 7, ed. E. Hecker, pp. 565-585, Raven Press, New York.
76. Wade, M.H., Trosko, J.E., and Schindler, M. (1986): Science, 232: 525-528.
77. Warner, A.E., Guthrie, S.C., and Gilula, N.B. (1984): Nature, 311: 127-131.
78. Weinstein, R.S., Merk, F.B., and Alroy, J. (1976): Adv. Cancer Res., 23: 23-89.
79. Weiss, R.A. (1970): Exp. Cell Res., 63: 1-18.
80. Welsch, F., Stedman, D.B., and Carson, J.L. (1985): Exp. Cell Res., 159: 91-102.
81. Williams, G.M., Telang, S., and Tong, C. (1981): Cancer Lett., 11: 339-344.
82. Willingham, M.C., Jay, G., and Pastan, I. (1979): Cell, 18: 125-134.
83. Yamasaki, H. (1984): In: Mechanisms of Tumor Promotion, vol. 4, ed. T.J. Slaga, pp. 1-26, CRC Press, Boca Raton.
84. Yamasaki, H., Aguelon-Pegouries, A-M., Enomoto, T., Martel, N., Furstenberger, G., and Marks, F. (1985): Carcinogenesis, 6: 1173-1179.
85. Yamasaki, H., Enomoto, T., Martel, N., Shiba, Y., and Kanno, Y. (1983): Exp. Cell Res., 146: 297-308.
86. Yamasaki, H., Enomoto, T., Shiba, Y., Kanno, Y., and Kakunaga, T. (1985): Cancer Res., 45: 637-641.
87. Yamasaki, H., Frixen, U., Mesnil, M., Aguelon, A-M., and Hollstein, M. (1986): Proc. Am. Assoc. Cancer Res., 27: 133.
88. Yancey, S.B., Edens, J.E., Trosko, J.E., Chang, C-C., and Revel, J-P. (1982): Exp. Cell Res., 139: 329-340.
89. Yotti, L.P., Chang, C-C., and Trosko, J.E. (1979): Science, 206: 1089-1091.
90. Zeilmaker, M.J., and Yamasaki, H. (1986): Cancer Res., 46: 6180-6186.

Tumor Promoters: Biological Approaches for
Mechanistic Studies and Assay Systems,
edited by Robert Langenbach et al.
Raven Press, New York © 1988.

INHIBITION OF METABOLIC COOPERATION IN V79 CELLS:
POTENTIAL CORRELATIONS WITH TUMOR PROMOTION

Eugene Elmore[1], Robert Langenbach[2], and Jeffrey S. Bohrman[3]

[1]Cellular and Molecular Toxicology Program,
Northrop Services, Inc. – Environmental Sciences.
Research Triangle Park, North Carolina 27709

[2]Toxicology Research and Testing Program,
National Institute of Environmental Health Sciences.
Research Triangle Park, North Carolina 27709

[3]Division of Biomedical and Behavioral Sciences,
Centers for Disease Control,
National Institute for Occupational Safety and Health.
Cincinnati, Ohio 45226

INTRODUCTION

Although much effort and expense has been used to correlate short-term "genotoxicity" assays with carcinogenesis, there are many classes of carcinogens that elude detection (32), i.e., chemicals that act indirectly or through non-genotoxic (epigenetic) mechanisms. However, the majority of these short-term assays will respond only when the chemical or its metabolites interact with the DNA of the test cell or organism. Chemically induced cancer appears to occur in at least two distinct stages: initiation, which is generally felt to be genetic in origin, and promotion, which may include both genetic and epigenetic mechanisms. Many carcinogens are considered complete carcinogens, i.e., having both tumor initiating and promoting activity. Assays designed to detect chemicals that act through epigenetic mechanisms may also detect carcinogens that act primarily through genetic mechanisms. Such assays may also distinguish between carcinogenic and noncarcinogenic genotoxic chemicals and thereby serve to complement genotoxicity assays by increasing the short-term tests' accuracy in detecting carcinogens (9).

Tumor promoters are chemicals or agents that promote the appearance of tumors in animals that were previously exposed to a single low carcinogen dose that would by itself not normally induce tumors. Tumor promoters were first defined from initiation and promotion studies on mouse skin (1). Recently, however, tumor promoters have also been identified using other organ systems (12, 29). Tumor promoters may act through a variety of mechanisms. One potential mechanism that has recently gained attention is the inhibition of cell-to-cell communication. Cell-to-cell communication is a property shared by many types of cells *in vivo*. It is important for the development and maintenance of normal cellular functions in a variety of tissues and organs because it regulates intercellular transfer of hormones, other regulatory molecules, and ions (19, 20).

The development of quantitative *in vitro* assays to detect tumor promoters and other toxicants that act through epigenetic mechanisms is of great importance since many environmentally important chemicals fall into this category. One such system, the Chinese hamster V79 cell metabolic cooperation assay (41), was reported to detect tumor promoters and other chemicals that may act through epigenetic mechanisms (8, 9, 10, 11, 15, 27, 33, 34, 35, 36, 38, 40, 41). The assay is based biologically on the chemically induced inhibition of gap junctional mediated intercellular communication (10, 40). In this assay, the inhibition of cell-to-cell communication is measured by determining the degree of cell killing that results when toxic 6-thioguanine (6-TG) monophosphate is transferred from wild type (6-TG^s) cells, which are capable of phosphorylating 6-TG, to 6-TG resistant (6-TG^r) cells, which are incapable of phosphorylating 6-TG. The 6-TG-monophosphate is further phosphorylated and incorporated into DNA and RNA resulting in cell death.

We will summarize the results of a study that evaluated the V79 metabolic cooperation assay (5). The data were collected using similar protocols and 23 coded chemicals of known tumor-promoting activity. The purposes of the study were to determine (1) the reproducibility of the assay in different laboratories, (2) the sources of potential variability, and (3) the response in the assay as compared to previous *in vitro* and *in vivo* observations.

THE METABOLIC COOPERATION ASSAY

The basic assay was adapted from Yotti et al. (41) and Tsushimoto et al. (37). Methods, test chemicals, and sources of all chemicals and cells used in this study are detailed elsewhere (4). Briefly, for each test chemical, preliminary assays were done to determine the relative cytotoxicity both at high and low cell densities. From the preliminary assays, five concentrations that permitted 70 to 100% survival in a colony forming efficiency assay were selected to use in the metabolic cooperation assay. The metabolic cooperation assay (Figure 1) was performed as follows: Culture medium containing 3% fetal bovine serum, 100 6-TG^r cells and 4×10^5 6-TG^s cells was dispensed into each 60 mm dish. Following an attachment period of 4 h, the appropriate concentration of test chemical or solvent was added to each dish

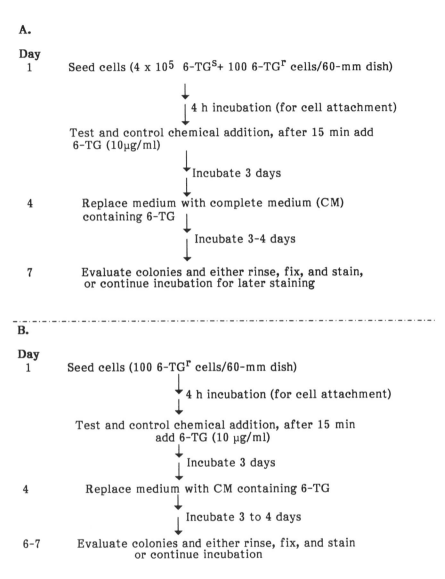

Figure 1. The Metabolic Cooperation Assay. Flowcharts showing both the Metabolic Cooporation (Recovery Efficiency) Assay (A) and the Parallel Cytotoxicity (Cloning Efficiency) Assay (B).

(20 dishes per concentration). After 15 min, 6-TG in culture medium was added to a final concentration of 10 µg/ml. After a 3-day incubation period, the medium containing test chemical or solvent and 6-TG was removed and replaced with fresh culture medium containing 10 µg/ml 6-TG but without test chemical and the incubation continued. On the sixth or seventh day, the dishes were removed and stained for counting. In the parallel cytotoxicity assay, all procedures were similar to those in the metabolic cooperation assay except that no 6-TGs cells were seeded with the 100 6-TGr cells. Each cytotoxicity and metabolic cooperation assay included medium, solvent, and positive (12-O-tetradecanoyl-phorbol-13-acetate [TPA], 4 ng/ml) controls.

The mean number of colonies per dish was calculated for each experimental group. Values from cells treated with test chemical in the metabolic cooperation assay were compared to the values from cells treated with solvent using only Dunnett's test (16). Data were analyzed relative to controls at the $p \leq 0.01$ confidence level. A chemical was classified as positive by a laboratory if it significantly inhibited metabolic cooperation at two concentration levels and if the cloning efficiencies at those concentrations in the concurrent cytotoxicity control were at least 70% of the solvent control. A chemical that did not significantly inhibit metabolic cooperation at any concentration was classified by a laboratory as negative. Chemicals that produced significant inhibition at only one concentration and/or showed significant inhibition only at a concentration(s) where the cytotoxicity exceeded 30% relative to the solvent control were classified by a laboratory as equivocal. The overall response with each chemical was based on individual laboratory responses. An overall chemical response was described as positive or negative when two of two, two of three, or all three laboratories agreed. A positive laboratory test and an equivocal laboratory test were considered positive. A negative laboratory test and one or two equivocal laboratory tests were considered negative.

INTERLABORATORY COMPARISONS

Data Summary

The laboratories participating in these studies used identical test chemicals, solvents, serum, medium, trypsin, culture dishes, and protocols, which differed only in nonessential procedures, to minimize variability. The statistical criteria, Dunnett's test and $\alpha=0.01$, were selected for evaluating the data, because in separate studies that used 10 dishes per condition, two control groups in the same assay were shown to differ from each other at $p \leq 0.05$ but not at $p \leq 0.01$ (5). The data from the 23 chemicals evaluated in this study are summarized in Table 1. Also presented in Table 1 are comparisons of these data with other reported *in vitro* metabolic cooperation results.

Phorbol esters with known promotional activity had similar responses in all laboratories in agreement with their previously reported *in vitro* responses (Table 1). Also, prescreening for cytotoxicity to permit the evaluation of the highest possible concentrations may have obscured some concentration response relationships especially for phorbol esters that effectively inhibit metabolic cooperation at concentrations producing little or no cytotoxicity in V79 cells. For example, TPA's maximum response occurs at 1 to 4 ng/ml (J.E. Trosko, personal communication) while concentrations evaluated ranged from 50 to 1250 ng/ml (Table 1).

Phenobarbital was reported to induce variable responses in different laboratories (8, 27, 35). The variability was also confirmed in this study when one laboratory recorded a negative response while the other two recorded positive responses. Amobarbital also produced a variable positive response similar to that observed with phenobarbital.

The multi-tissue promoters, butylated hydroxyanisole, butylated hydroxytoluene, and the bladder promoters, D(+)tryptophan, sodium cyclamate, and sodium saccharin, appeared to produce weak responses, agreeing with previous responses (22, 23, 34, 36, 38, 41). Interlaboratory variability was observed with most of the bladder promoters. This variability may be due to relatively weak activity in this class of chemicals or to some unidentified experimental variables. Concentrations required to produce a positive response differed between the bladder promoters and the phorbol esters. This was probably due to the presence of receptors for the phorbol esters (18). Thus, the relative concentration required to produce a response in the assay should be less with agents that have a high receptor-binding affinity. Butylated hydroxyanisole and butylated hydroxytoluene were active at similar concentrations. D(+)tryptophan produced a reproducible response in the 0.5 to 1 mg/ml range, while the sweeteners, sodium saccharin and sodium cyclamate, required up to 10 times this amount to produce weak activity in the assay. The "negative" control for sweeteners, sucrose, was positive only at 10 mg/ml or higher. Although a high sucrose diet has not been shown to promote tumors in the bladder, it has been shown to actively promote mammary tumors and liver foci (13, 17).

The peroxides were inactive in this study. The present data for benzoyl peroxide differ from a previous study (30). In this study, the lack of activity of peroxides may be due to the relative reactivity of these compounds in medium with a low serum concentration. Alternatively, the laboratory conditions used in this study may not have been conducive for producing the peroxide radicals that may be needed to activate the compounds. Generation of peroxide radicals can be affected by several parameters such as metal ion concentrations, oxygen concentrations, the presence of ionizing light, and the presence of antioxidants in the culture media or serum (26).

N-dodecane and 1-phenyldodecane promote tumors in mouse skin (3, 14, 25), but they were classified as overall negatives by the two laboratories. The concentrations of n-dodecane were limited by solubility, perhaps explaining this lack of cytotoxicity. 1-Phenyldodecane, however, was tested near the toxic limit. These chemicals may have lacked activity because they were weakly active compounds to begin with and not detected due to the variable response; or, as cocarcinogens, which act to enhance carcinogenic response during cotreatment, they may simply be inactive in this assay. The

TABLE 1: COMPARATIVE RESPONSES OF TEST CHEMICALS[a]

Compound	Laboratory Response			Overall Response	Lowest Effective Concentration[b]	Previous Metabolic Cooperation Results[c]	
	1	2	3			+ Response	− Response
4-0-Methyl-TPA	+[d]	+	+	+	.01	36	
TPA	+	+	+	+	0.05	27, 41	
Mezerien	+	+	+	+	0.1	36	
Catechol	+	+	ND	+	0.25	23, 24	
Ethyl phenylpropriolate	E	+	ND	+	0.25	ND	ND
Phorbol-12, 13-dibutyrate	+	+	+	+	1.0	36	
Butylated hydroxytoluene	+	+	−e	+	2.5	23, 36	
Butylated hydroxyanisole	+	+	−	+	2.5	ND	ND
Amobarbital	+	+	E	+	75	ND	ND
Phenobarbital	+	+	−	+	100	8, 15	38
D (+) tryptophan	+	+	+	+	250	ND	ND
Sodium saccharin	E	+	ND	+	5,000	36, 38	
Sucrose	+	+	ND	+	10,000	ND	ND
Pyrogallol	+	−	ND	E	(3)[f]	ND	ND
Phenol	+	−	ND	E	(25)		7, 21, 23, 24

(continued)

TABLE 1: (Continued)

Compound	Laboratory Response			Overall Response	Lowest Effective Concentration[b]	Previous Metabolic Cooperation Results[c]	
	1	2	3			+ Response	– Response
2, 4–Dinitro-fluorobenzene	–	–	–	–	(0.1)	39	
t–Butyl hydroperoxide	–	E	E	–	(2.0)	ND	ND
Benzoyl peroxide	–	–	–	–	(4.0)	30	ND
N–Dodecane	–	–	ND	–	(5)	ND	ND
Hydrogen peroxide	–	–	–	–	(7.5)		22
1–Phenyl dodecane	E	–	ND	–	(7.5)	ND	ND
Phorbol	–	–	–	–	(30)		28
Sodium cyclamate	–	E	+	E	(5,000)	22	

a – Table from Bohrman et al. (5). Responses are listed from highest to lowest activity.

b – The lowest effective concentration where statistically significant inhibition of metabolic concentration took place. Units in μg/ml. Numbers in parentheses indicate highest concentration tested.

c – Numbers indicate references cited.

d – Positive, two concentration levels were significantly (p ≤ 0.01) greater than solvent control, with a 70% or greater cloning efficiency in the cytotoxicity.

e – Negative, there was no significant difference from the solvent control value at any concentration tested

f – Numbers in parentheses indicate highest noneffective concentration tested in μg/ml.

ND– No data.

E – Equivocal. Neither laboratory or overall responses could be classified as positive or negative.

preliminary report of Bohrman et al. (6) supports the first hypothesis, since n-dodecane was weakly active in repeated assays.

Phenol was detected as positive in only one of two laboratory studies. Previous reports indicate that phenol was inactive in this assay (21, 23, 24, 25). The two metabolites of phenol, catechol and pyrogallol also showed some activity. Catechol was clearly the most active of the two. Both laboratories detected significant activity with catechol, although only one laboratory detected weak activity with pyrogallol. The finding with catechol agrees with a previous *in vitro* study (24).

Two other chemicals evaluated in this study were 2,4-dinitrofluorobenzene and ethyl phenylpropriolate. All three laboratories found dinitrofluorobenzene to be negative which contrasted with previous studies (39). The compound was evaluated to the limit of solubility. The response with ethyl phenylpropriolate suggested a positive response even though results from one laboratory were equivocal, which may indicate a weakly positive chemical similar to responses reported with phenobarbital (8, 27, 35).

Agreement Among Laboratories and With *In Vivo* Data

The response of chemicals tested in three laboratories agreed in all three laboratories for 9 of 15 chemicals. For the 23 chemicals tested in two laboratories, responses agreed for 16 chemicals.

In determining how *in vitro* and *in vivo* data agree, it is important to remember that *in vivo* responses vary widely within and between different organs and different species (5). In this comparison, we have considered any positive response *in vivo* to be positive irrespective of the target organ or species. With the exception of catechol and pyrogallol, all chemicals evaluated in this study have suggested *in vivo* tumor-promoting activity in at least one study (5). Of the 15 chemicals evaluated by three laboratories, 8 responded positively for a 53% agreement with *in vivo* data. Of the 23 chemicals evaluated in two or three laboratories, 12 responded positively, and 3 gave equivocal responses. Eleven of the 12 positive responses agreed with *in vivo* results. Catechol, which was negative *in vivo*, produced a positive response in the metabolic cooperation assay. The observed variability within and between laboratories for weakly active chemicals suggests that repeat assays may be required to confirm responses (5, 6, 8, 35, 38).

Two classes of compounds appear to escape detection in the V79 assays. These classes, the peroxides and the alkanes, were positive *in vivo* but negative *in vitro*. This may be due to their mechanisms of action or in the case of peroxides, their chemical reactivity. As with any system, it is useful if one can determine those classes of chemicals for which the assay is reliable. The studies on metabolites of phenol suggest that metabolism needs to be considered when evaluating chemicals that are known to be metabolized. However, it is possible that certain tumor promoters may act directly without being metabolized, even though they need metabolizing to become active in genotoxicity assays. Any single assay *in vitro* should not be expected to predict all potential mechanisms, and this is also true with the V79 metabolic cooperation assay. It is true that the general mechanism, inhibition of gap junction function, which makes the assay possible, is present in most organ systems; however, the chemically induced changes in cellular physiology that control the mechanism may not be identical in all organ systems (31).

SUMMARY AND FUTURE STUDIES

The number of mechanisms that may be involved in tumor promotion are unknown, and the role of gap junctional interruption in this process needs more study to evaluate the usefulness of this assay. In evaluating the data presented in this study, it should be considered that each laboratory performed only a single assay to determine whether a chemical was active in the assay. When testing a weakly active chemical in this assay, it is not uncommon to observe interlaboratory and intralaboratory variability (5, 6, 8). Therefore, independent repeat assays are needed to determine a chemical response. In the present study, the amount of collected data permits extensive statistical analysis to a degree not previously reported. However, it was still difficult to determine the statistical limits needed to avoid bias in the assays. Futhermore, information gained during the study indicated that criteria need to be established to determine the biological validity of an assay before determining statistical significance. For example, compounds that alter the pH of the medium or change the osmolarity may also affect gap junction function. Changes in pH of the culture medium alter the ionic balance within the cell, thereby changing intracellular pH. Intracellular pH can, in turn, alter gap junction function (31). As a minimum, assay conditions must be standardized to carefully control pH and osmolarity during chemical treatment (2).

In these studies and others (8, 28), the cytotoxicity limit for a valid experimental point was 70% clonal survival compared to the solvent control. To assess cytotoxicity, a cloning efficiency assay was used that measures the toxic effects at a cell density of 100 cells per 5 ml of medium. In contrast, the metabolic cooperation assay uses 400,100 cells per 5 ml of medium. Cytotoxicity, at either low or high cell density, could lead to inaccurate assessments of chemical activities in the metabolic cooperation assay. For some chemicals the toxic response at both densities appears to be identical; however, a clonal cytotoxicity assay is inadequate for assessing the potential toxicity of chemicals that are more or less active in mass cultures. For some chemicals, cytotoxicity seems to be reduced when cells are treated at high densities; thus, for these chemicals, it is possible to have higher recovery efficiencies than cloning efficiencies at identical chemical concentrations. The activities of those chemicals exhibiting this behavior may be missed by the V79 assay as it is presently conducted. The current protocol may need to be modified to control for this variable. With other chemicals, the cytotoxicity observed at cloning densities is less than that observed at high cell densities. This suggests that metabolism produces metabolites or other changes in medium components, resulting in cytotoxicity. Tumors can be promoted through a variety of mechanisms including cytotoxicity; therefore, it is necessary to consider *in vivo* data when selecting cytotoxic limits for a tumor-promoting assay.

In vitro systems are difficult to validate due to the shortage of adequately studied non-tumor promoters *in vivo*. Therefore, *in vivo* systems that screen for tumor promoters must be futher developed and their limits defined. This should provide adequate databases on tumor promoters and, of equal importance, nonpromoters for utilization in *in vitro* validation studies.

Since the events in carcinogenesis are complex, it is not surprising that assays which detect events associated with direct genetic damage are not capable of detecting all chemicals that cause cancer. Some of the chemicals that escape detection may act through epigenetic mechanisms. If short-term assays are to be more useful in identifying potential carcinogens, then systems which detect epigenetic chemicals must be developed. Thus, although validation of the V79 metabolic cooperation assay for tumor promoters is far from complete, the data gained from this study have helped identify potential sources of variation and indicate directions for future study.

ACKNOWLEDGMENTS

We would like to acknowledge the collaborators on the study reviewed in this chapter: Dr. Thomas R. Barfknecht, Pharmakon Research International, Dr. Dushyant K. Gulatti, Environmental Health Research and Testing and Dr. JeAnne Burg, National Institute for Occupational Safety and Health.

REFERENCES

1. Berenblum, I., and Shubik, P. (1947): *Brit. J. Cancer*, 1:383-391.
2. Binder, R.L., and Volpenhein, M.E. (1987): *Carcinogen*, 8:1257-1261.
3. Bingham, E., and Falk, H.F. (1969): *Arch. Environ. Health* 19:779-783.
4. Bingham, E., and Nord, P.J. (1977): *J. Natl. Cancer Inst.*, 58:1099-1101.
5. Bohrman, J.S., Burg, J., Elmore, E., Gulati, D.K., Barfknecht, T.R., Langenbach, R., and Niemeier, R.W. (Submitted): *Environ. Mol. Mutagen.*
6. Bohrman, J.S., Burg, J., Elmore, E., McGregor, D., and Langenbach, R. (1986): *In Vitro*, 22:36a.
7. Chen, T.H., Kavanagh, T.J., Chang, C.C., and Trosko, J.E. (1984): *Cell Biol. Toxicol.*, 1:155-171.
8. Elmore, E.L., Korytynski, E.A., and Smith, M.P. (1985): In: *Collaborative Study of Short Term Tests for Carcinogens, Volume 5, Progress in Mutation Research*, edited by J. Ashby, F.J. de Serres, M. Draper, M. Ishidate, Jr., B.H. Margolin, B.E. Matter, and M.D. Shelby, pp. 597-612. Elsevier Science Publishers, Amsterdam.
9. Elmore, E., Milman, H.A., and Wyatt, G.P. (In press): In: *Biochemical Mechanisms and Regulation of Intercellular Communication. Volume 14, Advances in Modern Envioronmental*

Toxicology, edited by H.A. Milman and E. Elmore, Princeton Scientific Publishing, Princeton.

10. Enomoto, T., Sasaki, Y., Kano, N., and Yamaski H. (1981): *Proc. Natl. Acad. Sci. USA*, 78:5628-5632.

11. Fitzgerald, D.J., and Murray, A.W. (1980): *Cancer Res.*, 40:2935-2937.

12. Hecker, E., Fusenig, N.E., Kunz, W., Marks, F., and Thielmann, H.W., editors (1982): *Cocarcinogenic and Biological Effects of Tumor Promoters: Carcinogenesis a Comprehensive Survey, Volume 7*. Raven Press, New York.

13. Hei, T.K., and Sudilovsky, O. (1985): *Cancer Res.*, 45:2700-2705.

14. Horton, A.W., Eshleman, D.N., Schiff, A.R., and Perman, W.H. (1976): *J. Natl. Cancer Inst.*, 56:387-391.

15. Jone, C., Trosko, J.E., Aylsworth, C.F., Parker, L., and Chang, C.C., (1985): *Carcinogen.*, 6:361-366.

16. Kirk, R.E. (1982): *Experimental Design*, 2nd edition, p.112. Brooks/Cole Publishing Co., New York.

17. Klurfield, D.M., Weber, M.M., and Kritchevsky, D. (1984): *Carcinogen.*, 5:423-425.

18. Leach, K.L., and Blumberg, P.M. (1985): *Cancer Res.* 45:1958-1963.

19. Loewenstein, W.R. (1979): *Biochem. Biophys. Acta*, 560:1-65.

20. Loewenstein, W.R. (1981): *Physiol. Rev.*, 61:829-913.

21. Malcolm, A.R., and Mills, L.J. (1983): *Ann. N.Y. Acad. Sci.*, 407:448-450.

22. Malcolm, A.R. and Mills, L.J. (1985): *New Approaches in Toxicity Testing and Their Application to Human Risk Assessment*, pp. 79-91. Raven Press, New York.

23. Malcolm, A.R., Mills, L.J., and McKenna, E.J. (1983): *Application of Biological Markers to Carcinogen Testing*, pp. 494-495. Plenum Press, New York.

24. Malcolm, A.R., Mills, L.J., and McKenna, E.J. (1985): *Cell Biol. Toxicol.*, 1:269-283.

25. Malcolm, A.R., Mills, L.J., and Trosko, J.E. (1985): In: *Carcinogenesis - A Comprehensive Survey, Volume 8, Cancer of Respiratory Tract: Predisposing Factors*, edited by M.J. Mass, D.J. Kaufman, J.M. Siegfried, V.E. Steele, and S. Nesnow, pp. 305-318. CRC Press, Boca Raton.

26. Marnett, L.J. (1987): *Carcinogen.* 8:1365-1373.

27. Murray, A.H., and Fitzgerald, D.J. (1979): *Biochem. Biophys. Res. Comm.*, 91:395-401.

28. Scott, J.K., Davidson, H., and Nelmes, A.J. (1985): In: *Collaborative Study of Short Term Tests for Carcinogens, Volume 5, Progress in Mutation Research*, edited by J. Ashby, F.J. de Serres, M. Draper, M. Ishidate, Jr., B.H. Margolin, B.E. Matter, and M.D. Shelby, pp. 613-618. Elsevier Science Publishers, Amsterdam.

29. Slaga, T.J. (1983): *Mechanisms of Tumor Promotion: Tumor Promotion in Internal Organs. Volume 1.* CRC Press, Boca Raton.

30. Slaga, T.J., Klein-Szanto, A.J.P., Triplett, L.L., Yotti, L.P., and Trosko, J.E. (1982): *Science*, 213:1023.

31. Spray, D.C. and Saez, J.C. (In press): In: *Biochemical Mechanisms and Regulation of Intercellular Communication. Volume 14,*

Advances in Modern Envioronmental Toxicology, edited by H.A. Milman and E. Elmore, Princeton Scientific Publishing, Princeton.

32. Tennant, R.W., Margolin, B.H., Shelby, M.D., Zeiger, E., Haseman, J.K., Spalding, J.W., Caspary, W., Resnick, M., Stasiewicz, S., Anderson, B., and Minor, R. (1987): *Science,* 236:933-941.

33. Trosko, J.E., and Chang C.C. (1984): *Pharmacol. Rev.,* 36:137s-144s.

34. Trosko, J.E., Dawson, B., Yotti, L.P., and Chang, C.C. (1980): *Nature,* 285:109-110.

35. Trosko, J.E., Yotti, L.P., Dawson, B., and Chang, C.C. (1981): In: *Short Term Tests for Chemical Carcinogens,* edited by H. Stich, pp. 410-427. Springer-Verlag, New York.

36. Trosko, J.E., Yotti, L.P., Warren, S.T., Tsushimoto, S., and Chang, C.C. (1982): In: *Carcinogenesis: Cocarcinogenesis and Biological Effects of Tumor Promoters, Volume 7,* edited by E. Hecker, N.E. Fusenig, W. Kunz, F. Marks, and H.W. Thielmann, pp. 565-585. Raven Press, New York.

37. Tsushimoto, G., Trosko, J.E. Chang, C.C. and Aust, S.D. (1982): *Carcinogen.,* 3:181-185.

38. Umeda, M., Noda, J., and Ono, T. (1980): *Gann,* 71:614-620.

39. Warren, S.T., Dolittle, D.J., Chang, C.C., Goodman, J.I., and Trosko, J.E. (1982): *Carcinogen.,* 3:139-145.

40. Yancey, S.B., Edens, J.E., Trosko, J.E., Chang, C.C. and Revel, J.P. (1982): *Expt. Cell Res.,* 139:329-240.

41. Yotti, L.P. Chang, C.C., and Trosko, J.E. (1979): *Science,* 206:1089-1091.3.

Tumor Promoters: Biological Approaches for
Mechanistic Studies and Assay Systems,
edited by Robert Langenbach et al.
Raven Press, New York © 1988.

DETECTION OF NEOPLASM PROMOTERS IN THE
HEPATOCYTE/LIVER EPITHELIAL CELL SYSTEM

Charles C. Tong and Gary M. Williams

Consultant, 177 Main Street,
Suite 268, Fort Lee, N.J. Ø7Ø24 (CCT) And
Naylor Dana Institute for Disease Prevention,
American Health Foundation, 1 Dana Road,
Valhalla, N.Y. 1Ø595 (GMW)

The cells in every tissue in a mature organism
are maintained in a differentiated state and under
controlled growth by a series of feed back
mechanisms (39,66). Contact inhibition and cellular
communication are important components of this
phenomenon (49). One form of contact dependent
intercellular communication is mediated by the gap
junctions (12,13,15). This kind of intercellular
communication is absent in malignant tissues
and/or transformed cells (9,1Ø,11,33,69,7Ø). These
reports not only establish the importance of
intercellular communication in homeostatic
mechanisms of growth control but also reveal that
the reduced level of communication can facilitate
an uncontrolled malignant growth. That is, the
inhibition of cellular communication can lead to a
phase of uncontrolled growth or neoplasm promotion
of neoplastic cells generated by exposure to
DNA-reactive carcinogens (74-76).

Intercellular communication also operates in
cells which are grown in vitro. Contact feeding
between cells grown in culture can be quantified
by co-culturing two genetically distinct cell types
under appropriate experimental conditions
(9,12,13). Contact feeding between co-cultured

161

cells occurs through intercellular gap junctions (18,28) which are evidently vital for cellular proliferation as well as differentiation during development and physiological adaptation.

Neoplasm promoters have been demonstrated to inhibit membrane mediated intercellular communication (36,59,61,73,79). Based on this principle. Trosko et al (61) have proposed that the phenomenon of metabolic cooperation inhibition can be applied as a useful screening test for carcinogens which act as tumor promoters. The assay emerged from the discovery that 12-0-tetradecanyl-phorbol-13-acetate (TPA),which is a powerful mouse tumor promoter, enhanced the recovery of UV-induced hypoxanthine guanine phosphoribosyl transferase negative (HGPRT) mutants in V79 chinese hamster lung cells (22,26,27,60). In these experiments a higher rate of recovery of HGPRT negative mutants was obtained. The phenomenon occurred because of the fact that the co-cultured wild type cells could not transport toxic metabolites to the mutant cells due to the inhibition of "metabolic cooperation" between the two cell types. Thus, based on the assumption that TPA like tumor promoters would inhibit intercellular metabolic cooperation, Trosko developed the assay with V79 chinese hamster lung cells and validated by testing many non-genotoxic agents which are suspected or known tumor promoters (62,63,64,65). Because of the lack of a substantial level of metabolic capability for the biotransformation of xenobiotics, the Trosko assay using V79 cells until recently can only detect activation independent agents (30). While the incorporation of the microsomal enzymes for activation has been attempted it is now generally accepted that intact cell metabolism more clearly resembles that of the in vivo situation (5,6,45,46).

The interest of our group in liver neoplasm promotion lead us to develop a liver-derived system in which to study liver neoplasm promoters (53,59,73,79,80). This assay involves co-culture of freshly isolated hepatocytes with HGPRT negative adult rat liver epithelial cells. The mutant cells when grown alone in the medium containing 6-thioguanine proliferate very well but die

passively when grown in co-cultures with freshly
isolated hepatocytes because of the toxic effect of
the nucleotide transferred from the enzyme
competent hepatocytes. This innovative modification
involving the use of freshly perfused hepatocytes
provides the assay with the much needed parameter
of intact cell metabolism which more closely
resembles that of the living organism and which is
absent in all the other systems developed to date.

   The following is a brief description of the
assay and some of the validation chemicals that
have been tested.

Rat liver cell cultures

   The 6-thioguanine resistant (TGr) strain of
adult rat liver epithelial cell (ARL) Line No. 14
was derived by selecting the hypoxanthine-guanine
phosphoribosyl transferase (HGPRT) deficient
mutants by exposure of the line to 6-thioguanine
(TG), as described previously (55,56,78). The TGr
strain was deficient in HGPRT. Primary cultures of
rat liver hepatocytes (HPCs) were obtained as
previously described (77).

Validation Chemicals

   The organochlorine pesticide,
1,1,1-Trichloro-2,2-bis(P-chlorophenyl)ethane
(DDT), chlordane and heptachlor were the three
selected chemicals initially used to standardize
the assay system. The oncogenic DDT (19,54) has
been studied extensively in our laboratory and was
not found to damage DNA or to be mutagenic in a
battery of in vito assays (52,57,72,73).

Metabolic cooperation studies

   ARL-14-TGr cells were plated at a density of 20
cells/cm2 in Williams Medium E supplemented with
10% calf serum (WMES). Twenty four hours later,
freshly isolated hepatocytes were plated onto the
same flasks and were given 3-5 hours for
attachment. These co-cultures were then exposed to

DDT in WMES for 4 hours before 6-thioguanine (TG)
at 10 ug/ml was added. The cells were grown for 2
days and were re-fed with WMES containing DDT and
TG. Three days later, the medium was replaced by
medium containing TG only. The cells were
maintanined for the next 4 days before they were
fixed with formalin and stained with crystal violet
for colony counting. By that time, only the
ARL-14-TGr colonies remained.

TABLE 1.   Inhibition of metabolic cooperation
            between hepatocytes and an ARL-TG(r)
            strain by a liver tumor promoter DDT

	TGr colonies/flask	
Condition	No hepatocytes	Hepatocytes (750,000)
ARL-14-TGr	126	−
+ TG	110	63
+ TG + DDT 10(−7)	103	86
+ TG + DDT 10(−6)	101	112
+ TG + DDT 10(−5)	105	117
+ TG + DDT 10(−4)	61	24

From (79).

As shown in Table 1, the colony forming
efficiency of HGPRT-deficient ARL-TGr cell is
comparable in control medium to that in TG
containing medium, i.e. 126 vs. 110. When
HGPRT-competent cells such as freshly isolated
hepatocytes (77), are co-cultivated with TGr cells
at ratios high enough to achieve significant
cell-to-cell contacts, the HGPRT-competent cells
metabolize the TG and transfer the mononucleotide
to the TGr cells by way of gap junctions (18),
thereby killing the TGr cells as well as
themselves. Consequently, as shown in Table 1, the
co-cultivation of hepatocytes with TGr cells in the
presence of TG reduced the colonies produced by TGr

cells from 110 to 63. As shown in Table 1, the addition of DDT to co-cultivated hepatocytes and TGr cells exposed to TG restored the recovery of TGr cells beginning at 10(-7)M and reaching 100% at 10(-6)M and 10(-5)M. DDT at 10(-4)M was toxic to ARL-14-TGr as shown by the reduced colony formation even in the absence of hepatocytes.

The next two organochlorine pesticides employed were Chlordane and Heptachlor.

Both chlordane and heptachlor were negative in the ARL-HGPRT mutagenesis assay, which is a sensitive system for detecting mutagenic potential of various compounds, includiing those which require metabolic activation (56). Earlier data on mutagenesis in another rat liver cell line and a human cell line also demonstrated a lack of mutagenic effect by these pesticides (52,57,73). Both chlordane and heptachlor were consistently inactive in the hepatocyte primary culture/DNA repair assay using hepatocytes from rat, mouse and hamster (32,72,73). Our data on lack of genotoxicity by chlordane and heptachlor in liver-derived systems is supported by other evidence of inactivity in various microbial assays (4,8,25,31,47,48,51) . Therefore, in spite of the reports by Ahmed et al (2,3) of production of DNA repair in human fibroblasts by chlordane and heptachlor and induction of ouabain resistant mutants in V-79 cells by chlordane, we consider it unlikely that the carcinogenicity of these two pesticides results from a genotoxic action.

In the assay of inhibition of intercellular communication, non-specific toxic effects to both the hepatocyte feeder and the target ARL cells must be excluded. The toxicity of the test chemicals on these ARL14 TGr target cells is routinely determined in the metabolic cooperation assay by measuring the inhibition of their colony forming efficiency after continuous exposure to increasing concentrations of the test compounds. To assay for toxicity to the hepatocyte feeder cells, they were

exposed to chlordane and hepatachlor for up to 72
hours, which represents the initial critical
interval of co-cultivation. The pesticides were
non-toxic to HPCs at up to 5x10(-4)M for chlordane
and 5x10(-5)M for heptachlor (not shown). Metabolic
cooperation was then measured at levels which were
non-toxic to both cell types.

In the co-cultivation system for measurement of
metabolic cooperation, HPCs at a ratio of 2500:1 to
mutant TGr cells reduced their colony formation by
more than 50% (Table 2), presumably through the
transfer of the toxic phosphoribosylated TG to the
mutant HGPRT deficient cells. Chlordane at
5x10(-6)M and heptachlor at 1x10(-6)M almost
completely restored the recovery of TGr colonies
indicating a profound inhibition of metabloic
cooperation.

TABLE 2.   Effect of chlordane and heptachlor on
           intercellular communication between rat
           liver cells.

Condition	TGr colonies per flask	
	No HPC(s)	1,250,000 HPC(s)
TGr alone	186	87
+ Chlordane 1x10(-7)	179	90
+ Chlordane 5x10(-7)	198	95
+ Chlordane 1x10(-6)	206	121
+ Chlordane 5x10(-6)	181	155
+ Chlordane 1x10(-5)	152	116
+ Chlordane 1x10(-4)	Toxic	
TGr alone	146	55
+ Heptachlor1x10(-7)	133	99
+ Heptachlor5x10(-7)	147	95
+ Heptachlor1x10(-6)	112	106
+ Heptachlor5x10(-6)	130	84
+ Heptachlor1x10(-5)	135	91
+ Heptachlor1x10(-4)	Toxic	

From (53).

Chlordane and heptachlor at the effective concentration of 10(-6)M did not affect the close cell to cell contacts between the polygonal hepatocytes and the mutant cells as determined by light microscopy (not shown). These observations suggest that the restoration of recovery of TGr cells was not due to disruption of the contacts between hepatocytes and mutant cells.

The transfer of phosphoribosylated TG to the mutant cells, which is necessary to kill them in the metabolic cooperation assay, would be reduced by decreased generation of the toxic nucleotide in hepatocytes. To preclude this effect as the basis for the inhibition of metabolic cooperation by the pesticides, their effect on the phosphoribosylation of guanine as a surrogate for TG was examined in hepatocytes. In a separate study (53), both chlordane and heptachlor produced no significant effect on the conversion of guanine to metabolites at the concentrations that were effective in inhibiting metabolic cooperation. These results clearly indicate that inhibition of the metabolism of TG in hepatocytes cannot be the basis for the restoration of TGr cells.

The next suspected promoter to be studied in our series of validation chemicals was polybrominated biphenyls (PBB). PBB have been demonstrated to have an enhancing effect on the development of liver neoplasms when administered after the liver carcinogen diethylnitrosamine (21). PBB did not elicit DNA repair synthesis in hepatocytes from mice, rats, or hamsters (80). The negative results with PBB corresponds to similar findings with hepatocarcinogenic polycyclic organochlorine compounds (32,73), providing strong evidence that these chemicals lack the capacity to damage DNA.

Additional evidence for a lack of genotoxicity was provided by the absence of mutagenicity of PBB in the ARL/HGPRT mutagenesis assay and the hepatocyte-mediated human fibroblast/HGPRT mutagenesis assay (59,80). As with DNA repair in hepatocytes, both of these systems have responded to genotoxic carcinogens, but not polycyclic organochlorine compounds (53,56,57,58,72,73). These findings expand considerably the available data (16,17) showing that PBB lack genotoxicity. As shown in Table 3, PBB inhibited intercellular communication between cultured rat liver cells,

TABLE 3.   Effect of PBB on metabolic cooperation
            between rat hepatocytes and ARL 14-TGr
            epithelial cells

Condition	TG colonies per flask	
	No Hepatocytes	1,000,000 Hepatocytes
ARL-14TGr + TG	194	31
+ TG + PBB 7.5x10(-5)	141	115
+ TG + PBB 10(-4)	172	47
+ TG + PBB 2.5x10(-4)	59	74
+ TG + PBB 5.0x10(-4)	Toxic	4
+ TG + PBB 7.5x10(-4)	Toxic	Toxic

From (80).

confirming the report of Trosko et al. (62) with
Chinese hamster V-79 lung cells. Therefore , it
seems probable that PBB, like the organochlorine
pesticides (53,72,74), are epigenetic carcinogens
of the promoter class.

    The next two compounds in this series of studies
were the food preservatives butylated
hydroxyanisole (BHA) and butylated hydroxytoluene
(BHT). BHA is an antioxidant that has been used
extensively in preserving foods from spoilage . BHA
has also been shown to inhibit the effects of
chemical carcinogens in a variety of organs
(20,68), largely through the induction of
detoxification enzyme systems (7,50). In a recent
study in this laboratory, 6000 ppm BHA or BHT in
the diet strongly inhibited the
hepatocarcinogenicity of aflatoxin B1 (83). BHA
nevertheless is a promoter of forestomach neoplasms
(75). Moreover, Ito and coworkers reported the
induction of squamous cell carcinoma in the
forestomach of rats fed 1.02% BHA in a pelleted
diet for 104 weeks (20). Subsequently, BHA was
found to induce benign papillomas in the
forestomach of hamsters that were fed either 1.04%
in pelleted diet or 1% in powdered diet for 24
weeks (20). No carcinogenic effect was observed in
a study in mice (84).

TABLE 4.   Inhibition of intercellular communication
            by butylated hydroxyanisole

Condition	Mutants recovered per flask		
	No Hepatocytes	750,000 Hepatocytes	Recovery %
ARL- TGr	195	130	67
+ DTT 10(-6)M	192	159	83
+ BHA 3.2x10(-7)M	185	177	96
+ BHA 1.6x10(-6)M	190	192	100

From (75).

BHA is not known to be genotoxic (1,23,42) and
in light of the unique pattern of tumor
induction, it seemed likely that its carcinogencity
might be exerted through epigenetic effects. To
shed further light on the mechanism of action of
BHA, we examined its potential genotoxicity and
epigenetic effects in a variety of in vitro systems
(75,76,82).

BHA induces hepatic enzyme systems and is
biotransformed in the liver (14) and, therefore,
several liver derived test systems were employed to
assay for genotoxic effects of BHA. In the
hepatocyte primary culture/DNA repair test (71),
BHA (mixed isomers) at concentrations of up to
10(-3) mg/ml did not induce DNA repair synthesis
and was non-mutagenic in 5 tester strains in the
Ames salmonella/microsome test at concentrations up
to 10 mg/plate, with or without a liver S9 fraction
. In a mammalian cell mutagenesis assay, using
adult rat liver epithelial cell cultures in which
mutations can be measured at the
hypoxanthine-guanine phosphoribosyl transferase
(HGPRT) locus (56), BHA was non-mutagenic at
concentrations up to 0.9 mg/ml , which was the
highest non-toxic dose. Also, at a concentration of
0.1 mg/ml, BHA did not induce sister chromatid
exchanges in Chinese hamster ovary cells. The
negative results, together with those in the
literature, strongly indicate that BHA is not DNA-
reactive, although there is evidence for protein
binding (14,40). As shown in Table 4, BHA was

TABLE 5. Inhibition of intercelluilar
          communication by butylated hydroxytoluene

Condition		Mutants recovered per flask		
		No Hepatocytes	750,000 Hepatocytes	Recovery %
ARL— TGr		193	124	64
+ DTT	10(-6)	192	159	83
+ BHT	3.2x10(-7)	205	144	70
+ BHT	1.6x10(-6)	211	159	75
+ BHT	8.0x10(-6)	215	187	87

From (76).

effective in blocking exchange between hepatocytes
and epithelial cells. In fact, the inhibition was
comaprable to that of DDT, a proven promoter and
inhibitor in this system (79).

Another important food preservative BHT was also
analysed in the same assay. BHT is a liver tumor
promoter (29,37).As expected, BHT also inhibited
metabolic cooperation in this cell system (Table
5).
Studies using our published procedures and the
rat liver epithelial line ARL14 6-thioguanine
resistant mutant obtained from our laboratory are
also being carried out in the laboratory of Dr.
Andrea Rogers—Back of the Microbiological
Associates, Inc. Dr. Rogers—Back was able to
confirm our observation using identical cell types
and have expanded the chemical data base as well
(41).

Other investigators have also made use of the
unique capability of the liver cell system in
evaluating the promoter potential of suspected
chemicals. In the lab. of Dr. Rolin—Limbosch and
colleague (43,44), the use of human hepatoma cell
lines was adopted . Of the several tumor lines
examined, only the SK-Hep-1 work effectively , ie,
was sensitive to metabolic cooperation. Of the
other two lines examined, the recovery of HGPRT
mutant derived from the Hep G2 and Hep 3 B did not
seem to be affected by the presence of 1000 fold
excess of their respective parental wild type
cells. In their studies, TPA was the most efficient

while the hormones testosterone, nor-testosterone and trembolone and the benzodiazepine tranquilizer ,diazepam and oxazepam and the barbiturate phenobarbital (PB) also inhibited metabolic cooperation but to a lesser degree. Several interesting observations came out of their studies.

First what they found was that using the typical clonogenic assay in which the inhibition is measured by the restoration of HGPRT- colonies, TPA and PB do not significantly inhibit metabolic cooperation up to the highest non-toxic concentrations allowed. However, using the autoradiographic technique which monitored the transfer of radioactive hypoxanthine, TPA and PB were shown to be effective. A major difference between these two assays, besides the obvious difference in the scoring of end point, was the length of exposure required. In the autoradiographic procedure, only 4 hours of exposure was adequate, thus permitting a higher concentration of TPA and PB to be used. More interesting is the fact that in those cultures that had been incubated in the presence of TPA or PB for more than 4 hours, e.g. 12 hours or 24 hours, the inhibitory effects of these agents were lost and the transfer of the labels resumed. This may incidentally explain the relative weak effect of PB in our earlier study using our liver derived cell system (73).

The inhibitory effect of TPA was also observed to be transient by Mesnel et al (34) using the dye transfer technique and by Walder and Lutzelschwab (67) using the autoradiographic assay in their rat liver epithelial cell systems. Walder and Lutzelschwab however reported negative result with Diazepam. In their study retinoic acid was positive. They were thus in agreement with a study reported by Pitt et al (1986) though Morel-Chaney et at (35) claimed that in their study, using the clonogenic assay, retinoic acid only enhanced the effect of TPA.

Still other investigators have used the unique metabolic capability of hepatocytes and incorporate them into various existing metabolic cooperation inhibition assay systems. One of which is the group from the Netherlands, in a proceeding from a Conference on the Concept & Theories in Carcinogenesis. Dr. Jonger and Dr. Temmink (24)

presented data incorporating into the V79 cell
system chicken embryo hepatocyte as the wild type
HGPRT+ cells. Their study using the
autoradiographic technique was able to detect the
inhibitory effect of both TPA and cigarette smoke
condensate in cellular communication. What they
have also observed was that the effect of TPA in
this system was also time dependent and its
inhibitory effect diminished and ultimately
disappeared when the cells were exposed to
prolonged period of TPA.

In summary, considerable evidence has been
accumulated to support the concept that the
inhibition of cellular communication can lead to a
phase of uncontrolled growth or neoplasm promotion.
Measurement of inhibition of intercellular
communication can thus be used to identify new
promoters. Trosko et al (63) e.g. showed that
polybrominated biphenyls were positive in cell
culture assays and, subsequently, promotion was
demonstrated (21). Likewise, our finding (53) that
chlordane and heptachlor inhibited intercellular
communication in cultured liver epithelial cells
had lead to them being demonstrated to be liver
tumor promoters (81). Our system using
metabolically competent liver cell appears capable
of contributing much to the understanding of tumor
promotion. Further studies however are required to
compare the relative merit and sensitivity of the
clonogenic approach versus that of the
autoradiographic approach. Another long term goal
may be the further development of the assay with
multispecies metabolic capability.

Reference

1.   Abe, S. and Sasaki, M. J.(1977): Natl. Cancer
       Inst., 58:1635-1640.

2.   Ahmed, F.E., Hart, R.W., and Lewis, N.J.(1977):
       Mutat Res., 42:161-174.

3.   Ahmed, F.E., Lewis, N.J. and Hart, R.W.(1977):
       Chem-Biol. Interactions, 19:369-374.

4.   Ashwood-Smith, M.J., Trevion, J. and Ring, R.
       (1972): Nature, 240:418-419.

5. Billings, R.E., McMahon, R.E., Ashmore, J. and
    Wagle, F.R.(1977): Drug Met. and Dispos.,
    5:518.

6. Casiciano, D.A.(1979): In: Banbury Report 2:
    Mammalian Cell Mutagenesis The Maturation
    of Test System, Eidted by A.W. Hsie, I.P.
    O'Neill and V.K. McElheny. pp.125. Cold
    Spring Harbor Laboratory, New York.

7. Cha, Y-N., and Heine, H.S. (1982):Cancer
    Research., 42:2609.

8. Chambers, C. and Dutta, S.K.(1976): Genetics,
    83:613.

9. Corsaro, C. M. and Migeon, B. R.(1975): Exptl.
    Cell Res., 95:39-46.

10. Corsaro, C. M. and Migeon, B. R.(1977): Proc.
    Natl. Acad. Sci. USA., 74:4476-4480.

11. Corsaro, C. M. and Migeon, B. R.(1977):
    Nature, 268:737-739.

12. Cox, R. D., Krauss, M. R. Balis, M. R. and
    Dancis, J.(1970): Proc. Natl. Acad. Sci.
    USA., 67:1573-1579.

13. Cox, R. D. Krauss, M. R. , Balis, M. R. and
    Dancis, J.(1972): Exptl. Cell. Res.,
    74:251-268.

14. Cummings, S.W., Ansari, G.A.S., Guengerich,
    F.P., Crouch, L.S. and Prough, R.A.
    (1985): Cancer Research, 45:5617.

15. Epstein, M. L. and Gilula, N. B.(1976): J. Cell
    Biol., 75:769.

16. Fisco, G.,and Wertz, G.F.(1976): Mutat Res.,
    38:388.

17. Garthoff, J.H., Friedman,L., Farber, T.M.,
    Locke, K.K., Sobatks, J.J., Green, S.,
    Hurley, N.E., Peters, E.L., Story, G.E.,
    Moreland, F.M., Graham, C.H., Key,J.E.,
    Taylor, M.J., Scabra, J. V., Rothlein,
    J.E.,Marks, E.M., Cerra, F.E.,Rodi, S.B.,
    and Sporn,E.M.(1977): Toxicol
    Environ Health, 3:769-796.

18. Gilula, N. B., Reeves, O.R. and Steinbach, A. (1972): Nature, 235:262-265.

19. Innes,J.R.M., Ulland, B.M., Valerio, M.C., Petrucelli, L.,Fishbein,L., Hart, E.R., Pattota, A.J., Bates, R.R., Falk, H.L., Gavt, J.J., Klein, M., Mitchell, I., and Peters, S.(1969): J.Natl. Cancer Inst., 42:1101-1114.

20. Ito, N., Fukushima, S. and Tsuda, H. (1985): CRC Critical Reviews in Toxicology, ol. 15, Issue 2, 109.

21. Jensen, R.K., Sleight, S.D., Goodman, J.I., Aust.,S.D. and Trosko, J.E.(1982): Carcinogenesis 3:1183-1186.

22. Jone, C., Trosko, J.E., Aylsworth, C.F., Parker, L. and Chang, C.C.(1985): Carcinogenesis, 6:361-365.

23. Joner, P.E.(1977): Acta Vet. Scand., 18:187.

24. Jonger, W.M.F. and Temmink, J.H.M.(1986): Cancer Letter, 30 (Suppl) S52.

25. Kada, T., Moriya, M. and Shirasu, Y.(1974): Mutat. Res., 26:243-248.

26. Lankas, G. R. Baxter, C. R. and Christian, R. T. (1977): Mutat. Res., 45:153-156.

27. Lankas, et al (1978): J. Toxicol. Environ. Health, 4:37-41.

28. Loewenstein, W. R.(1979):   Biochim. Biophys. Acta., 560:1-65.

29. Maeura, Y.D., Williams, G.M.(1984) Food and Cosmetic Toxicol, 22:191.

30. Malcolm, A.R., Mills, L.J. and Mckenna, E.J. (1985): Cell Biol and Toxicol, 1:.

31. Marshall, T.C., Dorough, H.W. and Swim, H.E. (1976): Food Chem., 24:560-563.

32. Maslansky, C.J. and Williams, G.M.(1981): J. Toxicol. Environ. Health, 8:121-130.

33. McNutt, N. S. and Weinstein, R.(1969):
    Science, 165:597-599.

34. Mesnil, M., Montesano, R. and Yamasaki, H.
    (1986): Expt'l Cell Res., 165:39-402.

35. Morel-Chaney, E., Aujard, C. and Lafarge-
    Frayssinet, C. (1986): Carcinogenesis,
    7:653-658.

36. Murray, A.W. and Fitzgerald, J. D.(1979):
    Biochim Biophys. Res. Comm. 91: 395-401.

37. Peraino, C.,Fry, R.J.M., Stffeldt, E. and
    Christopher, J.P.(1977): Fd, Cosmot.
    Toxicol, 15:93-96.

38. Pitt, J.D., Hamitton, A.E., Kam, E., Burk,
    R.R.and Murphy, J.P. (1986):
    Carcinogenesis, 7:1003-1010.

39. Potter, V. R.(1982): In: Progress in Nucleic
    Acid Research And Molecular Biology, edited
    by W.E. Cohn, Academic Press, New York.

40. Rahimtula, A.(1983): Chem.- Biol. Interact.,
    45:125.

41. Rogers-Back, A.M. and Clarke J.J. (1986):
    The Toxicobgist, 6:39.

42. Rogers, C.G., Nayak, B.,N. and Heroux-Metcalf,
    C.(1985): Cancer Lett., 27:61

43. Rolin-Limbosch, S., Vanhamme, L. and Szpirer C.
    (1986): Cancer Letter, 30 (Suppl) S51.

44. Rolin-Limbosch, S., Moen S. W.,and Szpirer C.
    (1986b): Carcinogenesis, 7:1235-1238.

45. Schmeltz, I., Trosk J. and Williams, G.M.
    (1978): Cancer Letters, 5:81-89.

46. Selkirk, J.R.(1977): Nature, 270:604.

47. Shirasu, Y., Moriya, M., Kato, K., Furuhashi,
    A. and Kada, T.(1976): Mutat. Res.,
    40:19-30.

48. Shirasu, Y., Moriya, M., Kato, K., Lienard, F.,
    Tezuka, H.Teramoto, S. and Kada, T.(1977):
    In: Origins of Human Cancer,edited by H.H.
    Hiatt, J.D. Watson and J.F. Winston, pp
    243-266, Cold Spring Harbor Lab., New York.

49. Subak-Sharpe, H.(1965): Exptl. Cell Res.,
    38:106-119.

50. Sydor, W., Lewis, K.F. and Yang, C.S. (1984):
    Cancer Research, 44:134

51. Tardiff, R.G., Carlson, G.P., and Simmon, V.
    (1976): In: Proc. Conf.Impact of Water
    Chlorinetion, pp.213-227,edited by T.L.
    Tolley, pp.213-227, Oak Ridge, Tennessee.

52. Telang, S., Tong, C., and Williams G.M.(1981):
    Environ,Mutagenesis, 3:359

53. Telang, S., Tong, C. and Williams, G.M.(1982):
    Carcinogenesis, 3:1175-1178.

54. Tomatis, L., Tursov, V., Day, N. and Charles,
    R.T. (1972): The effect of long-term
    exposure to DDT on CF-1 Mice. Int. J.
    Cancer, 10:489-506.

55. Tong, C. and Williams, G.M. (1978): Mutat Res.,
    58:339-352.

56. Tong, C., Williams, G.M. (1980): Mutation Res.,
    74:1-9.

57. Tong, C., Fazio, M. and Williams, G.M. (1981):
    Proc. Soc. Expt. Biol. Med., 167:572-575.

58. Tong, C., Laspia, M.F., Telang, S. and
    Williams, G.M. (1981): Environmental
    Mutagenesis, 4:477-487.

59. Tong, C., Telang, S. and Williams, G.M. (1983):
    Environmental Mutagenesis, 5:416.

60. Trosko, J.E., Chang, C.C., Yotti, 1.P. and
    Chu, E.(1977): Cancer Res. 37:188-193.

61. Trosko, J. E., Dawson, B., Yotti, L. P. and
    Chang, C. C. (1980): Nature 285:109-110.

62. Trosko, J. E., Yotti, L. P., Dawson, B. and
       Chang, C. C.(1981): In: Short Term Tests
       for Chemical Carcinogens, edited by H.
       Stich and R. H. C. San, pp. 420-427,
       Springer-Verlag, New York.

63. Trosko, J. E., Dawson, B. and Chang, C. C.
       (1981): Environ. Health Persp., 37:179-182.

64. Trosko, J.E., Jone, C. and Chang, C.C.
       (1983): Ann. N. Y. Acad. Sci. 407:316-327.

65. Tsushimoto, G., Trosko, J. E., Chang, C. C.,
       and Aust, S. D. (1982): Carcinogenesis,
       3:181-185.

66. Tubiana, M. and Frindel, E. (1982): J. Cell.
       Physiol. Suppl. 1:13.

67. Walder L., and Lutzelschwab R. (1984): Expt'l
       Cell Res., 152:66-67.

68. Wattenberg, L.W. (1978):J. Natl. Cancer Inst.,
       60:11

69. Weinstein, R. S., Merk, F. B. and Alroy,J.
       (1976): Adv. Cancer Res., 23:23-89 .

70. Weinstein, I. B., Wigler, M. and Pietropoole,
       C. (1977): In: Origins of Human Cancer,
       eduted by H. H. Hiatt, J. D. Watson, and J.
       F. Winston, pp. 751-772, Cold Spring Harbor
       Laboratory, New York.

71. Williams, G. M. (1977): Cancer Research,
       37:1845-1851.

72. Williams, G.M.(1979): In Advances in Medical
       Oncology, Research and Education Vol.1,
       pp.273-280, Carcinogenesis, edited by
       G.P.Margison Pergamon, New York.

73. Williams, G.M.(1980): Ann. N.Y. Acad. Sci.,
       349:273-282.

74. Williams, G.M.(1981): Food and Cosmetic
       Toxicology, 19:577-583.

75. Williams, G.M.(1986): Food & Chemical
       Toxicology in Press.

76. Williams, G.M. (1986): Proc. IV Int. Cong. Toxicology, Japan, in press.

77. Williams, G.M., Bermudez, E. and Scaramuzzino, D.(1977): In Vitro,13:809-817

78. Williams, G.M., Tong, C. and Berman, J.J. (1978): Mutat Research.,49:103-115.

79. Williams, G. M., Telang, S. and Tong, C. (1981): Cancer Lett., 11:339-344.

80. Williams, G. M., Tong, C., Telang, S.(1984): Environmental Res., 34:310-320.

81. Williams, G.M. and Numoto S.(1984): Carcinogenesis, 5:1689-1696.

82. Williams, G.M., Shimada, T., McQueen C., Tong, C. and Ved Brat S. (1984): The Toxicologist, 4:104.

83. Williams, G.M., Tanaka, T. and Maeura, Y. (1986): Carcinogenesis, 7:1043-1050.

84. Yokoro, K.(1981): Annual Report of the Cancer Research, Ministry of Health and Welfare, p.1013.

Tumor Promoters: Biological Approaches for Mechanistic Studies and Assay Systems, edited by Robert Langenbach et al. Raven Press, New York © 1988.

CHEMICO-BIOLOGICAL INTERACTIONS IN THE IMMUNOLOGIC

MODULATION OF INITIATED AND PROMOTED TRANSFORMATION

Charles H. Evans and Joseph A. DiPaolo

Laboratory of Biology
Division of Cancer Etiology
National Cancer Institute
Bethesda, Maryland 20892

Carcinogenesis develops in a dynamic biological milieu where it is subject to potential modification by a variety of chemical, physical and biological interactions resident in the target cell host-environment. Host interactions with the target cell in the multi-step transition to neoplastic transformation may be of an anti-carcinogenic or co-carcinogenic nature and when both are present they may produce an antagonistic and even neutralizing effect. As a result there may be a decrease, an increase or no change in the frequency of tumor appearance and it may be difficult to appreciate and define the presence of anti-carcinogenic and co-carcinogenic interactions in the complexity of the host environment. In addition to identifying agents capable of causing complete transformation, or initiating or promoting transformation *in vitro* carcinogenesis models capable of discriminating between the genetic and extra-genetic molecular events in the stages of carcinogenesis provide the means to study individually and collectively the chemico-biological interactions at the target cell level with the potential to prevent, reverse and even stimulate the carcinogenic process.

Transformation of guinea pig (7,12,15) fetal fibroblast-like cells (FIG. 1) and Syrian hamster (1,8,17) embryo fibroblast-like cells (FIG. 2) in cell culture are two useful models for identification of carcinogenic, anti- and co-carcinogenic biological, chemical and physical agents and for investigation of the genetic and biochemical pathways of their action. These two models also provide the opportunity to evaluate defined combinations of interactions *in vivo* as well as *in vitro* through the host-mediated combined *in vivo-in vitro* approach of initiating or inducing the complete carcinogenic process and the modulatory influence while the target cells are *in utero* followed by development including additional modulation of the transformation process *in vitro* after culture of the cells

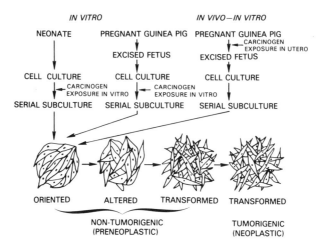

FIG. 1. Transformation of guinea pig fibroblast-like cells as a model for the study of carcinogenesis (7).

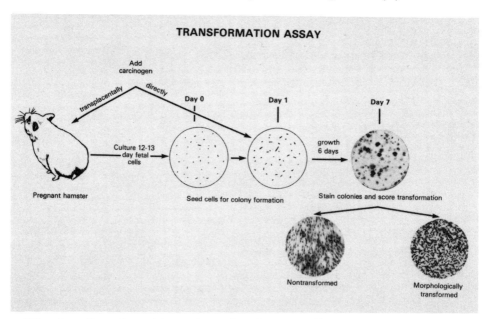

FIG. 2. Transformation of Syrian hamster fibroblast-like cells as a model system for the study of carcinogenesis (5).

(5,7,17,18). The two models also complement each other. The transition to neoplasia in guinea pig cells occurs in sequential extended stages (FIG. 3) spanning a continuum from two to twenty-four or more months between carcinogen insult and the expression of neoplastic transformation (7). By comparison, the transition to neoplasia in Syrian hamster cells is telescoped into a period as short as six weeks, the time required to observe morphologic transformation one week after carcinogen insult and to produce sufficient cells from a morphologically transformed colony of cells to administer to an appropriate host to demonstrate the ability of the transformed cells to form a progressively growing tumor (4).

THE STAGES OF CARCINOGENESIS

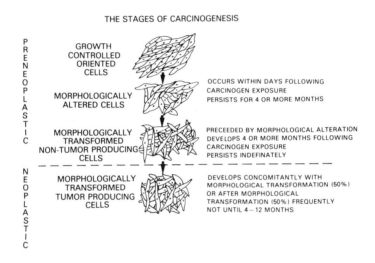

FIG. 3. Sequential stages in the transition of guinea pig cells to neoplastic transformation.

The long latent period characteristic of neoplastic transformation in guinea pig cells (FIG. 4) facilitates study of the genetic (12,21) and biochemical (20) changes developing in the target cell during the stages in the transition to neoplasia. On the other hand transformation of Syrian hamster cells by chemical carcinogen or radiation provides a model for more facile quantitative and rapid evaluation of co-carcinogenic (1,3) and anti-carcinogenic (7,9,12) chemico-biological interactions in terms of the potential of the interactions to influence the transition to neoplasia. Both models are valuable in defining the modulatory action of naturally occurring host biochemical (6,14) and immunologic (3,8,9,12,15,17,18) components for the carcinogenic process.

THE STAGES OF CARCINOGENESIS

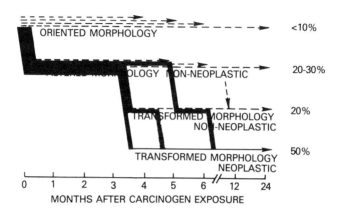

FIG. 4. Pathways to neoplasia in the transformation of guinea pig cells.

One area of aggregate and complex potential interactions where chemical carcinogen and radiation induced transformation of guinea pig and of Syrian hamster cells is useful is in the analysis of normal physiological mechanisms such as the immune system in terms of their ability to modify the development of carcinogenesis (FIG. 5). Investigations using both model systems have identified a new lymphokine, recently named leukoregulin (19), as one normal host biological component that possesses potent anti-carcinogenic activity. Leukoregulin is produced by activated lymphocytes and its direct acting anti-cancer actions include the ability to induce in target cells an anti-carcinogenic state without associated toxicity, to increase the sensitivity of pre-neoplastic as well as neoplastic cells to natural killer lymphocyte cytotoxicity, and to inhibit DNA synthesis in pre-neoplastic and neoplastic cells. Leukoregulin frequently copurifies with lymphotoxin, another lymphokine, and until recently, due to the frequent co-purification of the two lymphokines, the anti-cancer actions of leukoregulin were attributed to lymphotoxin (16,19). Leukoregulin and its anti-cancer actions can now be separated from lymphotoxin, interferon and other lymphokines by sequential fractionation on the basis of the differences in the isoelectric points, molecular weights, and other physicochemical properties of the individual immunologic hormones (16,19). In guinea pig cells the sensitivity to the DNA synthesis inhibitory action of leukoregulin frequently develops in close association with the expression of neoplastic transformation (12). However,

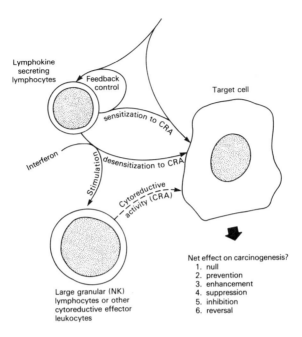

FIG. 5. Potential interactions of components of the immune system with the target cell that can modulate the development of carcinogenesis.

sensitivity to leukoregulin can develop in pre-neoplastic cells in both nonpromoted (12) and promoted (15) transformation. The sensitivity of target cells to the DNA synthesis inhibitory and natural killer lymphocyte sensitizing actions of leukoregulin also generally develops in guinea pig cells in close association with activation of the N-*ras* oncogene which, like neoplastic transformation, is expressed in an active form in guinea pig cells two to twelve or more months after carcinogen exposure and commencement of the transition to neoplasia (21).

Chemical carcinogen as well as ultraviolet- and x-radiation induced transformation of Syrian hamster cells can be prevented by exposure of the cells to leukoregulin from forty-eight hours before to forty-eight hours after carcinogen interaction (3,8). Prevention or inhibition of transformation when cells are exposed to leukoregulin after initiation of carcinogenesis occurs with an efficiency in terms of the specific activity of leukoregulin at least 22 times greater than the lymphokine's ability to inhibit DNA synthesis in neoplastically transformed cells (8). Induction of the anti-carcinogenic state in the target cell occurs without altering target cell replication and is accompanied by increased incorporation of glucosamine into high molecular weight membrane associated glycoproteins while glucosamine incorporation and synthesis of high molecular weight glycoproteins decreases following leukoregulin treatment of neoplastically transformed cells (13). The anti-carcinogenic state in Syrian hamster target cells can be induced by leukoregulin *in vivo* as well as *in vitro* (17,18) and leukoregulin is one of the molecular mediators by which antigen or mitogen stimulated normal lymphocytes are able to directly prevent ultraviolet-radiation induced transformation in Syrian hamster cells (10,11). Co-carcinogenic transformation of Syrian hamster cells following transplacental exposure to diethylnitrosamine *in vivo* and subsequently to x-radiation *in vitro* can also be inhibited by exposure of the target cells to leukoregulin *in vivo* (17). Both ultraviolet-radiation non-promoted and 12-0-tetradecanoylphorbol-13-acetate (TPA) promoted transformation *in vitro* are also sensitive to the anti-carcinogenic action of leukoregulin (2). The combined *in vivo–in vitro* studies also reveal that, as with many hormone induced changes in target cell physiology, the leukoregulin anti-carcinogenic state is transient and the steps or stages in co-carcinogenic transformation are differentially sensitive to the modulatory action of leukoregulin (17).

The temporal and molecular characteristics of the modulation of ultraviolet- and x-radiation initiated and phorbol ester promoted stages of transformation resulting from target cell interaction with leukoregulin are further defined by *in vitro* studies of Syrian hamster cell morphologic transformation . Both non-promoted complete transformation and the initiated stage of transformation are twice as sensitive to inhibition by leukoregulin as is the TPA promoted stage of transformation (2). Leukoregulin pulse chase experiments further demonstrate that leukoregulin induces an anti-carcinogenic state in the target cell during the period from six to forty-eight hours after leukoregulin-target cell interaction emphasizing the critical temporal relationship between interaction of the target cell with the carcinogen and with the anti-carcinogenic lymphokine in the prevention of carcinogenesis (3). The presence of the simple sugar galactose, due to its ability to bind to the active site on the lymphokine and as a result block leukoregulin binding, is sufficient to further modulate the frequency of transformation (FIG. 6). This illustrates the complexity of chemico-biological interactions that may affect carcinogenesis and the ability of *in vitro* model systems to delineate the individual components.

Chemical and radiation induced complete, initiated, and promoted transformation of guinea pig and hamster fibroblast-like cells in culture provides many valuable avenues for identifying and studying the molecular pathways by which chemico-biological interactions cause, facilitate, inhibit, and prevent carcinogenesis. With their wide divergency in latent periods of neoplastic transformation yet similarities in sensitivity to transformation by diverse chemical carcinogens and radiation and to the anti-carcinogenic action by biologic agents such as leukoregulin these models provide unique systems for investigating the carcinogenic and anti-carcinogenic action

MODULATION OF LEUKOREGULIN PREVENTION
OF TPA-PROMOTED X-IRRADIATION
INITIATED TRANSFORMATION

Day 0	Day 1	Day 2	Day 3	Day 4	Day 5	Day 6	Day 7	Av. Trans-formation/dish	Transformation (%)	Inhibition (%)
Seed							Stain			
			No Treatment					0	0	
			X					0	0	
			X + TPA					5.3	17	
LR			X + TPA					2.8	6.7	61
LR + Gal			X + TPA					4.2	12.6	26
LR			X + TPA + Gal					1.5	3.7	78

300 HEC were treated with leukoregulin (LR) (25 units/ml) for 3 days and on day 3 exposed to 240 R X-radiation. TPA (80 nm) was added on day 3 for 4 days. Galactose (2 mM) was present during the first 3 or final 4 days.

FIG. 6. Chemico-biological interactions modulating the TPA promotion of x-radiation initiated transformation of Syrian hamster fibroblast-like cells.

of environmental agents and host components in relation to the stages in the transition from the growth controlled to the neoplastic state. The ability to include *in vivo* as well as *in vitro* exposure to initiating, promoting, and other types of carcinogenic agents in evaluating the events and pathways in the carcinogenic process provides a powerful approach to investigate chemico-biological interactions in each stage of carcinogenesis. The continued use and development of transformation in guinea pig and Syrian hamster cells in investigating the many chemico-biological interactions that can occur in the complexity of the host environment will be increasingly valuable to elucidating the fundamental molecular pathways in the initiation, promotion, and progression of carcinogenesis and in the continued evaluation of genotoxic and epigenetic carcinogenic agents.

REFERENCES

1. DiPaolo, J. A., DeMarinis, A. J., Evans, C. H., and Doniger, J. (1981): *Cancer Lett.*, 14:243-249.
2. DiPaolo, J. A., Evans, C. H., DeMarinis, A. J., and Doniger, J. (1982): *Int. J. Cancer*, 30:781-786.
3. DiPaolo, J. A., Evans, C. H., DeMarinis, A. J., and Doniger, J. (1984): *Cancer Res.*, 44:1465-1471.

4. DiPaolo, J.A., Nelson, R.L. and Donovan, P.J. (1969): *Science*, 165:917-918.
5. DiPaolo, J. A., Nelson, R. L., Donovan, P. J., and Evans, C. H. (1973): *Arch. Path.*, 95:380-385.
6. Evans, C. H., and Boynton, A. L. (1983): *Cancer Lett.*, 15:271-279.
7. Evans, C. H. and DiPaolo, J. A. (1975): *Cancer Res.*, 35:1035-1044.
8. Evans, C.H. and DiPaolo, J.A. (1981): *Int. J. Cancer*, 27:45-49.
9. Evans, C. H. and DiPaolo, J. A. (1982): *J. Natl Cancer Inst.*, 69:1175-1182.
10. Evans, C. H., DiPaolo, J. A., Heinbaugh, J. A., and DeMarinis, A. J. (1982): *J. Natl Cancer Inst.*, 69:737-741.
11. Evans, C. H., Heinbaugh, J. A., and DiPaolo, J. A. (1983): *Cell. Immunol.*, 76:295-303.
12. Evans, C. H., Rabin, E. S., and DiPaolo, J. A. (1977): *Cancer Res.*, 37:898-903.
13. Fuhrer, J. P. and Evans, C. H. (1983): *Cancer Lett.*, 19:283-292.
14. Greiner, J. W. and Evans, C. H. (1982): *Cancer Res.*, 42:4014-4017.
15. Ransom, J. H. and Evans, C. H. (1982): *Int. J. Cancer*, 29:451-458.
16. Ransom, J. H. and Evans, C. H. (1983): *Cancer Res.*, 43:5222-5227.
17. Ransom, J. H., Evans, C. H., and DiPaolo, J. A. (1982): *J. Natl Cancer Inst.*, 69:741-744.
18. Ransom, J. H., Evans, C. H., Jones, A. E., Zoon, R. A., and DiPaolo, J. A. (1983): *Cancer Immunol. Immunother.*, 15:126-130.
19. Ransom, J. H., Evans, C. H., McCabe, R. P., Pomato, N., Heinbaugh, J. A., Chin, M., and Hanna, M. G., Jr. (1985): *Cancer Res.*, 45:851-862.
20. Sisskin, E. E., Weinstein, I. B., Evans, C. H., and DiPaolo, J. A. (1980): *Int. J. Cancer*, 26:331-336.
21. Sukamar, S., Pulciani, S., Doniger, J., DiPaolo, J. A., Evans, C. H., Zbar, B., and Barbacid, M. (1984): *Science*, 223:1197-1199.

Tumor Promoters: Biological Approaches for Mechanistic Studies and Assay Systems,
edited by Robert Langenbach et al.
Raven Press, New York © 1988.

MECHANISMS OF TRANSFORMATION

AND PROMOTION OF SYRIAN HAMSTER EMBRYO CELLS

Tore Sanner and Edgar Rivedal

Lab for Environmental and Occupational Cancer,
Institute for Cancer Research, The Norwegian Radium
Hospital, Montebello, N-0310 Oslo 3, Norway

The induction of a transformed cell phenotype in vitro is appealing because the derived morphology and behaviour bear a striking resemblance with the malignant cell phenotype in vivo. It seems likely that many of the steps involved in the formation of a tumor may be reflected in in vitro cell transformation.

The Syrian hamster embryo (SHE) cell transformation assay has primarily been developed by the groups of DiPaolo (6,7) and Pienta (13). The sensitivity of the test has recently been increased by introducing a new step in the assay where the medium and test chemical are renewed some days prior to scoring of the colonies (16).

In the present communication some of our studies on the mechanism of formation of morphologically transformed colonies and on the use of the assay in studies of promoters will be reviewed.

EXPERIMENTAL PROCEDURE

Primary cultures of Syrian hamster (Wright, Chelmsford, Essex, UK) embryos at 14 days of gestation were prepared and cryopreserved in liquid nitrogen as described by Pienta et al (13). The SHE cell bioassay procedure previously described was used with small modifications (13,20). The assay is started by reconstitution of the feeder cells from liquid nitrogen. The cells are X-irradiated at confluence with 4.500 rad, and 6×10^4 cells are plated in 60 mm

Petri dishes. 150 target cells are seeded on the feeder layer the next day. The test chemical is added 24 h later. The medium is removed after a certain time period, usually 4 days, the dishes rinsed and fresh medium with new chemicals are added to the dishes. The colonies are fixed, stained with Giemsa and inspected for morphological transformation 8 days after seeding of the target cells.

In the normal colonies, the cells are growing in monolayer and are nicely oriented side by side. The clear growth pattern has disappeared in the morphologically transformed colonies. Morphological transformation is scored on the basis of altered colony morphology consisting of criss-crossing and piling-up of cells not observed in the control dishes (5,13).

RESULTS AND DISCUSSION

Two-Stage Transformation Experiments

Recently, we examined different phorbol esters for their ability to enhance the transformation frequency of cells preexposed to BaP[*] (16). Table 1 shows some of the results with the phorbol esters as well as some other substances previously studied in two-stage mouse skin carcinogenesis. No enhancement of the transformation frequency was observed with PMM, 4α-PDD and 4-O-Me-TPA which are inactive in mouse skin carcinogenesis (4). On the other hand, the presence of PDD and TPA during the second incubation period strongly enhanced the transformation frequency. Thus, the phorbol esters which are promoters in mouse skin carcinogenesis (4) do also enhance the frequency of morphological transformation when given subsequently to BaP. Mezerein and retinoic acid which have been shown to promote the induction of tumors in mouse skin experiments (10,23) did likewise enhance the transformation frequencies (16).

----

[*]Abbreviations: BaP, benzo(a)pyrene; PMM, phorbol-12-monomyristate; 4α-PDD, 4α-phorbol-12,13-didecanoate; 4-O-Me-TPA, 4-O-methyl-12-O-tetradecanoyl phorbol-13-acetate; PDD, phorbol-12,13-didecanoate; TPA, 12-O-tetradecanoyl phorbol-13-acetate; FCS, fetal calf serum; NCS, newborn calf serum.

TABLE 1 Transformation of SHE cells by sequential exposure to BaP and mouse skin tumor promoters and non-promoters.

Additions		Cloning efficiency (% of control)	Total no of trans-formed colonies	Transfor-mation frequency (%)
Period 1 (3 days)	Period 2 (4 days)			
None	None	100	0	0
BaP(0.05)	None	103	1	0.2
None	PMM(1)	97	2	0.3
BaP(0.5)	PMM(1)	79	5	1.2
None	4α-PDD(1)	103	0	0
BaP	4α-PDD(1)	79	2	0.4
None	4-O-Me-TPA(1)	103	0	0
BaP(0.05)	4-O-Me-TPA(1)	86	4	0.9
None	PDD(0.1)	97	9	1.6
BaP(0.05)	PDD(0.1)	83	45	8.7
None	TPA(0.1)	97	12	1.8
BaP(0.05)	TPA(0.1)	76	54	13.6
None	Mezerein(0.05)	66	10	3.1
BaP(0.05)	Mezerein(0.05)	56	16	5.9
None	Retinoic ac(0.5)	83	2	0.8
BaP(0.05)	Retinoic ac(0.5)	96	26	5.2
None	BaP(0.01)	78	5	1.5
TPA(0.05)	None	67	1	0.3
TPA(0.05)	BaP(0.01)	61	6	2.3

6-12 dishes were evaluated for each experimental point. The cloning efficiency in the control was 29%. In the experiments with mezerein the cells were incubated with the promoter for only 2 days and then left for 2 days with only medium prior to staining. The transformation frequency is calculated as the number of transformed colonies divided by the total number of surviving colonies multiplied by 100. The numbers in parenthesis gives the concentrations in μg/ml. Retinoic ac represents trans-retinoic acid.

The results (Table 1) show that when TPA is present in the first period with BaP in the second period, the transformation frequency is not significantly increased compared to that obtained with BaP alone. This is in accordance with the generally accepted definition of promotion. TPA present during the first period with no addition during the second period did not induce any significant number of transformed colonies, while both TPA and PDD increased the number of transformed colonies when present during the second period. The significance of this will be discussed later.

TABLE 2 <u>Modulation of the promoter effect of TPA on</u> <u>morphological transformation of SHE cells.</u>

Additions		Cloning efficiency (% of control)	Total no of trans- formed colonies	Transform- ation frequency (%)
Period 1 (3 days)	Period 2 (4 days)			
None	None	100	0	0
BaP	None	108	3	0.6
None	TPA	75	4	1.2
BaP	TPA	58	20	10.2
BaP	TPA+hydrocortisone (0.250 µM)	63	2	0.8
BaP	TPA+dexamethasone (0.025 µM)	58	5	1.5
BaP	TPA+caffeine (515 µM)	78	5	3.1
BaP	TPA+theophylline (278 µM)	53	0	0
BaP + dexamethasone (0.250 µM)	TPA	63	42	11.7
BaP + theophylline (278 µM)	TPA	98	9	9.2

Conditions as in Table 1. The cloning efficiency in the control was 24%. In all experiments the concentration of BaP was 0.05 µg/ml (0.20 µM) and the concentration of TPA 0.05 µg/ml (0.08 µM).

The modulation of the promoter effect of TPA by glucocorticoids and phosphodiesterase inhibitors are shown in Table 2. Both glucocorticoids as hydrocortisone and dexamethasone and phosphodiesterase inhibitors as caffeine and theophylline abolished the promoter activity of TPA when present together with TPA. It is of interest that when dexamethasone or caffeine were present in the first incubation period with BaP they had no effect on the transformation frequency (14,17). The present results agree with that found in two-stage mouse skin carcinogenesis (1,3,22).

The data presented indicate that with the sequential incubation procedure the SHE transformation system responds to promoters and inhibitors of the promoter activity of TPA in a similar way as the two-stage mouse skin carcinogenesis assay. Thus, one may be tempted to draw the conclusion that the SHE cell transformation system is well suited for studies of tumor promoters. However, what are we actually measuring? Is there any reason to assume that the 8 day SHE transformation assay can distinguish between two stages which reflect the initiation and promotion of mouse skin carcinogenesis? Before discussing this problem we shall briefly consider the mechanisms of transformation of SHE cells and focus on some factors modulating the transformation frequency.

Mechanisms of cell transformation

Genotoxic substances may induce transformation by interaction with DNA. Evidence for the involvement of oncogenes have been obtained by Thomassen et al (24). In addition to the cooperative action of the v-Ha-ras and v-myc oncogenes, at least one other change is necessary for neoplastic transformation of normal SHE cells.
Extensive studies on the mechanism of transformation by a number of non-genotoxic substances have been carried out by the group of Carl Barrett (2,11). They found that the compounds caused different types of chromosome changes and suggested that morphological transformation of SHE cells may be caused by chromosomal changes not involving gene mutation.
Substances which cause liver tumors in animals by increased peroxisome proliferation do also transform SHE cells. We have just started a study in order to try to elucidate the mechanism of cell transformation by such substances.

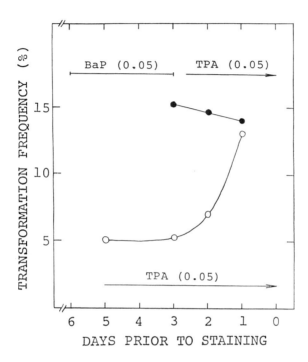

Fig. 1. Effect of TPA addition different days prior to staining on the transformation frequency.

    The results in Table 1 demonstrated that TPA alone could induce morphological transformation of SHE cells. The results in Fig 1 show the effect of addition of TPA to the dishes different days prior to staining. It is apparent that the later TPA was added, the greater was the observed transformation frequency. The greatest effect was obtained when TPA was added only one day prior to staining of the dishes. The fact that the transformation frequency decreases when TPA is added earlier is probably due to metabolic destruction of the compound. The finding that TPA is able to induce morphologically transformed colonies very fast is of interest. It is not likely that this effect could be caused by any interaction with DNA or chromosomal changes. The upper curve shows the results obtained from an initiation - promotion experiment.

BaP was added as initiator, the transformation frequency appeared to be independent of the time for addition of TPA as in the two-stage mouse skin experiments.

Together with Drs Yamasaki and Enomoto we have studied the effect of TPA on cell communication (18). The results showed that TPA inhibited cell communication in a SHE cell line which is sensitive to induction of transformation by TPA, while TPA had no effect on the communication in two SHE cell lines where TPA did not affect the formation of transformed colonies. The formation of morphologically transformed colonies in the presence of TPA are presumably related to inhibition of cell communication (18,26).

If cells from a morphologically transformed colony are seeded on a new Petri dish with a feeder layer, the colonies formed appear normal. Thus, when cells from a transformed colony grow in fresh medium, their growth pattern can not be distinguished from that of cells from normal colonies.

On the other hand, if transformed colonies are cloned and subsequently grown in 25 cm^2 flasks it is possible to derive permanent cell lines. In an experiment where morphologically transformed colonies after sequential exposure to BaP and TPA were cloned, cell lines were obtained from 2 out of 8 morphologically transformed colonies. Cells from normal colonies on the same dish as well as cells from 6 of the morphologically transformed colonies senescenced after 4-18 passages following cloning. On the average they survived about 8 passages. The two morphologically transformed colonies that developed into cell lines gave rise to colony formation in soft agar. Our finding that only a certain fraction of the morphologically transformed colonies will develop into cell lines are in accordance with previous unpublished data by Dr Pienta. DiPaolo et al (6) have previously found that nearly all of their morphologically transformed colonies developed into tumorigenic cell lines. In their experiment an extra selection of morphologically transformed colonies were included after reseeding of the originally transformed colony in a medium without carcinogen. Thus, the difference between the result of DiPaolo and our results may depend on the experimental procedure used.

It is apparent that several mechanisms may be involved in the formation of a morphologically transformed colony, and moreover, that some colonies may be reversibly transformed, while others may be affected by permanent changes and be able to develop into a tumorigenic cell line. From the morphology of the colony it is not possible to tell anything about the mechanisms involved in the transformation or whether the transformation is reversible or not. The possibility exist that the fraction of reversibly transformed colonies depend on the mechanisms involved in the transformation and thus on the transforming substance. This is a problem which we are at present studying.

Modulation of Transformation by Serum Factors

Fetal calf serum is of essential importance in studies of transformation of SHE cells. If newborn calf serum is added to the transformation assay mixture, the formation of transformed colonies is inhibited (Table 3). However, if the serum is passed through an affinity chromatography column of Sepharose coupled gelatin, the inhibitory effect disappears. On the other hand, the eluted gelatin binding material inhibit the transformation. We have identified the inhibitory factor in NCS to be fibronectin (15).

TABLE 3 Effect of NCS on morphological transformation of SHE cells.

Serum added in 2nd exposure period	Cloning efficiency (%)	No of trans- formed colonies	Transfor- mation frequency (%)
20% FCS	28	13	5.2
20% FCS + 10% NCS	22	2	1.0
20% FCS + 10% NCS flow through[a]	26	19	8.1
20% FCS + gelatin binding material (50 ug/ml)[b]	25	5	2.2

Experimental procedure is explained in table 1. The cells were treated with 0.05 ug/ml BaP during the first period and with 0.05 ug/ml TPA in the second period.
[a]NCS flow through from affinity chromatography on Sepharose coupled gelatin.
[b]Gelatin binding material from NCS.

Fetal calf serum is necessary for induction of transformed colonies in the SHE cell transformation system. FCS passed through an Affigel blue column, will not longer support the induction of morpho- logically transformed colonies. If the column is eluted with 50% ethylene glycol and the eluate is added to the medium, it will stimulate the formation of morphologically transformed colonies. We are working on the identification of the substance. It has properties similar to PDGF.

The data in Table 2 showed that glucocorticoids inhibit the promotion by TPA. We have previously found that dexamethasone also reverses morphologically transformed colonies back to normal appearance and that this is a rapid phenomenon (14). Thus, 24 h following the addition of the steroid, more than 90% of the transformed colonies were restored to normal morphology. A decrease in the number of morphologi- cally transformed colonies could be observed as early as 6 h after addition of dexamethasone. The mechanism underlying the effect of glucocorticoids is unknown. It has been suggested, however, that glucocorticoids could increase the content of membrane structural proteins like fibronectin, thereby restoring the extra cellular matrix (9). Reduction of membrane proteolytic enzymes has also been suggested as a possible mechanism (19). Moreover, it is known that steroid hormones counteract a number of changes induced by the tumor promoter TPA (21) and that dexamethasone reverse the inhibitory effect of TPA on cell communication (25). The ability of the phosphodiesterase inhibitors to abolish the promoting effect of TPA is probably due to inhibition of TPA induced processes (8).

The present results clearly demonstrate that the transformation frequency do not only depend on the added chemical, but are modulated by a number of factors. Several substances which are present in the serum influence the transformation. This may be one reason why the transformation frequency observed are so dependent on the serum.

Identification of promoters

Table 4 shows the results obtained with some substances which we have tested in experiments with sequential exposure using BaP as initiator. Cigarette smoke extract may be expected to be a promoter both from animal experiments as well as epidemiological studies. Also coal tar and creosote is expected from animal studies to possess promoter activities.

It has been suggested that many of the carcinogenic metals may possess higher promoter activity than initiating activity and than this may be one of the causes for the difficulties in inducing tumors in animal experiments except after injection. The data presented here with nickel sulphate and cadmium acetate support the idea that these metals may act as promoters. It should also be mentioned that epidemiological studies in early nickel refinery workers suggest a late stage effect for nasal sinus cancer (12). Please also notice that with BaP which is normally used as initiator and which is a well known complete carcinogen a significant promoter activity is obtained.

TABLE 4 Promotion of SHE cell transformation by different substances after sequential exposure.

Additions		Cloning efficiency (% of control)	Total no of trans- formed colonies	Transfor- mation frequency (%)
Period 1 (3 days)	Period 2 (4 days)			
None	None	100	0	0
BaP	None	69	2	0.5
None	Cigarette smoke extract (5)	104	0	0
BaP	Cigarette smoke extract (5)	81	19	3.8
None	Coal tar (20)	106	0	0
BaP	Coal tar (20)	67	3	1.0
None	Creosote (20)	106	0	0
BaP	Creosote (20)	47	4	2.0
None	$NiSO_4 \cdot 6H_2O$ (5)	81	2	0.3
BaP	$NiSO_4 \cdot 6H_2O$ (5)	93	17	4.9
None	$CdAc_2 \cdot 2H_2O$ (0.5)	81	7	1.4
BaP	$CdAc_2 \cdot 2H_2O$ (0.5)	78	24	5.7
None	BaP (0.01)	77	5	1.5
BaP	BaP (0.01)	76	24	8.6

Experimental conditions as in table 1. Cloning efficiency in controls 24 - 32%. Concentration of BaP as initiator 0.05 ug/ml. The numbers in parenthesis gives the concentrations in ug/ml.

TABLE 5 Morphological transformation of SHE cells by substances with promoter properties.

Addition	Cloning efficiency (% of control)	Total no of trans- formed colonies	Transfor- mation frequency (%)
None	100	0	0
trans-Retinoic acid (9)	103	3	1.0
Cigarette smoke extract (5)	100	2	0.3
$NiSO_4$ $6H_2O$ (5)	63	9	3.0
Phenobarbital (100)	103	9	2.1
Coal tar (40)	84	5	2.1
Mineral oil[a] (67)	81	3	1.5
Motor engine oil (new) (288)	69	4	1.2
Motor engine oil[b] (used) (1440)	50	3	1.3
Motor engine oil (rerefined) (288)	77	5	1.4
Bitumen from road dust (15)	72	7	3.9

Experimental procedure as in table 1 except that the same chemical was present during the two periods. Cloning efficiency in controls 24 - 32%. The numbers in parenthesis gives the concentrations in µg/ml.
[a]Contains 31% (by weight) aromatic hydrocarbons and 69% saturated hydrocarbons, boiling range 200-400°C, viscosity 13.2 mm^2 sec^{-1} at 20° C.
[b]Used for 9.000 km in 4-strike gasoline engine.

Table 5 shows experiments where most of the substances shown in Table 4 were tested for transform- ing activity when present alone during the whole assay period. Trans-retinoic acid, cigarette smoke extract, nickel sulphate and coal tar which we have shown to act as promoters in the assay with BaP as initiator do also induce transformation alone. In addition, some compounds which are known to be promoters or may be expected to act as promoters such as phenobarbital, mineral oil, motor engine oil, unused as well as rerefined oil, and bitumen from road dust, all induce transformation in the SHE transformation system.

When discussing whether the SHE cell transformation system can be used in assay for promoters, it is important to consider the definition of promotion and promoters. Should the terms initiation and promotion be used as operationally terms for substances that when tested in a certain manner give enhancement of tumor induction or cell transformation, or should the terms be used in relation to specific processes in carcinogenesis. Independent of what is decided in the future concerning the terms initiation and promotion, it is important to realize that there are no substances with only initiation or promotion activity.

The crucial point for the use of the SHE cell transformation system in testing of chemicals is whether a sufficiently good correlation exists between substances inducing tumors in animals and giving transformation of SHE cells. The results from long-term animal experiments give no information of the mechanism of tumor induction and do not tell whether a specific substance act primarily by stimulating initiation or promotion processes. Similar with the SHE cell transformation system. Formation of trans-formed colonies suggests that the compound may cause tumors but additional experiments are needed in order to obtain information on the mechanisms of action of a compound.

With substances expected to act as promoters, the transformation frequencies found in the SHE cell transformation system with sequential exposure were 2 - 3 times higher with cells preexposed to BaP than when the substance under study was present in both incubation periods. Thus, the SHE cell transformation system may be useful in studies of promoters.

REFERENCES

1. Armuth, V., and Berenblum, I. (1981): Carcinogenesis, 2:977-979.
2. Barret, J.C., Thomassen, D.G., and Hesterberg, T.W. (1983): Ann. NY Acad. Sci., 407:291-301.

3. Belman, S., and Troll, W. (1974): Cancer Res., 34:3446-3455.
4. Diamond, L., O´Brian, T.G., and Bairdk, W.M. (1980): Adv. Cancer Res., 32:1-74.
5. DiPaolo, J.A., and Casto, B.C. (1979): Cancer Res., 39:1008-1013.
6. DiPaolo, J.A., Donovan, P., and Nelson, R. (1969): J. Natl. Cancer Inst., 42: 867-874.
7. DiPaolo, J.A., Nelson, R.L., and Donovan, P.J. (1971): Cancer Res., 31:1118-1127.
8. Enomoto, T., Martel, N., Kanno, Y., and Yamasaki, H. (1984): J. Cell. Physiol., 121:323-333.
9. Furcht, L.T., Mosher, D.F., Wendelschafer-Crabb, G., and Foidart, J.M. (1979): Cancer Res., 39:2077-2083.
10. Hennings, H., Wenk, M.L., and Donahue, R. (1982): Cancer Lett., 16:1-5.
11. Oshimura, M., Hesterberg, T.W., Tsutsui, T., and Barret, J.C. (1984): Cancer Res., 44:5017-5022.
12. Peto, J. (1984): In: Models, Mechanisms and Etiology of Tumour Promotion. IARC Scientific Publications No 56, edited by M.Börzsönyi, N.E.Day, K.Lapis, and H.Yamasaki, pp 359-371, IARC, Lyon.
13. Pienta, R.J., Poiley, J.A., Lebherz, W.B. (1977): Int. J. Cancer 19:642-655.
14. Rivedal, E. (1982): Cancer Lett., 15:105-113.
15. Rivedal, E. (1982): Cancer Lett., 17:9-17.
16. Rivedal, E., and Sanner, T. (1982): Cancer Lett., 17:1-8.
17. Rivedal, E., Sanner, T. (1985): Cancer Lett., 28:9-17.
18. Rivedal, E., Sanner, T., Enomoto, T., and Yamasaki, H. (1985): Carcinogenesis, 6:899-902.
19. Roblin, R., and Yong, P.L. (1980): Cancer Res., 40:2706-2713.
20. Sanner, T., and Rivedal, E. (1985): In: Progress in Mutation Research Vol 5. Evaluation of Short-Term Tests for Carcinogens., edited by J.Ashby et al., pp 665-671, Elsevier, Amsterdam.
21. Slaga, T.J. (1980): In: Carcinogenesis, Vol.5, Modifiers of Chemical Carcinogenesis, edited by T.J.Slaga, pp 111-126, Raven Press, New York.
22. Slaga, T.J. (1980): In: Carcinogenesis, Vol.5, Modifiers of Chemical Carcinogenesis, edited by T.J.Slaga, pp 111-126, Raven Press, New York.
23. Slaga, T.J., Fischer, S.M., Nelson, K., and Gleason, G.L. (1980): Proc. Natl. Acad. Sci., 77:3659-3663.
24. Thomassen, D.G., Gilmer, T.M., Oshimura, M., Annab, L.A., and Barret, J.C. (1985): In: Carcino-

genesis, Vol.9, Mammalian Cell Transformation, Mechanisms of Carcinogenesis and Assays for Carcinogens, edited by J.C.Barret and R.W.Tennant, pp 41-49, Raven Press, New York.

25. Yamasaki, H., and Enomoto, T. (1985): In: Carcinogenesis, Vol.9, Mammalian Cell Transformation, Mechanisms of Carcinogenesis and Assays for Carcinogens, edited by J.C.Barret and R.W.Tennant, pp 179-194, Raven Press, New York.

26. Yamasaki, H., Enomoto, T., Shiba, Y., Vanno, Y., and Kalunaga, T. (1985): Cancer Res., 45:637-641.

Tumor Promoters: Biological Approaches for
Mechanistic Studies and Assay Systems,
edited by Robert Langenbach et al.
Raven Press, New York © 1988.

IMPLICATIONS FOR MECHANISMS OF TUMOR PROMOTION
AND ITS INHIBITION BY VARIOUS AGENTS FROM STUDIES OF
IN VITRO TRANSFORMATION

Ann R. Kennedy

Department of Cancer Biology
Harvard School of Public Health
665 Huntington Avenue
Boston, MA 02115

INTRODUCTION

We have been performing transformation studies to elucidate the mechanisms involved in promotion in vitro for many years, as described in detail in other publications (6-8, 17,18,21,22,25,29,30). Of great importance to the elucidation of such mechanism(s) is a determination of the time when promoting agents have their enhancing effect on the transformation process. Our previous studies suggested that promoting agents such as 12-0-tetradecanoyl-phorbol-acetate (TPA) have their primary effect on "initiated" proliferating, cell populations (6,8,17,22). Although our previous results suggested that the application of TPA to confluent "initiated" cells did not lead to promotion in vitro (17,22), our past studies did not address the question of whether promotion in vitro could occur for initiated cells exposed to TPA during confluence and later allowed to express themselves as transformed foci in the absence of TPA treatment. Further studies performed to address this question are described in detail here.

Much information about mechanisms of promotion in vitro can be gathered from studies utilizing agents which are antagonistic to promotion. We have now studied many different agents which modify transformation in vitro as well as the TPA enhancement of carcinogen induced transformation in vitro; these studies have been described in detail elsewhere (1,2,5-10,12,15,16,18,24-29,33,36,37). In our studies, the most effective inhibitors of late stages of radiation induced transformation in vitro have been certain protease inhibitors and antioxidants. The data presented here suggest that these different classes of anticarcinogenic agents do not affect the transformation process in the same manner. Many other investigators have also observed that transformation in vitro is a highly modifiable process; studies of other investigators which are relevant to our own studies discussed in this report are cited in each of the individual referenced articles concerning different aspects of the modifying agents being investigated.   The intent of this article is to summarize the information from our own studies on the different manners in which several modifying agents affect transformation in vitro.

METHODS AND RESULTS

The experiments reported here were performed with the C3H10T½ (clone 8) transformation assay system, which has been used extensively in our laboratory for studies of radiation-induced transformation in vitro. Stock cultures were maintained in 60-mm Petri dishes and were passed by subculturing at a 1:20 dilution every 7 days. The cells used were in passages 9-14. They were grown in a humidified 5% CO_2 atmosphere at 37ºC in Eagle's basal medium supplemented with 10% heat-inactivated fetal bovine serum and gentamycin. Plating efficiencies were determined from 3 dishes seeded with a cell density one fifth that of the dishes used for the transformation assay; these cultures were terminated at 10 days. The various treatment toxicities were considered in the design of the experiments such that all dishes used for the transformation assays contained (initially) approximately 300 viable cells per dish. The concentrations and sources of the chemical compounds used in the studies reported here were as follows: TPA (lot 028, Consolidated Midland Co., Brewster, New York) 0.1 µg/ml; antipain was provided by Dr. Walter Troll and the U.S. Japan Cooperative Cancer Research Program.   Vitamin E (d-ɑ- tocopherol succinate Type IV) and dimethylsulfoxide (DMSO) were obtained from the Sigma Chemical Co. (St. Louis, MO).

Previous studies of ours on radiation transformation indicate that transformation is a multi-step process: the first step is a frequent alteration occurring in a large fraction of irradiated cells, while a later step, leading directly to malignant transformation, is a rare event which occurs randomly during cellular proliferation (with an approximate   frequency   of 10^{-6} per   cell   per   generation) (6,11,13,14,17,19,20).   Recent results have suggested that at least 3 steps are involved in the induction of radiation transformation in C3H10T½ cells (8).   In the typical radiation transformation experiment, a sufficient number of cells are seeded into Petri dishes such that approximately 300 viable cells result (considering the plating efficiency of the cells and the toxicity of the treatment); these cells then proliferate until confluence is reached at 10 days to 2 weeks postirradiation (at approximately 2×10^6 cells/dish). The dishes then remain in confluence for approximately 4 weeks until transformed foci, overlying the confluent monolayer, can be scored. Our previous studies suggested that it was during the growth phase of the culture, when the second step in transformation occurs randomly, that tumor-promoting agents, such as TPA, could enhance transformation (17,22). Other studies indicated that TPA did not have the ability to enhance radiation transformation when applied to confluent cell populations in the routine radiation transformation assay period (22). We did observe that TPA could enhance radiation transformation when added to cultures at a late time, however, as long as it was added to proliferating cells (22). These experiments are described schematically in Fig. 1.

Whether TPA treatment was effective at enhancing transformation only if present while cells were proliferating was not answered definitively with the experimental designs described above, however, as we did not determine whether promotion in vitro could occur if initiated cells were allowed to proliferate after a period of TPA treatment during which the cells were in confluence. We have now determined whether promotion in vitro can occur with the protocol described above, as shown in Table 1. In this study, the

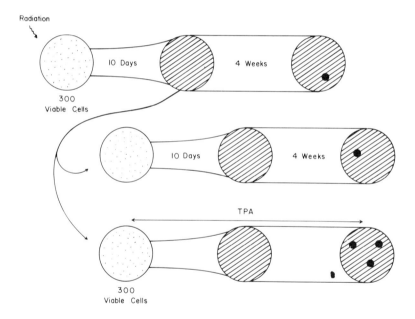

Figure 1: Promotion in vitro by TPA can occur at long time periods after carcinogen exposure (13 cell divisions post-irradiation). Cells were irradiated and then allowed to undergo 13 cell divisions until confluence was reached, at which time the cultures were trypsinized and subcultured to approximately 300 viable cells per dish. It was observed that TPA could effectively promote radiation transformation when present after subculturing occurred -i.e., when present during the second cycle of 13 cell divisions until confluence was reached and the 4 week period during which the transformed phenotype is displayed. These studies have been described in detail elsewhere (22).

Table 1. Promotion in vitro does not occur when x-irradiated cells are allowed to proliferate after a period (one week) of TPA treatment during which the cells are in confluence. (See text for experimental details)

Treatment	Plating Efficiency	Total Number of Surviving Cells (Initially[a] or Reseeded[b])	Total Number of Foci Observed (Types 2+3)	Fraction of Dishes Containing Transformed Foci (Types 2+3)
1. Controls-No Treatment	43.8%	4818[a]	0	0/11
2. 100 rads	42.3%	5076[a]	0	0/12
3. 100 rads+ TPA Treatment-routine protocol	42.5%	5100[a]	11	6/12=0.50
4. Irradiated, subcultured cells with and without TPA treatment during confluence				
A. Dishes which received TPA treatment during confluence	19.4%	7332[b]	1	1/47=0.02
B. Dishes which did not receive TPA treatment during confluence	23.0%	8256[b]	0	0/48

protocol for 100 rads+ TPA treatment involves the growth (13 divisions) to confluence of approximately 300 viable cells (per dish) which have been irradiated and treated with TPA (3 times per week) and maintained as for the routine radiation transformation experiments (as described above). In treatment group 4, the cultures were irradiated as in the routine protocol described above and allowed to grow to confluence. These cultures were then kept in confluence for one week, during which time some of the cultures were exposed to TPA (with three additions of TPA to cultures during the week in confluence). After the week in confluence, each of 100 dishes (50 dishes with the TPA treatments, 50 dishes without) was trypsinized and reseeded into a new dish at approximately 300 cells/dish. The cells were again allowed to proliferate to confluence (approximately 13 cell divisions) and remain in confluence for 4 weeks until foci could be scored. It can be observed in Table 1 that neither of the subcultured groups of dishes showed an enhancement of radiation transformation in vitro by TPA; enhancement was observed in the same experiment in the treatment group utilizing the routine protocol (Group 3) and has previously been observed for subcultured dishes (in other studies [22]) in which TPA treatment was given to proliferating initiated cells (as shown schematically in Figure 1). A 100 rad x-ray treatment has previously been shown to "initiate" the cells (17,21) and a one week treatment with TPA (3 treatments per week) has previously been shown to be sufficient to observe promotion in vitro when TPA was given to proliferating initiated cells (17,19,22); thus, promotion in vitro should have occurred in the study utilizing the experimental design described above if TPA could act on confluent cells subsequently allowed to proliferate. As promotion in vitro did not occur under the conditions described for the results shown in Table 1, it can be concluded that TPA must be applied to proliferating cells to have its enhancing effect on radiation transformation in vitro.

Several of our experiments utilizing inhibitors of the later steps in the tranformation process are summarized in Table 2; details of our studies of the agents utilized in these studies have been described elsewhere (1,5,7,8,10,12,15,18,24,25,33,36,37). While several aspects of each of these agents have been studied in the referenced papers, the intent of this discussion is to focus on the different manners in which these agents inhibit radiation transformation in the same assay system.

In our experiments, the two classes of agents which we have studied in the greatest depth are the protease inhibitors (anticarcinogenic protease inhibitors include antipain, the soybean-derived, Bowman-Birk inhibitor, etc.) and antioxidants, such as catalase, DMSO, Vitamin E, etc. As can be observed in Table 2, the protease inhibitors have an irreversible effect on the transformation process, while antioxidants have a reversible effect (i.e., transformants appear when these agents are removed from the carcinogen-treated cultures). In general, the effects of specific compounds within these broad classifications of agents are similar,

Table 2

NATURE OF THE SUPPRESSIVE EFFECTS OF VARIOUS INHIBITORS
OF THE LATER STAGE(S) OF TRANSFORMATION IN VITRO

Inhibitor of Transformation	Nature of Suppressive Effect*	Suppression of X-ray Transformation	TPA Enhancement of X-ray Transformation
Certain Protease Inhibitors	Irreversible	+++	+++
Catalase	Reversible	—	++
Dimethyl Sulfoxide	Reversible	+++	++
Vitamin E	Reversible	++	—

* Refers to whether transformants appear when the compound is removed from irradiated cultures (with or without additional treatment(s) of the cultures with TPA).

although there are some differences. For example, within the antioxidant classification, DMSO (24) and catalase (6,10,12,25,30) affect the TPA enhancement of transformation in vitro, while Vitamin E (33 and unpublished data) does not (see Table 2).

Although various protease inhibitors have very different potencies in their ability to suppress radiation induced transformation in vitro (see reference 8), the effects observed for these agents have been similar. Protease inhibitors affect the transformation process in an irreversible fashion (5-8,15,18,36), treatment with these agents is still effective even if exposure is delayed for long time periods of time after carcinogen exposure (5,6,8,18,36), and TPA has no effect on carcinogen-treated cells after they have been exposed to protease inhibitors (according to a known "anticarcinogenic" treatment protocol) (8). These major effects of protease inhibitors are described schematically in Figs. 2 and 3. From our work with protease inhibitors, we have hypothesized that these agents are able to reverse the initiated state of carcinogen-treated cells (8).

As shown in Fig. 4, antioxidants, such as DMSO and Vitamin E, do not appear to reverse the initiated state of carcinogen-treated C3H10T½ cells. In experiments similar in design to those utilized in our previous protease inhibitor studies, the removal of Vitamin E or DMSO from irradiated cultures (previously exposed to these

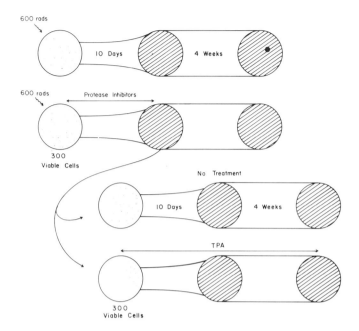

Figure 2: Protease inhibitors affect proliferating initiated cells, and have an irreversible effect on the transformation process. If protease inhibitors are applied to proliferating initiated cells, transformed foci do not occur in the routine transformation assay (as shown in line 2 of the figure) or in a subculture -type assay in which the carcinogen-treated cells are subcultured and exposed to TPA (or not exposed to TPA) during subsequent growth of the cultures to confluence and maintenance in confluence for the usual four-week period (lines 3 and 4 of the figure). These results suggest that protease inhibitors have reversed the initiated state of the carcinogen-treated cells, as discussed in detail in reference 8.

compounds according to a protocol in which their anticarcinogenic effects are known to occur) leads to the appearance of transformed foci when the cultures are subsequently subcultured and maintained without the presence of Vitamin E or DMSO. Our results suggest that both DMSO (24) and Vitamin E (33) affect a very late step in the transformation process, but are not capable of reverting cells to the "un-initiated" condition which existed before carcinogen exposure.

Our current concepts on the nature of carcinogen induced transformation in C3H10T½ cells are shown schematically in Fig. 5. As can be observed in Fig. 5, we believe that there is a major difference in the effects of protease inhibitors and antioxidants on carcinogen induced transformation in vitro. While protease inhibitors

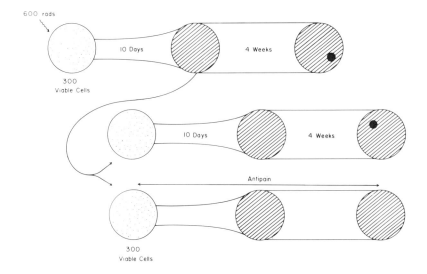

Figure 3: Protease inhibitors can suppress radiation transformation when applied to cultures as late as 10 days and 13 cell divisions after carcinogen exposure. As shown in lines 1 and 2 of the figure, subculture of the irradiated cells at confluence leads to approximately the same yield of transformed foci as observed for dishes which are not subcultured (8,14,22). If protease inhibitors are applied to subcultured dishes, transformed foci do not appear (as shown in line 3 of the figure); this result is the same as that observed when protease inhibitors are applied to cells soon after carcinogen exposure (as shown in Fig. 2 (line 2)).

appear to revert cells back to their original condition after carcinogen exposure, antioxidants (such as Vitamin E and DMSO) appear to be reverting cells to an intermediate state which can be promoted subsequently by TPA. Some our current concepts on the mechanisms of action of agents which modify carcinogen-induced transformation in vitro are described elsewhere (3-8, 12, 17,23,24,26,30-35). More detailed studies on the mechanisms of action of anticarcinogenic agents which affect promotion in vitro are currently being performed in our laboratory.

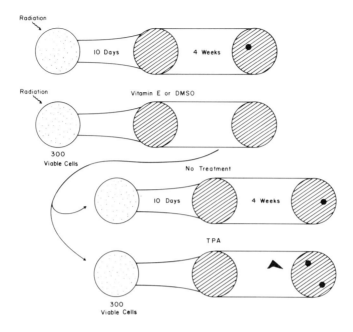

Figure 4: The design of the studies shown schematically in this figure is similar to those described in Figures 1-3. As can be observed in line 2 of this figure, Vitamin E and DMSO have the ability to suppress radiation transformation when present during the entire radiation transformation asssay period. If the irradiated cultures are subcultured, however, and maintained without the presence of DMSO or Vitamin E (and either with or without TPA), transformed foci appear. These results suggest that Vitamin E and DMSO have not reversed the initiated state of the cells.

Postulated Scheme for the Induction of
Malignant Transformation in vitro

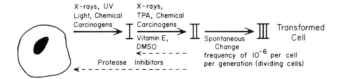

Figure 5: Our current concepts on the steps involved in the induction of transformation in C3H10T½ cells. Evidence for each of these postulated steps, and their possible modification by various agents, is discussed in the text.

ACKNOWLEDGEMENTS

The research presented or summarized in this report was supported by NIH Grants CA22704, CA34680 and ES-00002. I thank Marilyn Collins and Babette Radner for excellent technical assistance in these studies.

REFERENCES

1. Baturay, N.Z., and Kennedy, A.R. (1986): Cell Biol. Toxicol., 2:21-32.

2. Baturay, N.Z., Targovnik, H.S., Reynolds, R.J., and Kennedy, A.R. (1985): Carcinogenesis, 6:465-468.

3. Billings, P.C., Carew, J.A., Keller-McGandy, C.E., Goldberg, A., and Kennedy, A.R. (1986): Proc. Natl. Acad. Sci. (submitted)- ("A new serine protease activity in C3H10T½ cells which is inhibited by anticarcinogenic protease inhibitors").

4. Chang, J.D., Billings, P., and Kennedy, A.R. (1985): Biochem. Biophys. Res. Comm., 133:830-835.

5. Kennedy, A.R. (1982): Carcinogenesis, 3:1093-1095.

6. Kennedy, A.R. (1984): In: Mechanisms of Tumor Promotion, Vol. III, "Tumor Promotion and Carcinogenesis In Vitro" edited by T.J. Slaga, pp. 13-55. CRC Press, Inc.

7. Kennedy, A.R. (1984): In: Vitamins, Nutrition and Cancer, edited by K.N. Prasad, pp. 166-179. S. Karger AG, Basel.

8. Kennedy, A.R. (1985): Carcinogenesis, 6:1441-1446.

9. Kennedy, A.R. (1985): Cancer Letters, 29:289-292.

10. Kennedy, A.R. (1985): In: Vitamins and Cancer- Human Cancer Prevention by Vitamins and Micronutrients, edited by F.L. Meyskens and K.N. Prasad, pp. 51-64. The Humana Press, Inc., Clifton, New Jersey.

11. Kennedy, A.R. (1985): In: Carcinogenesis: A Comprehensive Survey Volume 9: Mammalian Cell Transformation: Mechanisms of Carcinogenesis and Assays for Carcinogens, edited by J.C. Barrett and R.W. Tennant, pp. 355-364. Raven Press, New York.

12. Kennedy, A.R. (1986): In: Oxygen and Sulfur Radicals in Chemistry and Medicine, edited by A. Breccia, M.A.J. Rodgers, and G. Semerano, pp. 201-209. Edizioni Scientifiche, "Lo Scarabeo", Bologna, Italy.

13. Kennedy, A.R., Cairns, J., and J.B. Little. (1984): Nature, 307:85-86.

14. Kennedy, A.R., Fox, M., Murphy, G., and Little, J.B. (1980): Proc. Natl. Acad. Sci. U.S.A. 77:7262-7266.

15. Kennedy, A.R., and Little, J.B. (1978): Nature, 276:825-826.

16. Kennedy, A.R., and Little, J.B. (1980): Int. J. Radiat. Biol., 38:465-468.

17. Kennedy, A.R., and Little, J.B. (1980): Carcinogenesis, 1:1039-1047.

18. Kennedy, A.R., and Little, J.B. (1981): Cancer Res. 41:2103-2108.

19. Kennedy, A.R., and Little, J.B. (1981): In: Cancer: Achievements, Challenges and Prospects for the 1980s, edited by J.H. Burchenal and H.F. Oettgen, pp. 491-500. Grune and Stratton Inc.

20. Kennedy, A.R., and Little, J.B. (1984): Radiation Res. 99:228-248.

21. Kennedy, A.R., Mondal, S., Heidelberger, C., and Little, J.B. (1978): Cancer Res., 38:439-443.

22. Kennedy, A.R., Murphy, G., and Little, J.B. (1980): Cancer Res., 40:1915-1920.

23. Kennedy, A.R., Radner, B., and Nagasawa, H. (1984): Proc. Natl. Acad. Sci., USA 81:1827-1830.

24. Kennedy, A.R. and Symons, M.C.R. (1987): Carcinogenesis (in press). ("Water Structure vs. "Radical Scavenger" theories as explanations for the suppressive effects of DMSO and related compounds on radiation induced transformation in vitro").

25. Kennedy, A.R., Troll, W., and Little, J.B. (1984): Carcinogenesis, 5:1213-1218.

26. Kennedy, A.R., and Umans, R.S. (1986) Eur. J. Cancer and Clin. Onc., (in press). ("Effects of testosterone and dihydrotestosterone on malignant transformation in C3H10T½ cells").

27. Kennedy, A.R., and Weichselbaum, R.R. (1981): Carcinogenesis, 2:67-69.

28. Kennedy, A.R., and Weichselbaum, R.R. (1981): Nature, 294:97-98.

29. Little, J.B., and Kennedy, A.R. (1982): In: Carcinogenesis, Vol. 7, edited by E. Hecker et al., pp. 243-257. Raven Press, New York.

30. Little, J.B., Kennedy, A.R., and H. Nagasawa. (1983) In: Radioprotectors and Anticarcinogens, edited by O.F. Nygaard and M.G. Simic, pp. 487-493. Academic Press, New York.

31. Long, S., Quigley, J., Troll, W., and Kennedy, A.R. (1981): Carcinogenesis, 2:933-936.

32. Radner, B.S., and Kennedy, A.R. (1984): Cancer Letters, 25:139-144.

33. Radner, B.S., and Kennedy, A.R. (1986): Cancer Letters, 32:25-32.

34. Umans, R.S., Radner, B., and Kennedy, A.R. (1985): Fed. Europ. Biochem. Soc., 193:27-30.

35. Umans, R.S., Weichselbaum, R.R., Johnson, C.M., and Kennedy, A.R. (1984): Carcinogenesis, 5:1355-1357.

36. Yavelow, J., Collins, M., Birk, Y., Troll, W., and Kennedy, A.R. (1985) Proc. Natl. Acad. Sci., USA 82:5395-5399.

37. Yavelow, J., Finlay, T.H., Kennedy, A.R., and Troll, W. (1983) Cancer Res., 43:2454-2459.

Tumor Promoters: Biological Approaches for
Mechanistic Studies and Assay Systems,
edited by Robert Langenbach et al.
Raven Press, New York © 1988.

ENHANCEMENT OF C3H/10T1/2 CELL TRANSFORMATION

BY TUMOR PROMOTERS

Craig J. Boreiko

Department of Genetic Toxicology
Chemical Industry Institute of Toxicology
Research Triangle Park, NC   27709

BACKGROUND

C3H/10T1/2 clone 8 is an aneuploid cell line of mouse embryo fibroblasts with firm density-dependent controls upon cell proliferation (18). As a result, C3H/10T1/2 cells inoculated into a cell culture dish grow to form an evenly staining monolayer of cells and then enter a quiescent resting state. The carcinogen-induced transformation of these fibroblasts is accompanied by characteristic alterations in cell morphology and growth control that impart an ability to proliferate at confluence. This permits use of C3H/10T1/2 cells in a focus formation cell transformation assay approximately six weeks in duration (14,19). In this assay carcinogen treatment of low density C3H/10T1/2 cultures is followed by prolonged incubation at confluence and the subsequent formation of large foci of actively growing transformed cells. These foci (figure 1) are quite distinct from the background monolayer of quiescent nontransformed cells and can be scored with relative ease.

The morphological transformation of C3H/10T1/2 mouse embryo fibroblasts is enhanced by the presence of tumor promoters such as the phorbol ester 12-O-tetradecanoylphorbol-13-acetate (TPA). Moreover, numerous aspects of this enhancement process mirror initiation and promotion on mouse skin (4,5,17). The ability to mimic what are presumed to be essential features of multistage carcinogenesis indicates that the C3H/10T1/2 system could have applications for the identification and study of chemicals with tumor promoting potential.

PROMOTION IN CULTURE

As reviewed previously (4,5,17), the operational mechanics of the C3H/10T1/2 system are not unlike those established for mouse skin

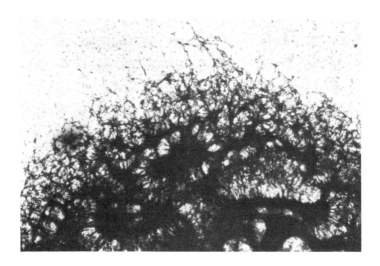

FIG. 1: Photomicrograph of a fixed and stained C3H/10T1/2 culture at the termination of a cell transformation experiment. Shown is the periphery of a type III transformed focus. The polar, darkly staining, actively growing focus cells are quite distinct from the surrounding monolayer of quiescent nontransformed cells. Cytoplasmic staining in the nontransformed cells is very light and only the cell nuclei are clearly visible.

initiation and promotion. In and of themselves, promoters have little transforming activity. However, they enhance focus formation in cultures previously exposed to an "initiating" dose of a carcinogen. Dose response kinetics for promoter action are usually characterized by "all-or-none" dose response plateaus. In almost all instances, promoting activity is evident at chemical concentrations that lack overt cytotoxicity as measured by reductions in plating efficiency or growth rate. Finally, the foci produced by promotion with TPA are unstable and revert upon the withdrawal of TPA from the medium (20). This "regression" phenomenon is not unlike that described for TPA-dependent papillomas on mouse skin (10).

A variety of compounds can enhance C3H/10T1/2 focus formation. The spectrum of activity produced by different chemicals suggests that the C3H/10T1/2 system might be most sensitive to the effects of chemicals observed to possess stage II promoting activity on mouse skin (4). For example, TPA and mezerein are potent promoters of transformation while 4-O-methyl-TPA lacks promoting activity (9). Activity is also observed with a variety of chemicals suspected of exerting promoting effects in tissues other than mouse skin (4,17).

The multiple similarities between promotion in C3H/10T1/2 cultures and mouse skin suggest that the C3H/10T1/2 promotion system could be applied as a routine screen for tumor promoters. Unfortunately, use of the system in its present form for such a purpose is probably not feasible. The promotion assay is subject to variation with a number of cell culture variables, the successful control of which is difficult, time-consuming, and costly (13). Until variability with factors such as serum lot can be limited, the C3H/10T1/2 system is not likely to provide a portable, cost-effective, or practical routine screen for putative tumor promoters.

Although technically difficult, the C3H/10T1/2 promotion system has obvious basic research applications. Moreover, use of the system for examination of selected classes of compounds can be justified. For example, recent studies have demonstrated that the potent carcinogen and tumor promoter 2,3,7,8-tetrachlorodibenzo-p-dioxin (TCDD) lacks initiating or transforming activity in the C3H/10T1/2 system. However, TCDD is an extraordinarily potent promoter of transformation that elicits responses at concentrations as low as 4 pM (1). Other dioxin isomers elicit C3H/10T1/2 promotion assay responses at concentrations that are concordant with their in vivo carcinogenic activity (2). Although still technically difficult, promotion studies with dioxin isomers generally do not suffer from the extreme serum lot specificity that complicates study of phorbol-related compounds. The C3H/10T1/2 system may thus be suited for the identification and study of carcinogenic dioxin isomers. Studies are underway to determine if other polyhalogenated hydrocarbons are also amenable to evaluation.

Alternate Assay Endpoints

The pleiotropic effects of tumor promoters have complicated efforts to develop biologically relevant in vitro assays for tumor promoting activity. Diverse and often opposing cellular responses can be elicited in a variety of cultured cell types as a consequence of exposure to a given tumor promoter. In many instances, the ability of the cultured cells under study to respond to the biologically relevant (promoting) properties of test chemicals is not known. Since C3H/10T1/2 cells respond to the presence of tumor promoters with the enhancement of focus formation processes presumed to be of importance to neoplasia, they should be a relevant cell type for in vitro studies of other relevant promoter-induced effects. Surrogate assay endpoints that supplant the labor intensive transformation assay, although of less certain mechanistic significance, could be desirable for screening purposes.

Effects upon intercellular communication have been proposed to mediate the process of promotion in a variety of experimental systems (21). The feasiblity of monitoring chemically induced effects upon intercellular communication as an assay for tumor promoting activity in C3H/10T1/2 cultures was thus investigated. Initial experiments used an autoradiographic method for monitoring the exchange of tritiated uridine molecules between cells (11). In this procedure, a small number of "donor" cells growing on coverslips were prelabelled with tritiated uridine, washed, and then cocultivated with a large excess of unlabelled "recipient" cells. Following cocultivation, donor-recipient cell preparations were processed for autoradiography and analyzed for the transfer of radiolabel (silver grains) from heavily labelled donors to surrounding recipients.

Extensive transfer of uridine label occurred between cocultivated donor and recipient cells and indicated that significant levels of intercellular communication probably occurred within C3H/10T1/2 cultures. Moreover, the addition of TPA to the medium of donor and recipient cells at the time of cocultivation produced a marked ($\geq$ 80%) inhibition of label transfer (11). Subsequent studies (9) indicated that the ability of phorbol-related compounds (phorbol, 4-O-methyl-TPA and mezerein) to promote transformation correlated with their ability to inhibit uridine exchange. Inhibition of intercellular communication, as measured by inhibition of uridine exchange, may thus have predictive value for screening the promoting potential of these types of compounds.

Several aspects of results obtained with the uridine exchange assay were disquieting. Although TCDD is a potent promoter of transformation (1), it did not inhibit uridine exchange between cells (9). Furthermore, the inhibition of label transfer by both mezerein (9) and TPA (11) appeared to be transient. Preexposure of donor and recipient cells to either compound for 12 or more hours prior to execution of the assay rendered the cells refractory to the effects of challenge with a second dose of compound. The transient nature of this inhibition was not consistent with the continuous and prolonged exposure regimen needed to both induce focus formation (13) and to maintain the transformed phenotype (20) in promotion studies with TPA. The relevance of inhibited uridine exchange to the actual mechanism of promotion was thus uncertain.

Unfortunately, the uridine exchange assay need not provide an accurate representation of alterations in intercellular communication during an actual promotion experiment. For example, the uridine exchange assay entails trypsinization steps and brief cocultivation periods that may not be comparable to the conditions within monolayers of quiescent cells confluent for several weeks. In more recent studies (7,8), we have used procedures for the microinjection of Lucifer yellow dye into cells to monitor alterations in intercellular communication during actual C3H/10T1/2 promotion experiments. Although cell density in early stages of a promotion assay is quite low, intercellular communication appears to occur freely between cells in contact. The addition of TPA to the cultures on day 5 produces pronounced morphological alterations and an inhibition of Lucifer yellow dye transfer (figure 2). Preliminary studies indicate that this inhibition can be elicited by very low concentrations of TPA ($<$ 1 ng/ml) comparable to that required for inhibition in the uridine exchange assay (8). Dye transfer within TPA-treated cultures resumes within 24 hr (by day

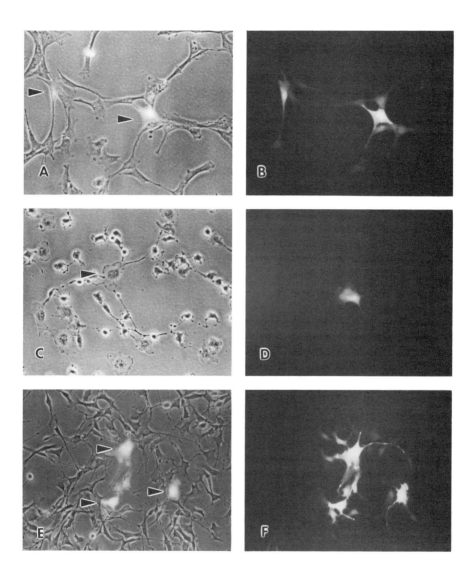

FIG. 2: Photomicrographs depicting alterations in intercellular communication in early stages of promotion experiments. Cells indicated by the arrows have been microinjected with Lucifer yellow dye. Cell density is low at early stages of the assay (A), but under fluorescence microscopy (B) dye transfer between sparse nontransformed cells is evident. TPA addition on day 5 produces rapid alteration in cell morphology (C) and inhibition of dye transfer (D). Twenty-four hr later, morphology (E) and dye coupling (F) have essentially returned to normal.

6) and is accompanied by the return of nearly normal cell morphologies. Similar transient effects have been observed in studies of BALB/c 3T3 cells (12).

Combined with results of other microinjection studies, which indicated that TCDD does not inhibit intercellular communication between the C3H/10T1/2 cells (7,8), these experiments suggest that the uridine exchange assay provides an accurate representation of chemically induced effects upon intercellular communication in the early stages of a transformation assay. Validation of the transient nature of TPA's initial effects upon intercellular communication reinforces earlier concerns with respect to the mechanistic relevance of promoter assays that rely upon a detection of a rapid, short-term inhibition of communication. Although such an inhibition may bear a correlative relationship to the promoting activity of some classes of promoters, the early inhibition in and of itself is probably of minimal importance in the promotion of C3H/10T1/2 cell transformation.

Alterations in intercellular communication in later stages of transformation assays may play a role in promotion in the BALB/c 3T3 cell transformation system (22). Whether this is true of the C3H/10T1/2 system is not clear. Extensive intercellular communication occurs between confluent C3H/10T1/2 cells and the formation of foci is associated with a generalized disruption of dye-coupling between transformed and nontransformed cells (7). This disruption is evident in foci produced by promotion with either TPA or TCDD, and during transformation resulting from a single application of a transforming agent such as 3-methylcholanthrene. Disruptions of communication thus accompany, and may facilitate, the C3H/10T1/2 focus formation process. However, intercellular communication between confluent nontransformed C3H/10T1/2 cells is not inhibited by the presence of either TPA or TCDD (7). If

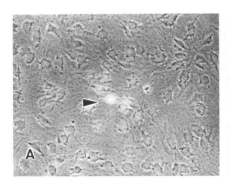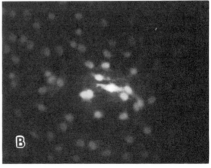

FIG. 3: Phase contrast (A) and fluorescence (B) photomicrographs showing extensive dye coupling in the presence of 100 pM TCDD at day 16 of a promotion assay. A single monolayer cell has been injected (arrow).

promoter-induced effects upon intercellular communication are mechanistically linked to C3H/10T1/2 promotion, this inhibition is either specific to the interaction of transformed and nontransformed cells and/or is expressed at the beginning phases of focus formation in freshly confluent cultures.

Mechanisms Responsible for Enhanced Focus Formation

The process of focus formation is complex and subject to modulation by a variety of chemical agents (3,5,16) and physical factors such as replating or cell density (3,15,17). Not all of these modulating forces need be relevant to in vivo carcinogenesis (6). Although there is a tendency to discuss "the" mechanism of promotion, there are probably multiple mechanisms by which focus formation can be enhanced in a C3H/10T1/2 culture. For example, the work of Bertram and colleagues (3) has indicated that nontransformed cells have the ability to suppress the growth of transformed cells into foci. Factors that modify this interaction (eg effects upon intercellular communication) could modulate the efficiency with which transformed cells develop into foci and lead to what are interpreted as promoting or "anti-promoting" effects. The studies of Kennedy (17) and Bertram (3) and colleagues have also indicated that the events which result in the conversion of a nontransformed cell to a transformed cell can be complex and multistep. Within this framework, factors that facilitate cellular events necessary for the conversion of nontransformed cells to transformed state could function as promoters of transformation.

Whether one, or both of the above mechanisms underlie responses in the C3H/10T1/2 promotion system remains to be determined. Most telling in this regard is the reversible fashion in which TPA promotes focus formation (20). Withdrawal of TPA from the medium supplied a focus produced by promotion with TPA will usually result in rapid regression of the focus. This regression process indicates that TPA promotion yields foci composed of cells that require the continued presence of TPA for the expression of a transformed phenotype. This is quite unlike the stable nature of foci produced by transformation with compounds such as methylcholanthrene and indicates that TPA does not function by merely increasing the efficiency with which transformed foci develop into foci. Rather, TPA must be producing qualitative changes that facilitate or permit the expression of transformation in individual cells.

In contrast, foci produced by TCDD promotion appear to be as stable as those generated by direct transformation with agents such as 3-methylcholanthrene. As noted in the previous sections, there are additional subtle differences between TPA and TCDD promotion. TPA has early effects upon intercellular communication. TCDD exerts its effects in the absence of any detectable alterations in dye coupling. TPA promotion is highly serum lot specific, TCDD promotion is less so. These differences are probable indicators that promoters of focus formation accomplish their effects by diverse mechanistic pathways. Moreover, it is equally possible that promotion in different transformation systems reflect fundamentally different mechanistic events. The precise relationship of any of these mechanistic pathways to in vivo carcinogenesis remains to be determined.

CONCLUSIONS

The C3H/10T1/2 cell transformation system has an intriguing ability to mimic phenomena analogous to initiation and promotion on mouse skin. Unfortunately, the complexity of the system is such that use for the routine screening of chemicals for tumor promoting potential is not feasible. Rather, the system is best suited for basic research purposes and for the screening of limited classes of compounds. Dioxins may represent a class of environmentally significant chemicals, difficult to study by most other in vitro systems, for which use of the C3H/10T1/2 system may be cost-effective.

Efforts to develop surrogate assay endpoints to supplant the labor-intensive transformation assay have been only partially successful. Inhibition of intercellular communication may be diagnostic of the action of some classes of compounds (phorbol esters) but not of others (dioxins). The mechanistic links between effects upon intercellular communication and promotion by phorbol esters are unclear. Assays for early effects upon intercellular communication (e.g. uridine exchange) do not reflect effects upon intercellular communication during the chronic treatment protocol of a promotion experiment. Some caution is thus indicated in interpreting the results of intercellular communication assays.

As demonstrated by both the diversity of mechanistic models proposed to explain in vitro promotion phenomena and the multiple discrete differences in the effects of phorbol esters and dioxins, the mechanism(s) by which tumor promoters enhance transformation are probably diverse. Use of the C3H/10T1/2 system for the study of promoters must proceed with the caveat that the single assay endpoint of enhanced focus formation can probably result by multiple pathways. Not all of these pathways need be relevant to the carcinogenic process in an intact animal.

REFERENCES

1. Abernethy, D.J., Greenlee, W.F., Huband, J.C., and Boreiko, C.J. (1985): Carcinogenesis, 6:651-653.
2. Abernethy, D.J., Huband, J.C., and Boreiko, C.J. (1985): Proc. Am. Assoc. Cancer Res., 26:130.
3. Bertram, J.S. (1985): In: Carcinogenesis - A Comprehensive Survey, vol 9, Mammalian Cell Transformation, edited by J.C. Barrett and R. Tennant, pp. 327-336. Raven Press, New York.

4. Boreiko, C.J. (1985): In: Carcinogenesis - A Comprehensive Survey, vol. 8, Cancer of the Respiratory Tract, edited by M.J. Mass, D.G. Kaufman, J.M. Siegfried, V.E. Steele, and S. Nesnow, pp. 329-340. Raven Press, New York.

5. Boreiko. C.J. (1985): In: Carcinogenesis - A Comprehensive Survey, vol 9, Mammalian Cell Transformation, edited by J.C. Barrett and R. Tennant, pp. 153-165. Raven Press, New York.

6. Boreiko, C.J. (1987): Banbury Reports, 25: in press.

7. Boreiko, C.J., Abernethy, D.J., and Stedman, D.B. (1987): Carcinogenesis, 8:321-325.

8. Boreiko, C.J., Abernethy, D.J., and Stedman, D.B. (1986): Proc. Am. Assoc. Cancer Res., 27:133.

9. Boreiko, C.J., Abernethy, D.J., Sanchez, J.H., and Dorman, B.H. (1986): Carcinogenesis, 7:1095-1099.

10. Burns, F.J., Vanderlaan, M., Sivak, A. and Albert, R.E. (1976): Cancer Res., 36:1422-1427.

11. Dorman, B.H., Butterworth, B.E., and Boreiko, C.J. (1983): Carcinogenesis, 4:1109-1115.

12. Enomoto, T. and Yamasaki, H. (1985): Cancer Res., 45:2681-2688.

13. Frazelle, J.H., Abernethy, D.J., and Boreiko, C.J. (1983): Carcinogenesis, 4:709-715.

14. Heidelberger, C., Freeman, A.E., Pienta, R.J., Sivak, A., Bertram, J.S., Casto, B.C., Dunkel, V.C., Francis, M.W., Kakunaga, T., Little, J.B., and Schechtman, L.M., (1983): Mutat. Res., 114:283-385.

15. Huband, J.C., Abernethy, D.J., and Boreiko, C.J. (1985): Cancer Res., 45:6314-6321.

16. Kennedy, A.R. (1984): In: Mechanisms of Tumor Promotion, vol. 3, Tumor Promotion and Carcinogenesis In Vitro, edited by T.J. Slaga, pp. 13-56. CRC Press, Boca Raton, Florida.

17. Kennedy, A.R. (1985): In: Carcinogenesis - A Comprehensive Survey, vol 9, Mammalian Cell Transformation, edited by J.C. Barrett and R. Tennant, pp. 355-364. Raven Press, New York.

18. Reznikoff, C.A., Bertram, J.S., Brankow, D.W., and Heidelberger, C. (1973): Cancer Res., 33:3239-3249.

19. Reznikoff, C.A., Brankow, D.W., and Heidelberger, C. (1973): Cancer Res., 33:3231-3238.

20. Sanchez, J.H., Abernethy. D.J., and Boreiko, C.J. (1986): Carcinogenesis, 7:1793-1796.

21. Trosko, J.E. and Chang, C. (1984): In: Mechanisms of Tumor Promotion, vol. 4, Cellular Responses to Tumor Promoters, edited by T.J. Slaga, pp. 119-145. CRC Press, Boca Raton, Florida.

22. Yamasaki, H. and Enomoto, T. (1985): In: Carcinogenesis - A Comprehensive Survey, vol. 9, Mammalian Cell Transformation, edited by J.C. Barrett and R.W. Tennant, pp. 179-194. Raven Press, New York.

Tumor Promoters: Biological Approaches for Mechanistic Studies and Assay Systems,
edited by Robert Langenbach et al.
Raven Press, New York © 1988.

THE ROLE OF RETINOIDS AS INHIBITORS OF TUMOR PROMOTION[1]

John S. Bertram

Cancer Research Center of Hawaii
University of Hawaii
Honolulu, Hawaii 96813

INTRODUCTION

Growing interest and concern over the public health implications of exposure to promoters is being matched by increasing efforts to understand the biological and biochemical mechanisms of promoter action. Unfortunately, much of this research is hindered by the phenomenological nature of the process of promotion. Promoters by definition exert their effects on carcinogen-initiated cells, and these effects may, or may not be, qualitatively or quantitatively different from the effects of promoters on non-initiated cells. An initiated cell represents an intermediate stage between normal and transformed; it is presumably genetically abnormal, since its state can be maintained stably over long time periods, yet it is phenotypically non-transformed, requiring the action of a promoter to expose its characteristics (7). Thus, initiated cells are inextricably linked to promoters and vice versa, one requiring the other for identification. Herein lies one problem; carcinogen-exposure of normal cells forms initiated cells only rarely. These are cryptic and typically not available for direct study. A second major problem in the study of promoter-action on initiated cells is that in attempting to compare the properties of normal cells, or of carcinogen-initiated cultures, with those of transformed cells resulting from exposure to promoters, the investigator must allow the rare transformant time to replicate in order to be recognized and to supply sufficient cells for analysis. During this time period, many secondary events may take place which can obscure the promoter-specific events.

In recognition of these problems and of the importance of studying the promotional phase of carcinogenesis, much of my group's efforts have been directed towards the development

_____
[1]Supported by Grant CA 39947 from the US National Cancer Institute

of defined in vitro models and have focused on the actions of retinoids, which in most biological systems function as anti-promoters.

Retinoids as Inhibitors of Promotion

In the C3H/10T1/2 (10T1/2) system of mouse embryo fibroblasts, neoplastic transformation can be induced by a variety of chemical and physical carcinogens. Morphologically transformed cells first appear some 4 weeks after carcinogen exposure, approximately 3 weeks after both control and treated cultures have attained a stable contact-inhibited monolayer. These refractile, polar cells are not sensitive to post-confluence growth control and divide to form a focus of transformed cells which can be recognized macroscopically after a further week in culture. Cells from type III foci are tumorigenic in immunosuppressed syngeneic hosts as rapidly as they can be tested (27). Transformation in this system thus occurs after a latent period of 4 weeks without the necessity of applying a classical tumor promoter such as TPA. Whether transformation in fact occurs without promotion is doubtful, since Mordan (personal communication) has recently shown that transformation does not occur in the absence of platelet-derived growth factors, normally supplied by the serum component of the medium. However proliferation per se is not inhibited suggesting that growth factors have promoting ability.

The addition of non-toxic concentrations of natural or certain synthetic retinoids to carcinogen-treated cultures, as long as 21 days after carcinogen-exposure, was found to give rise to the suppression of formation of transformed foci in a dose-dependent manner (Fig. 1). Moreover, removal of retinoids from carcinogen-treated cell cultures resulted in the appearance of transformed foci some 3-5 weeks later, demonstrating that retinoids were reversibly inhibiting the ability of the putative initiated cells present in the cultures from undergoing morphological transformation. That retinoids are not inhibiting expression per se was established by the demonstration that retinoids did not inhibit the growth of transformed cells, or their ability to form transformed foci on a contact inhibited 10T1/2 monolayer. In fact their growth was enhanced in these mixed cultures (2).

Based on these observations we hypothesized that retinoids were acting to stabilize initiated cells. If this is correct, it should be possible to isolate such stabilized cells from a carcinogen-treated population. This we achieved (23), and the possession of this cell line has made possible much of the work to be described here.

Properties of Retinoid-Stabilized Carcinogen-Initiated Cells

Because carcinogen-treated cultures of 10T1/2 cells appear

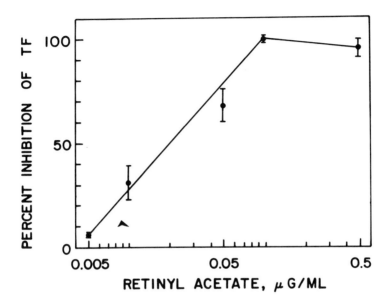

FIGURE 1. Concentration-response relationship for the inhibition by RA of MCA-induced neoplastic transformation. Starting 7 days after MCA exposure, cultures were treated weekly with the appropriate concentration of RA for 4 weeks and then scored for transformed foci. The percentage of inhibition of TF was calculated in relation to cultures that received MCA plus acetone. Values represent the mean of measurements from 2 experiments. The data was calculated as follows. The total number of transformed foci (types II and III) in each of 2 experiments, each utilizing 12 dishes/data point, were determined, and the TF was calculated from the formula

$$TF = \frac{\text{mean no. of transformed foci/dish}}{\text{mean no. surviving cells/dish}} \times 100$$

The number of surviving cells obtained from the experiments to determine PE was typically 20% of cells plated and was not reduced by retinoid treatment. The TF for each data point was then expressed as a percentage of the MCA-only-treated controls. The mean and S.E. were then calculated from the data obtained in the 2 experiments. The MCA-treated controls gave a TF of 1.0 ± 0.1 throughout the experiments reported here, or approximately 2 foci/dish (48 foci/data point)from the above equation. Bars, S.E.

phenotypically normal prior to transformation (22) and do not have a growth advantage over 10T1/2 cells (12), the INIT/10T1/2 cells isolated by selective cloning of methylcholanthrene-treated cultures in the presence of retinyl acetate were expected to be essentially identical in microscopic appearance and growth rate to retinyl acetate treated parental 10T1/2 cells. This was confirmed, only after removal of retinyl acetate and a 3-4 week latent period, were differences apparent. At this time in INIT/10T1/2 cultures, multiple regions of the monolayer began to proliferate and to form transformed foci. Because of the overlapping nature of the foci, the transformation frequency could not be estimated; in other experiments in which colonies of initiated cells were surrounded by co-cultured 10T1/2 cells it was found that about 60% of clonogenic initiated cells would form type II or III foci. The INIT/10T1/2 cell line is also tumorigenic in nude mice after a latent period of 6-8 weeks. This latent period could be extended up to at least 16 weeks by dietary administration of the synthetic retinoid 4-hydroxyphenyl retinamide, indicating that endogenous plasma retinol levels in the nude mouse are not sufficient to suppress neoplastic transformation of these cells (23).

Modulation of Transformation of INIT/10T1/2 Cells

Tumor promoters

The inhibitory effects of retinyl acetate on transformation can be partially antagonized by exposure to TPA. This action is observed not as an increase in number of clonogenic INIT/10T1/2 cells forming transformed foci, but as an acceleration of the rate at which foci develop (Table 1).

TABLE 1.   Promotion of neoplastic transformation of INIT/10T1/2 cells by TPA

Treatment	Foci/dish			
	Day 21		Day 32	
	no./dish	%[a]	no./dish	%[a]
Control	4.1 ± 0.8	33.1	12.4 ± 1.7	100.0
RAC	0	0	0	0
TPA	12.1 ± 1.4	97.6	13.3 ± 1.8	107.2
RAC + TPA	0	0	5.7 ± 2.5	44.1

[a]Mean number of Types II and III foci/dish/mean number of clonogenic cells forming Types II and III foci in control cultures on day 32. The plating efficiency of INIT/10T1/2 cells was 20%.

Thus, in the absence of TPA only 33% of potentially transformed cells had formed foci 21 d after seeding without retinyl acetate, while in the presence of TPA essentially 100% of such cells had produced foci at that time. Concurrent administration of TPA and retinyl acetate produced intermediate effects, especially noticeable at day 32 post-seeding when only 44% of potentially transformed cells had produced foci in TPA/RAC treated cultures. This contrasts with 0% foci in RAC only cultures and 100% foci in TPA or control cultures. This mutual antagonism suggests that TPA and RAC may be affecting common pathways.

Colony Size Effects

We had earlier reported the paradoxical finding that, as the seeding density of 10T1/2 cells was increased, carcinogen treatment resulted in progressively lower transformation frequencies (27). This suggested to us that either the proportion of cells being initiated was decreasing or that expression of these initiated cells as transformed foci was progressively being inhibited. Recently others using X-rays as initiating agent, had noted the same effect, and had come to the provocative conclusion that the results were explicable if it were assumed that all carcinogen-exposed cells became initiated, and that the probability of transformation was determined by the number of generations undergone by each initiated cell (16). Thus, low seeding densities allow many divisions prior to confluence and thus enhance the probability that a daughter cell will undergo transformation.

Clearly, resolution of the mechanism behind this paradoxical behavior of 10T1/2 cells in response to seeding density is vital to meaningful quantitative studies of transformation in this widely used system; less clear at the time was the realization that this behavior could shed light on an important property of tumor promoters: that of interfering with intercellular communication.

The possession of an initiated clone of 10T1/2 cells put us in the position of being able to set up reconstruction experiments utilizing mixtures of INIT/10T1/2 and 10T1/2 cells, and of thus accurately quantitating and manipulating the various variables in cell density experiments. Principal among these are: the ratio of initiated/non-initiated cells; the colony size attained by an initiated cell, which is inextricably linked to the cell generations accumulated by that initiated cell in that culture; the total number of generations accumulated by an initiated cell which is not equal to the previous variable if re-seeding of cultures is performed; and the number of initiated cells/culture.

Our results clearly demonstrated that in reconstruction experiments, the INIT/10T1/2 cells behaved as did *de novo* initiated cells. That is as the seeding density of a culture containing 100 initiated cells was increased, by increasing the number of co-cultured 10T1/2 cells, so the transformation frequency decreased. At high seeding densities, which allowed the initiated cells to produce colonies of fewer than 40 cells, the transformation frequency was very low (1%), while when colonies of above approximately 1000 cells were allowed to form by seeding at low initial densities, transformation frequencies increased to the maximum of 60% (Fig. 2). In this experiment, all the variables listed above were altered by each experimental manipulation and the results did not identify a single variable as contributing to the response. In a separate experiment, the effect of total generations accumulated by the initiated cells was found not to contribute to the variation in transformation frequency observed (24).

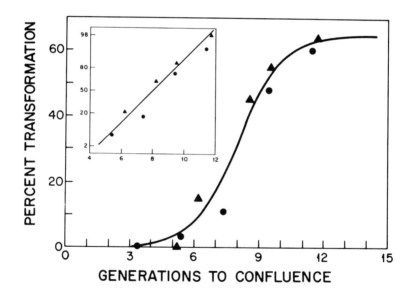

FIGURE 2. Influence of the number of generations to confluence of initiated cells plated without reseeding on the efficiency of transformation. Because cultures were not reseeded the number of generations to confluence is directly related to the colony size attained by the initiated cell. Inset, probit analysis of these data. As described, 60% transformation is the maximum value attainable by these cells ● and ▲ indicate separate experiments.

The results thus far obtained indicated clearly the requirement for large colonies for efficient expression of transformation. However, the results might simply reflect an increased probability of transformation as a consequence of the increased numbers of initiated cells contained in these large colonies. To control for this variable, we plated serial dilutions of a mixture of INIT/10T1/2 and 10T1/2 cells. Because the final saturation density is constant regardless of seeding density, and since both cell types have the same growth rate, it will be apparent that the relative proportions of initiated and normal cells at confluence will be the same as at the time of seeding. All cultures at confluence will contain the same number of INIT/10T1/2 cells; they will, however, differ in their distribution. Cultures seeded at high density (undiluted) will contain many small colonies; those seeded at lower densities (diluted) will contain fewer but larger colonies, with the mathematical product

Colony number X cells/colony = constant

These considerations also apply to the co-cultured 10T1/2 cells.

Serial dilution of the mixed cell suspension produced no significant variation in the number of transformed foci in cultures receiving 1:4 to 1:64 dilutions (Table 2), in spite of a 16-fold variation in the numbers of initiated cells seeded. These results are similar to those reported by Kennedy et al. (16) using de novo X-ray induced transformation (i.e. a constant yield of transformants is produced regardless of the initial numbers of cells at risk). However for cultures seeded at high density in which initiated cells were only able to produce small colonies (maximum 11, minimum 4 cells/colony), no transformed foci developed in any of 10 dishes. The uncertainty about the colony size reflects uncertainty of the true plating efficiency at these high seeding levels. Because the number of viable initiated cells plated, and thus the number of potentially transformed foci is known in these reconstruction experiments, one can calculate the true transformation frequency (TF). This is seen to increase from zero to a maximum of 65% in dishes seeded sparsely and yielding colonies larger than about 1000 cells (Table 2). This is believed to be the maximum frequency attained by this initiated cell line.

Thus is it clear that the calculated transformation frequency can only provide a valid estimate of the number of original initiating events if seeding densities are chosen that allow the expression of transformation in all competent colonies. At higher seeding densities progressively fewer colonies achieve transformation as demonstrated by the progressively declining values of the TF. In this model the constant yield of transformed foci/dish seen with dilution in the reconstruction experiments, and with increasing numbers of cells at risk in the de novo transformation experiments, is due to a balance between the increased number of potentially

TABLE 2. Effect of serial dilution of a mixed cell-suspension of 10T1/2 cells and INIT/10T1/2 cells on the transformation of INIT/10T1/2 cells

Dilution	Total cells seeded	Viable INIT/10T1/2 cells seeded[b]	Foci/dish	% of transformation	Generations to confluence	Cells/colony at confluence[e]
1:0	2.5×10^5	1205	0	0	3.4	4-11
1:4	6×10^4	301	10.5 ± 1.7[f]	3.5	5.4	42
1:16	1.5×10^4	75	8.3 ± 1.2	11.0	7.4	169
1:64	4×10^3	19	9.1 ± 1.8	48.0	9.4	676
1:256	1×10^3	5	3.0 ± 0.0	60.0	11.4	2702

[a] Calculated from plating efficiency of 100 cells from the mixed cell suspension.

[b] Calculated from plating efficiency of 100 INIT/10T1/2 cells.

[c] Percentage of viable INIT/10T1/2 cells seeded which formed types II and III foci.

[d] Calculated from plating efficiency of 100 cells from the undiluted suspension of INIT/10T1/2 plus 10T1/2 cells and the saturation density of the cells.

[e] Calculated from the formula

$$Cells/colony = 2^N$$

where N equals the number of cell generations to confluence.

[f] Mean $\pm$ S.D.

transformed   cells,   and   the   decreased   probability   of
transformation   forced   by   the   smaller   colony   sizes   at   high
density.

Mechanisms for Suppression of Neoplastic Transformation: The Cell/Cell Communication Model

Our earlier studies of factors modulating the transformation
frequency of carcinogen-treated 10T1/2 cultures provided the
conceptual framework for this model. As noted above, our
original studies had shown that seeding density had profound
effects on the observed transformation frequency (26). We
later demonstrated that suppression of transformation occurred
upon increasing the saturation density of cultures by elevating
serum levels in the growth medium (2). Furthermore we
demonstrated that at permissive concentrations of serum no
transformed foci developed in carcinogen-treated cultures which
had been treated with agents such as forskolin and/or
inhibitors of cAMP phosphodiesterase which cause elevation of
intracellular cAMP levels (3,5). Drug removal, or lower serum
concentrations, resulted in the rapid appearance of transformed
foci. Two additional findings are worthy of note; first, even
established neoplastically transformed cells can be prevented
from producing foci when seeded onto a confluent monolayer of
10T1/2 cells when treated with agents elevating cAMP levels;
second the effect requires intimate cell/cell contact (5).
Because of the known ability of cAMP to increase gap-junctional
communication in many cell types (10), we proposed that
suppression of the expression of transformation was being
mediated by the transfer of growth inhibitory signals from
post-confluent, G1 growth inhibited 10T1/2 cells to initiated
cells, preventing their transformation, or to transformed
cells, preventing the expression of the transformed phenotype.

In this model, transformation will be facilitated by an
agent or procedure that inhibits heterologous communication, or
prevents the intimate contact of an initiated or transformed
cell with a contact-inhibited 10T1/2 cell. Agents having this
ability are the tumor promoters, which in many cell types
including 10T1/2 cells, inhibit communication (8, 30, 31), and
retinoic acid, which will also inhibit communication in many
systems (8, 25). The effects of colony size on the
transformation of initiated cells described above could also be
explained by this model, since centrally located cells in large
colonies should be effectively isolated from direct contact
with surrounding 10T1/2 cells, whereas cells located in small
colonies, in which transformation is inhibited, should be in
more intimate contact with 10T1/2 cells.

Test of the Communication Model of Inhibition
of Expression of Neoplastic Transformation

To test this hypothesis, we collaborated with Dr. Werner
Loewenstein, the co-discoverer of gap-junctional communication
(19), who had also proposed that one logical function for the
gap-junction would be the exchange of growth regulatory signals
between contacting cells (18). In this study, we compared the
communication capacity (measured by the transfer of a
fluorescent dye from a microinjected transformed cell to
contacting 10T1/2 neighbors) of a series of selected cell lines
transformed by methylcholanthrene. Some responded to elevation
of cAMP in mixed culture by a dose dependent decrease of
proliferation, measured as a decrease in colony size and
number, others failed to respond to this stimulus. We found
that for the responsive cells, there existed an excellent
correlation between the ability for heterologous communication
between transformed and non-transformed cells, and the observed
inhibition of colony formation. In contrast, the
non-responsive cells were found to exhibit high basal levels of
communication, but this could not be further stimulated by
elevation of cAMP (21).

The association between communication and inhibition of
proliferation of the neoplastic cell was additionally
strengthened by the observation that both retinoic acid and
retinol inhibited heterologous communication, and inhibited the
constitutive and cAMP induced growth inhibition, without
inhibiting the elevation of cAMP induced by adenylate cyclase
stimulation or phosphodiesterase inhibition. While this action
of retinoids is at first glance surprising, it must be noted
that these measurements are of heterologous communication. The
report by Yamasaki's group that retinoids enhance communication
was restricted to a study of homologous communication (31).
Others have shown that retinoic acid will inhibit communication
(5) and this effect may be related to the enhancement of in
vitro carcinogenesis in 10T1/2 (4) and keratinocyte cultures
(17), and the enhancement of tumor formation in vivo (11).
Work is in progress to determine the effects of retinoids on
homologous communication between 10T1/2 cells and between
initiated cells.

Role of Tumor Promoters in Modulating Communication

Although our studies did not examine classical promoters
such as TPA for their effects on growth control and
communication, Borieko has shown that TPA will profoundly
inhibit heterologous communication between 10T1/2 cells and
their transformed counterparts (6). Furthermore, Mordan
(personal communication) has examined the influence of TPA on
the colony size dependence for transformation of INIT/10T1/2
cells, using the protocol described above, and has found TPA to

reduce the minimum colony size required for efficient transformation, as would be predicted for a compound reducing communication. Additional evidence for the role of communication in modulating the expression of transformation comes from the work of Hershman and Brankow (14). In these studies, UV modulation of 10T1/2 cells was shown to induce a cellular phenotype whose transformed potential is completely suppressed by contact with non-transformed 10T1/2 cells. This suppression can be relieved by addition of TPA or by removal of 10T1/2 cells. The action of TPA as an inhibitor of communication fits well with the role for promoters in mouse skin carcinogenesis by Hennings and Yuspa (13). In this model, promoters function by allowing clonal outgrowth of initiated cells thereby, producing a larger cell population in which rare secondary events may occur.

Control of Junctional Permeability

It is currently accepted that the transfer of ions and small molecules between contacting cells occurs by means of gap junctions, which are recognizable by freeze-fracture electron microscopy as an array of particles each exhibiting a hexagonal structure and a central pore of sufficient size (15-20 A) to allow transfer of the largest molecules shown to be capable of passage (1200-1400 daltons) (18). A major component of the isolated gap junction is a 27 Kd protein (26). Antibodies to this protein have been shown to localize approximately in regions of intercellular contacts, furthermore microinjection of this antibody into communicating cells blocks communication (15).

It is presently not known how communication is regulated, though of the three agents widely demonstrated to alter communication (i.e. Ca^{++}, TPA, and cAMP), all can exert their effects directly or indirectly at the level of protein phosphorylation. The p27 component of the gap junction is phosphorylated in intact cells but only to a low level (28), casting doubt on the physiological relevance of this finding. In this context, Loewenstein's group has demonstrated that junctional competence can be regained in a cAMP kinase deficient line of cells by addition of exogenous kinase to these cells (29). This group has also demonstrated that a very early event that occurs upon returning a Ts mutant of Rous sarcoma virus infected cells to the permissive temperature is the loss of junctional communication between these cells (1), suggesting that activation of pp60[src], a tyrosine-specific protein kinase, leads to phosphorylation of a gap-junctional associated protein. It thus appears that phosphorylation by protein kinase C, activated by TPA, or by pp60[src] will block communication, while phosphorylation by cAMP kinase,·which has different substrate specificity than protein kinase C, will open the channel and allow communication.

The role of the retinoids in modulating communication is presently unclear and requires clarification of their effects on heterologous vs. homologous communication as mentioned above. However, it may be relevant that in the INIT/10T1/2 system, we have recently shown retinyl acetate to decrease the phosphorylation state of two as yet unidentified proteins (20). It is thus possible that the observed antagonism between retinoids and TPA may be exerted at the level of protein phosphorylation.

REFERENCES

1. Azarnia R. and Loewenstein W.R. (1984): J. Memb. Biol., 82:191-205.

2. Bertram J.S. (1977): Cancer Res., 37:514-523.

3. Bertram, J.S. (1979): Cancer Res., 39:3502-3508.

4. Bertram, J.S. (1980): Cancer Res., 40:3141-3146.

5. Bertram, J.S. and Faletto, M.B. (1985): Cancer Res., 45:1945-1952.

6. Boreiko, C.J. Abernethy, D.J., Sanchez, J.H. and Dorman, B.H. (1986): Carcinogenesis, 7:1095-1099.

7. Boutwell, R.K. (1964): Prog. Exp. Tumor Res. 4:207-205.

8. Davidson, J.S., Baumgarten, I.M. and Harley, E.H. (1985): Carcinogenesis, 6:645-650.

9. Enomoto, T., Martel, N., Kanno, Y. and Yamasaki, H. (1984): J. Cell. Physiol., 121:323-333.

10. Flagg-Newton, J.L., Dahl, G. and Loewenstein, W.R. (1981): J. Memb. Biol., 63:105-121.

11. Forbes, P.D., Urbach, F. and Davis, R.E. (1979): Cancer Lett., 7:85-90.

12. Haber, D.A., Fox, D.A., Dynan, W.S. and Thilly, W.G. (1977): Cancer Res., 37:1644-1648.

13. Hennings, H. and Yuspa, S.H. (1984): J. Natl. Cancer Inst., 74:735-740.

14. Hershman, H. and Brankow, D.W. (1986): Science, 234:1385-1388.

15. Hertzberg, E.L., Spray, D.C. and Bennett, M.V.L. (1985): Proc. Natl. Acad. Sci. USA, 82:2412-2416.

16. Kennedy, A.R., Fox, M., Murphy G., and Little, J.B. (1980): Proc. Natl. Acad. Sci. USA, 77:7262-7266.

17. Kulesz-Martin, M., Blumenson, L. and Lisafeld, B. (1986): Carcinogenesis, 7:1425-1429.

18. Loewenstein, W.R. (1979): Biochim. Biophys. Acta, 560:1-65.

19. Loewenstein, W.R. and Kanno, Y. (1984): J. Cell. Biol., 22:565-586.

20. Martner, J.E. and Bertram, J.S. (1986): Carcinogenesis, 7:1301-1308.

21. Mehta, P.P., Bertram, J.S. and Loewenstein, W.R. (1985): Cell, 44:187-196.

22. Merriman, R.L. and Bertram, J.S. (1979): Cancer Res. 39:1661-1666.

23. Mordan, L.J., Bergin, L.M., Budnick, J.E.L., Meegan, R.R. and Bertram, J.S. (1982):Carcinogenesis, 3:279-285.

24. Mordan, L.J., Martner, J.E. and Bertram, J.S. (1983): Cancer Res., 43:4062-4067.

25. Pitts, J.D., Hamilton, A.E., Kam, E., Burk, R.R., and Murphy, J.P. (1986): Carcinogenesis, 7:1003-1010.

26. Revel, J.P., Nicholson, B.J. and Yancey, S.B. (1985): Ann. Rev. Physiol., 47:263-279.

27. Reznikoff, C.A., Bertram, J.S., Brankow, D.W., and Heidelberger, C. (1973): Cancer Res., 33:3239-3249.

28. Saez, J.C., Spray, D.C., Nairn, A.C., Hertzberg, E., Greengard, P. and Bennett, M.V.L. (1986): Proc. Natl. Acad. Sci. USA, 83:2473-2477.

29. Weiner, E.C. and Loewenstein, W.R. (1983): Nature, 305:433-435.

30. Yamasaki, H., Aguelon-Pegouries, A.-M., Enomoto, T., Martel, N., Furstenberger, G. and Marks, F. (1985): Carcinogenesis, 6:1173-1179.

31. Yamasaki, H., Enomoto, T. (1985): In: Carcinogenesis, Vol. 9, edited by J.C. Barrett and R.W. Tennant, pp. 179-194. Raven Press, New York.

Tumor Promoters: Biological Approaches for
Mechanistic Studies and Assay Systems,
edited by Robert Langenbach et al.
Raven Press, New York © 1988.

COMPARISON OF TRANSFORMATION SYSTEMS FOR
DETECTING TUMOR PROMOTORS

Alice S. Tu

Life Sciences Section
Arthur D. Little, Inc.
Acorn Park, Cambridge, MA 02140

INITIATION-PROMOTION EXPERIMENTAL SYSTEMS

The concept of a two stage initiation-promotion carcinogenic process was put forth over forty years ago with experimental support from the mouse skin model (1,2). This experimental system is characterized by several unique features. Neither the application of a small dose of carcinogen (initiating agent) to the mouse skin nor the multiple applications of a tumor promotor alone causes tumors. However, many tumors developed if the tumor promoter is applied to skin that has been initiated. Reversing the order of treatment did not result in tumors. Moreover, the effect of the initiator appears to be permanent while the effect of the promotor is reversible to a certain extent. Thus defined, only the initiating phase is consistent with the irreversible somatic mutation theory of cancer. The promoting phase is manifested by a reversible, epigenetic mode of action. While the exact mechanism of action and the role of promotion in the overall process of carcinogenesis remain to be elucidated, there is increasing evidence to demonstrate that the initiation-promotion process can be extended beyond the mouse skin model to other organs. For example, several agents have been shown to enhance tumor formation in epithelial tissues of the lung (32,33), liver (22,23), colon (17,19) and bladder (4,10).

Parallel to the development of in vivo model systems for studying tumor promotion, a number of in vitro cell culture systems have also been reported recently. The in vitro systems include a variety of cell types such as rodent fibroblastic cells (14,16,26,30), mouse epidermal cells (5), rat tracheal cells (29), human bronchial (31) and endometrial stromal cells (25). The availability of the in vitro model systems permits more in-depth dissection on the biological effects of tumor promotors at the cellular, biochemical and molecular levels. Some of the pleiotropic effects of tumor promotors, such as that on cell proliferation, differentiation and intercellular communication, on membrane and receptor interactions and on the synthesis and metabolism of specific proteins (e.g., polyamines, ornithine decarboxylase, and arachidonic acid) have been discussed extensively (6,8,28, also this volume). This chapter examines the in vitro model systems from a different perspective, namely, their potential utility as screening assays for detecting tumor promotors. The current status of three cell transformation assays for tumor promotors using the Syrian hamster embryo (SHE) cells, the BALB/c-3T3 and the C3H-10T½ cells are reviewed. A number of key issues that need to be considered for tumor promotion assays in general are discussed.

IN VITRO TRANSFORMATION - PROMOTION ASSAYS

The rationale of using transformation assays to detect promoters are multifold. First, the in vitro cell transformation assays measure the ability of chemicals to induce morphological transformation of nontransformed cells to a transformed, preneoplastic state. Morphologically transformed cells generally progress to be tumorigenic in appropriate host animals. Thus this endpoint is believed to be relevant for studying carcinogenesis. Second, there is a substantial data base on the use of the rodent cell transformation assays to detect chemical carcinogens (9). Third, in contrast to some transformation assays which measure the chemical effect on viral transformation, these three transformation assays apparently measure the direct effect of chemical to induce morphological transformation. Finally, a two-stage chemical transformation analogous to the initiation-promotion phases of the mouse skin model has been demonstrated in all three systems (11,16,21).

A typical initiation-promotion assay protocol of the three transformation systems is shown in Figure 1. Although the procedure of the three assay systems are similiar in that initiator and test promotor are sequentially added, there are inherent differences among the three target cells to suggest that the mechanism underlying the morphological transformation of these three systems may differ. For example, the SHE cells are normal diploid low passage mixed cell population while both the BALB/c-3T3 and C3H-10T½ cells are established cell lines with hyperdiploid karyotypes. Morphological transformation is detected clonally in the SHE cells but is measured as transformed foci of cells over a background monolayer in the two cell lines. The short assay duration of the SHE system limits the length of time that a test promotor can be exposed to the target

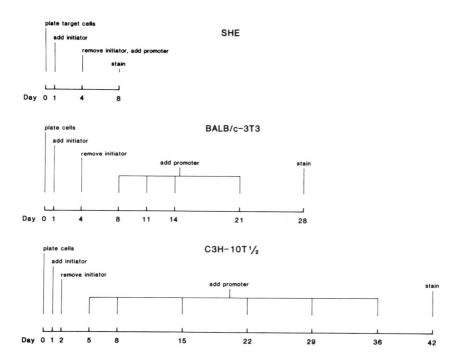

FIG 1.   Initiation-promotion assay protocol of the three cell transformation systems.

cells.   While there are more similarities between the two mouse fibroblast cell lines, the accumulated data suggest that these two cell lines may have varied sensitivity to chemicals.   There is also evidence which suggests that different clonal populations of BALB/c-3T3 cells have varied responsiveness to transformation by chemicals (12,27).   Whether this observation can be extended to tumor promotors remains to be determined.

Thus far, there is little distinction made between initiating agents and complete carcinogens in the in vitro transformation systems.   In fact, most of the initiating agents used in the promotion assay are suboptimal concentrations of potent in vivo "complete" carcinogens which transform cells at higher concentrations without addition of promoters.   These include physical agents such as X-ray or UV and chemical agents either requiring metabolic activation (e.g., 3-methylcholanthrene, MCA) or direct-acting alkylating agents (e.g., N-methyl-N'-nitro-N-nitrosoguanidine, MNNG).

Like most in vivo systems, 12-0-tetradecanoyl-phorbol-13-acetate (TPA) is the model tumor promotor used to demonstrate that the cell transformation assays are responsive to a 2-stage promotion protocol. The results in Tables 1 and 2 illustrate the reproducibility of such responsiveness in the C3H-10T½ and the BALB/c-3T3 systems, respectively. The data also show some of the differences between these two transformation systems. For example, the C3H-10T½ cells rarely exhibit any spontaneous transformation, while the population of BALB/c-3T3 cells that is used in our laboratory consistently show a low but measurable spontaneous transformation frequency. Continuous treatment of the C3H-10T½ cells with TPA but without any initiator generally does not induce any transformed foci. In contrast, treatment of

TABLE 1. Responsiveness of C3H-10T½ Cells to Promotion by TPA

Initiator (μg/ml)	Promotor (μg/ml)	Foci/Dishes (Dishes w/ Foci)
Experiment 1		
None	None	0/20 (0/20)
MNNG (0.50)	None	0/20 (0/20)
None	TPA (0.25)	0/20 (0/20)
MNNG (0.50)	TPA (0.25)	5/20 (3/20)
Experiment 2		
None	None	0/20 (0/20)
MNNG (0.50)	None	0/20 (0/20)
None	TPA (0.25)	0/20 (0/20)
MNNG (0.50)	TPA (0.25)	5/19 (4/19)
Experiment 3		
None	None	0/20 (0/20)
MNNG (0.50)	None	1/20 (1/20)
None	TPA (0.25)	0/20 (0/20)
MNNG (0.50)	TPA (0.25)	5/20 (5/20)

TABLE 2. Responsiveness of BALB/c-3T3 Cells to Promotion by TPA

Initiator (μg/ml)	Promotor (μg/ml)	Foci/Dishes (Dishes w/ Foci)
	Experiment 1	
None	None	1/20 (1/20)
MCA (0.01)	None	3/20 (2/20)
None	TPA (0.002)	7/20 (5/20)
MCA (0.01)	TPA (0.002)	15/15 (6/15)
	Experiment 2	
None	None	2/20 (2/20)
MCA (0.01)	None	1/20 (1/20)
None	TPA (0.002)	4/20 (3/20)
MCA (0.01)	TPA (0.002)	7/20 (6/20)
	Experiment 3	
None	None	1/19 (1/19)
MCA (0.01)	None	3/20 (3/20)
None	TPA (0.002)	4/20 (4/20)
MCA (0.01)	TPA (0.002)	10/20 (8/20)

the BALB/c-3T3 cells with TPA alone in a promotor protocol results frequently in a small increase of transformed foci over that of spontaneous transformation frequency. On the other hand, the BALB/c-3T3 cells appear to be more sensitive to enhanced transformation by TPA than the C3H-10T½ cells in producing a higher frequency of transformants at a lower concentration of TPA.

The number of chemicals that have been tested in the promotion protocol of the three transformation assays is still quite small. Nevertheless, several agents with demonstrated tumor promotion activity in mouse skin and other in vivo systems have been shown to enhance morphological transformation of carcinogen-initiated cells in vitro. In addition, carcinogens such as saccharin and diethylstibestrol which typically exhibited no genotoxic activity have produced a positive response in the in vitro promotion assays (Table 3). These results suggest that using an initiation-promotion protocol, the three morphological transformation assay systems can indeed detect some chemicals with properties of tumor promoters.

TABLE 3.　Examples of Positive Chemicals in a Promotion Assay Protocol of the C3H-10T½, BALB/c-3T3 and SHE Transformation Systems

C3H-10T½	BALB/c-3T3	SHE
TPA	TPA	TPA
Mezerein	12-0-retinyl phorbol-13-acetate	PDD
Telocidin	Phorbol-12,13-didecanoate (PDD)	1α,25-dihydroxy-vitamin D_3
Cigarette Smoke Condensate (CSC)	Merzerein	CSC
Anthralin	Telocidin	Nickel Sulfate
Saccharin	1α,25-dihydroxy vitamin D_3	Cadmium Acetate
Epidermal Growth Factor (EGF)	CSC	Potassium Chromate
Diethylstibestrol	Anthralin	Coal Tar
Bile Acids	Saccharin	Mezerein
2,3,7,8-tetrachloro-dibenzo-p-dioxin	Insulin	Retinoic Acid
Roussin's Red	EGF	Creosote
Formaldehyde		
Cortisone		
Dexamethasone		
Butyrated Hydroxytoluene		

PRACTICAL AND THEORETICAL CONSIDERATIONS

Despite the encouraging results, the potential utility of the cell culture assays for detecting tumor promoters is hampered by a number of technical and theoretical limitations that are generally not applicable to their use for screening chemical carcinogens. Since the promotion phenomenon is an arbitary definition of the experimental system, it is likely that a tumor promotor defined in one system may have a different mechanistic basis than that of another, even among the in vitro transformation systems. By operational definition, several terminologies may be applicable to the same chemical. For example, benzo(a)pyrene (B(a)P) can be defined by four different terms in the SHE transformation system by virtue of the sequence to which it is exposed to the target cells in the experimental procedure (Figure 2). In other instances, contradictory responses may be exhibited by a chemical. Dexamethasone, which has been shown to have promotion activity in the C3H-10T½ cells (15), was demonstrated to have an inhibitory effect in the same system when exposed to the cells prior to the addition of a carcinogen (13).

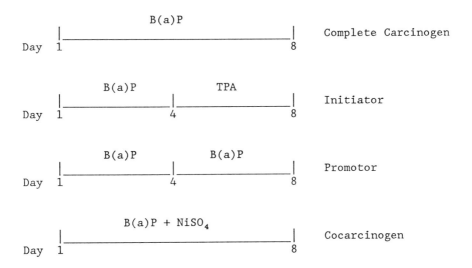

FIG 2. Several definitions of Benzo(a)pyrene as a consequence of different treatment schedule in the SHE clonal transformation assay

In the transformation assays, promotion is measured by an enhancement of transformation frequency above the background level of transformation. The BALB/c-3T3 cells exhibit a consistent frequency of spontaneous transformation. In addition, an increase in transformed foci is often observed when the cells are treated with either the initiator or the test promoter alone. This phenomenon has created a difficulty in judging for an enhanced transformation response, since it is not clear how the transformation frequencies of the three different sets of control (untreated, initiator-treated and promoter-treated) should be taken into account in the interpretation of results.

On the other hand, the induced transformation frequency of the C3H-10T½ cells is generally quite low. Many experimental modifications have been used to improve the transformation response. These include synchronizing the target cells (3), varying the target cell density (7), increasing the exposure time (20), delaying treatment of the test chemical after the target cells are seeded (18) or replating the target cells after confluency to amplify the response (24). The fact that the development of transformed foci is subject to manipulation by various experimental variables suggests that not all factors resulting in enhanced transformation are of relevance to carcinogenesis. To sort out the biological events significant to tumor promotion based on a morphological transformation phenomonen which is not well understood may prove to be a formidable task.

Thus, it is premature at this point in time to consider any of the in vitro systems for routine assay of tumor promoters. Clearly, however, these cell culture assays serve as valuable tools for studying factors which regulate/modulate cell growth and gene expression. Perhaps in time, when the initiation and promotion process can be more vigorously defined and when the in vitro transformation process is better understood in perspective of in vivo carcinogenesis, these assays would serve a useful purpose for screening tumor promoters.

REFERENCES

1. Berenblum, I. (1929): *J. Pathol. Bacteriol., 32:* 425-434.
2. Berenblum, I., and Shubik, P. (1947): *Br. J. Cancer, 1:* 383-391.
3. Bertram, J.S., and Heidelberger, C. (1974): *Cancer Res., 34:* 526-537.
4. Cohen, S.M., Arai, M., Jacobs, J.B., and Friedell, G.H. (1979): *Cancer Res., 39:* 207-217.
5. Colburn, N.H., Koehler, B., and Nelson, K.A. (1980): *Teratogenesis, Carcinogenesis, Mutagenesis, 1:* 87-96.

6. Fujiki, H., Hecker, E., Moore, R.E., Sugimura, T., and Weinstein, I.B., editors (1984): *Cellular Interactions by Environmental Tumor Promotors*. Japan Scientific Societies Press, Japan, and V.N.U. Science Press BV, The Netherlands.

7. Haber, D.A., Fox, D.A., Dynan, W.S. and Thilly, W.G. (1977): *Cancer Res.*, *37:* 1644-1648.

8. Hecker, E., Fusenig, N.E., Kunz, W., Marks, F., and Thielman, H.W., editors (1982): *Cocarcinogenesis and Biological Effects of Tumor Promoters*. Raven Press, New York.

9. Heidelberger, C., Freeman, A.E., Pienta, R.J., Sivak, A., Bertram, J.S., Castro, B.C., Dunkel, V.C., Francis, M.W., Kakunaga, T., Little, J.B., and Schechtman, L.M. (1983): *Mutat. Res.*, *114:* 283-385.

10. Hicks, R.M. (1980): *Br. Med. Bull.*, *36:* 39-46.

11. Hirakawa, T., Kakunaga, T., Fujiki, H., and Sugimura, T. (1982): *Science, 216:* 527-529.

12. Kakunaga, T., and Crow, J.D. (1980): *Science, 209:* 505-507.

13. Kuszynski, C., Somogyi, A. and Langenbach, R. (1982): *Cancer Letters, 15:* 215-221.

14. Lasne, C., Gentil, A., and Chouroulinkov, I. (1974): *Nature, 247:* 490-491.

15. Little, J.B., and Kennedy, A.R. (1982): In: *Caocarcinogenesis and Biological Effects of Tumor Promoters*, edited by E. Hecker, N.E. Fusenig, W. Kunz, F. Marks and H.W. Theilman, pp. 243-257. Raven Press, New York.

16. Mondal, S., Brankow, D.W., and Heidelberger, C. (1976): *Cancer Res.*, *36:* 2254-2260.

17. Narisawa, T., Magadia, N.E., Weisburger, J.H., and Wynder, E.L. (1974): *J. Natl. Cancer Inst.*, *53:* 1093-1097.

18. Nesnow, S., Garland, H. and Curtis, G. (1982): *Carcinogenesis, 3:* 377-380.

19. Nigro, N.D., Singh, D.V., Campbell, R.L., and Pak, M.S. (1975): *J. Natl. Cancer Inst.*, *54:* 429-442.

20. Oshiro, Y., and Balwierz, P.S. (1982): *Environ. Mutagenesis, 4:* 105-108.

21. Papescu, N.C., Amsbaugh, S.C., and DiPaolo, J.A. (1980): *Proc. Natl. Acad. Sci.*, *74:* 7282-7286.

22. Peraino, C., Fry, R.J.M., Staffeldt, E., and Kisieleski, W.E. (1973): *Cancer Res.*, *33:* 701-705.

23. Pitot, H.C., and Sirica, A.E. (1980): *Biochem. Biophys. Acta.*, *605:* 191-215.

24. Schechtman, L.M. Personal Communication.

25. Siegfrield, J.M., and Kaufman, D.G. (1983): *Int. J. Cancer, 32:* 423-429.

26. Sivak, A., and Van Duuren, B.L. (1970): *J. Natl. Cancer Inst.*, *44:* 1091-1097.

27. Sivak, A., and Tu, A.S. (1980): In: *The Predictive Value of Short-Term Screening Tests in Carcinogenicity Evaluation*, edited by G.M. Williams, R. Kroes, H.W. Waaijers, and K.W. van de Poll, pp. 171-190. Elsevier/N. Holland Press, The Netherlands.

28. Slaga, J.T., Sivak, A., and Boutwell, R.K., editors (1978): *Mechanisms of Tumor Promotion and Cocarcinogenesis.* Raven Press, New York.

29. Steele, V.E., Marchok, A.C., and Nettlesheim, P. (1978): *Cancer Res., 38:* 3563-3565.

30. Trosko, J.E., Yotti, L.P., Dawson, B., and Chang, C.C. (1981): In: *Short Term Tests for Chemical Carcinogens*, edited by H. Stitch and R.H.C. San, pp. 420-427. Springer-Verlag, New York.

31. Willey, J.C., Saladino, A.J., Ozanne, C., Lechner, J.F., and Harris, C.C. (1984): *Carcinogenesis, 5:* 209-215.

32. Witschi, H.P., and Lock, S. (1979): *Toxicol. Appl. Pharmacol., 50:* 391-400.

33. Witschi, H.P. (1981): *Toxicology, 21:* 95-104.

Tumor Promoters: Biological Approaches for
Mechanistic Studies and Assay Systems,
edited by Robert Langenbach et al.
Raven Press, New York © 1988.

THE POTENTIAL ROLE OF CELL

DIFFERENTIATION IN CARCINOGENESIS

E. Huberman

Division of Biological and Medical Research
Argonne National Laboratory
9700 South Cass Avenue
Argonne, IL 60439-4833

Carcinogenesis is considered to be a multistage process, each stage of which can be affected by physiological and environmental factors including chemicals, radiation, and viruses (15). From an experimental point of view, we can separate the process into three steps: initiation, promotion, and progression (10,15,31,32). The first step is the conversion of a normal cell into an initiated (preneoplastic) cell, while the second step entails the growth of the initiated cell into a benign tumor. The final step, progression, covers both the transformation of the preneoplastic cell into a malignant cell and its subsequent multiplication into a malignant tumor that may cause the death of the host.

THE CONTROL OF CELL DIFFERENTIATION IN CARCINOGENESIS

The hallmarks of cancer cells are uncontrolled cell replication and blocked differentiation processes. Consequently, hypotheses about carcinogenesis should, as part of their premise, include alterations in events that affect cell growth and maturation. In the present paper, I propose a working hypothesis of carcinogenesis, especially of its promotion step. I suggest that tumor formation may, in principle, result from continuous expression of growth facilitating genes that, as a result of some types of changes, was placed under the control of genes that are expressed during normal cell differentiation. In addition, I will describe some experiments dealing with the way some tumor promoters induce differentiation processes in cultured human cells and relate these results to the working hypothesis.

Cells in our body produce and respond to growth and differentiation-inducing factors (6,26,35). It is believed that stem

cells begin to mature after the interaction of a specific
"inducer" of differentiation with its appropriate cellular
receptor. Following this interaction, a series of cellular
signals are transmitted from the receptor to the genome causing,
within a short time, the activation and expression of specific
genes, presumably regulatory genes. The products of these early
activated genes cause, through positive or negative controls
(e.g., through a "trans"-acting process or ligand receptor
interaction), a sequential expression of genes that code for the
different growth and maturation functions, initially causing
cell growth (required for self-renewal) and then induction of
cell maturation. In the case of the maturation pathway, the
"inducer" causes the expression of Gene A, which in turn activates
Gene B, which in turn activates Gene C. In turn, Gene C activates
Gene D and so forth. Furthermore, the products of some of these
genes may also represent the various functions that constitute
the differentiated state. It is also expected that the product
of one or more of the genes that are expressed at a later part
of the maturation process will cause the suppression of the
growth facilitating gene(s) (designated as G in Fig. 1), thus
causing a terminal differentiated state.

Tumor initiation is thought to involve specific irreversible genetic change(s) in a normal stem cell (10,15,31,32). One
of these changes may involve a mutational event (e.g., base pair
substitution or addition or deletion of a base or a sequence of
bases) in a critical gene (e.g., Gene C in Fig. 2) that is part
of the normal sequence of genes whose expression results in the
terminally differentiated state. Thus, following the interaction of a cell with the appropriate "inducer" of differentiation, such a mutation may prevent the completion of the

NORMAL CELL

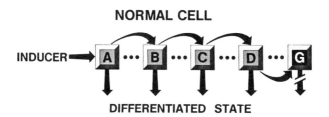

DIFFERENTIATED STATE

FIG. 1. Diagram showing normal cell maturation pathway. The
        "inducer" of differentiation interacts with its
        receptor and causes the expression of Gene A, which in
        turn activates Gene B, which in turn activates
        Gene C. In turn, Gene C activates Gene D. Gene D
        inactivates the gene that facilitates growth, Gene G.
        The resulting situation is expression of Genes A, B, C,
        and D, all of which code for cell maturation functions,
        and suppression of the growth facilitating gene,
        Gene G. The resulting phenotype will be that of a
        terminally differentiated cell.

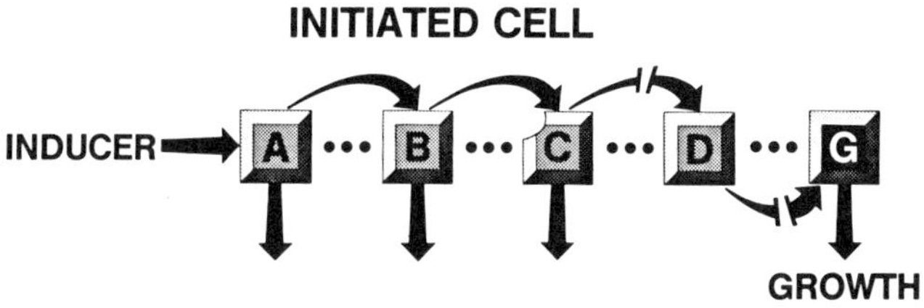

INITIATED CELL

FIG. 2. Diagram showing the differentiation of an initiated
cell. As in Fig. 1, the inducers cause the expression
of Gene A, which in turn activates Gene B, which in
turn acts on a mutated Gene C. This gene does not
activate Gene D. In turn, Gene D does not inactivate
Gene G. Thus, we have expression of Genes A, B, C, and
G, but not D. The resulting phenotype will be that of
a partially differentiated continuously growing cell.

maturation process, resulting in a cell that exhibits partial
maturation and continuous cell growth (Fig. 2). A similar
situation can also occur following a loss of a gene(s) or gene
rearrangement in which a growth control gene—for example, a
protooncogene (4)—may become part of the sequence of the
activated genes that code for the maturation functions (Fig. 3).
As in the previous case, initial interaction with the "inducer"
will cause the activation of the sequence of genes that result
in a mature phenotype. However, this sequential gene activation
can be interrupted if a growth control gene(s) does not produce
the appropriate signal for completion of the process of differentiation (Fig. 3). Again, such a cell will express some early
functions of cell maturation and will grow continuously. When
cells with the genetic alterations described above are induced
to differentiate, the degree of maturation of these cells will
obviously depend on the location of the genetic change in the
sequence of the genes that code for the maturation markers.
Those occurring early in the process will result in poorly
differentiated cells whereas those that take place at a later
stage will produce cells that exhibit a more mature phenotype.
    There are probably different types of inducers that cause
the same or a similar maturation phenotype in an affected stem
cell. Some of these inducers may activate genes that are
located beyond the gene that is altered during initiation; consequently, these cells may still be able to mature. Perhaps
this is the reason why some inducers of cell differentiation can
cause maturation of cultured tumor cells (7,16-18,22,26,27,
33-35,40). Yet this maturation may not be complete because some
genes that are part of the cascade of genes activated during
cell differentiation were skipped.
    The changes induced during tumor initiation in the cascade
of genes that control cell differentiation most probably involve

INITIATED CELL

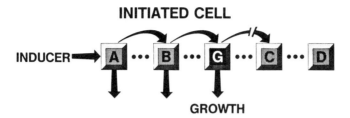

FIG. 3.   Another diagram showing a different differentiation
sequence in an initiated cell. As in Fig. 1, the
inducer activates Genes A and B, as well as the trans-
located growth-facilitating gene, Gene G. Because
Gene G is not capable of activating Gene C, this gene
and Gene D are not expressed. Because of inactivation
of gene D, there is also no suppression of the growth-
facilitating gene G as is described in Fig. 1. The
resulting phenotype is that of a partially differentiated continuously growing cell.

gene inactivation. To obtain continuous cell growth after an
interaction with the appropriate "inducer," as described before,
the genetic alterations occurring during initiation have to take
place in both alleles of the affected gene (e.g., as a result of
a clastogenic event) or in the unaffected allele of a gene that
is already heterozygous for the affected locus because of a
previous mutation, as in the case of retinoblastoma in children
(20,28).

    The suggestion that inactivation of genes that control cell
differentiation is part of the process that leads to malignant
cell transformation is compatible with experiments showing that
fusion of tumor cells with normal or nonmalignant cells or
introduction of specific chromosomes from normal cells into
tumor cells results in the suppression of malignancy (36,38,41).
The chromosomes from the normal or nonmalignant cells presumably
contain unaffected genes that have been inactivated in the tumor
cells during tumor initiation. This suggestion can also explain
why tumor cells usually do not grow in vitro. The culture
medium presumably lacks sufficient amounts of the specific
"inducer" of differentiation.

    The hypothesis described here suggests that natural tumor
promotion may result from an interaction of an initiated cell
with a continuously produced "inducer" of differentiation;
alternatively, promotion may result from an increased production
of a usually suppressed "inducer," perhaps due to aging (e.g.,
during menopause) or other physiological changes. These
"inducers" may cause a clonal expansion of the initiated cells
through the expression of growth-facilitating genes (4), which
as a result of prior gene mutation, gene loss, or gene
rearrangement (during tumor initiation) have been placed under

the control of genes that regulate normal cell differentiation. This step should result in the production of benign
tumors that will stop growing when the promotional stimulus is
removed. The same premise explains why environmental tumor
promoters introduced into the body through air, food, or skin
contact, should either cause the production of specific
"inducers" or be by themselves potent "inducers." In recent
years, studies with cultured cells have shown that some classes
of tumor promoters (e.g., phorbol diesters, teleocidins, or
2,3,7,8-tetrachlorodibenzo-p-dioxin) can act as potent inducers
of cell differentiation (15,17,21,40).

The next step in carcinogenesis, i.e., tumor progression,
may also entail changes (1,12,19) in the arrangement (e.g., gene
amplification) or structure of genes that control cell growth
(protooncogenes), resulting in increased cell replication
(Fig. 4).

Unlike the genes that control cell differentiation, which
are usually inactivated or suppressed during initiation, those
control genes that facilitate cell growth during the other steps
most likely exhibit a dominant trait, as was shown for a number
of viral and transfectable cellular oncogenes (4). It is also
expected that during progression, additional changes may cause
this altered growth control gene to be exempt from the "inducer"
regulating effect, resulting in uncontrolled cell growth that is

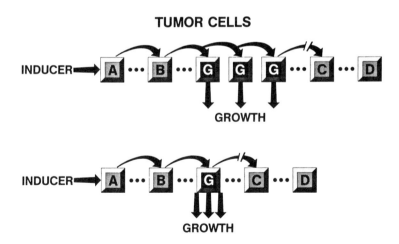

TUMOR CELLS

FIG. 4.   Diagrams showing development of tumor cells. This
          situation is similar to that shown in Fig. 3 except
          that the growth-facilitating gene, Gene G, is over-
          expressed because of gene amplification or gene
          restructuring (e.g., activation of a potent pro-
          moter). Genes A and B, but not C and D, are expressed
          and Gene G is overexpressed. This situation produces
          tumor cells that exhibit a partially differentiated
          phenotype with enhanced cell growth.

independent of the tumor-promoting stimulus [e.g., hormone-dependent tumors that lose this dependency with time (11)]. In this context, one should assume that tumor cells that grow in culture are selected for independence from the "inducer" effect unless such a factor exists in the serum that usually supplements tissue culture growth medium.

Let me, however, insert a caveat into my description of the role of "inducers" in the transformation of normal into malignant cells. Tumorigenesis may also result from events that encompass those described for both initiation and progression without necessarily requiring a promotion step, namely through genetic changes that cause an enhanced expression of growth control genes that are not dependent on the action of the "inducer."

INDUCTION OF DIFFERENTIATION IN HUMAN LEUKEMIA CELLS BY PHORBOL DIESTERS

Let me now explain the mode of action of tumor promoters as inducers of cell differentiation (17,18,22,25,29,33,34,39), keeping in mind the working hypothesis I have just described. We have been analyzing the various cellular and molecular events associated with induction of differentiation in the human promyelocytic HL-60 leukemia cells, which are useful for such studies because they display markers of cell maturation (7). In these HL-60 cells, the tumor-promoting phorbol diester prototype, phorbol 12-myristate 13-acetate (PMA), induces a mature phenotype that resembles that of macrophages (16,12,33).

Induction of cell differentiation by phorbol diesters and some related chemicals begins when they bind to a high-affinity and saturable receptor (8,14,37), which is a calcium- and phospholipid-dependent kinase (protein kinase C) (3,5,30). We have shown that in HL-60 cells this binding results in the phosphorylation of various cellular proteins, including some that reside in or around the nucleus (2). On the basis of these results, we have suggested that induction of cell differentiation by PMA may require the translocation (migration) of protein kinase C (PMA-receptor) from the cytosol to the cellular membranes (including nuclear membranes) where, through phosphorylation of regulatory proteins, the kinase causes alterations in gene expression (13).

To study the mechanism of PMA-induced cell differentiation and to analyze the role of protein kinase C translocation in this event, we used HL-60 cells that are either susceptible or resistant to PMA-induced cell differentiation (13). Treatment of cells from one of the variants designated HL-205 with a dose of PMA as low as 3 nM caused the cells to acquire a mature phenotype resembling that of macrophages, whereas cells from three other cell variants (HL-525, HL-534, and HL-402) remained undifferentiated even after treatment with PMA at a dose as high as 3 μM. The mature phenotype in the differentiation-susceptible HL-205 cells was defined by an increase in cell reactivity with monoclonal antibodies to maturation-specific cell surface

markers (9), staining for nonspecific esterase activity (42),
acquisition of a morphologically mature phenotype (Table 1), and
attachment of the cells to the surface of tissue culture dishes.
All of these properties are typical of peripheral macrophages
and monocytes. We also tested the response of the four cell
variants to another inducer of cell differentiation, 1α,25-dihy-
droxycholecalciferol [1,25(OH)$_2$D$_3$]. Treatment of cells from the
PMA-susceptible HL-205 variant and from the PMA-resistant HL-525
and HL-534 variants with 1,25(OH)$_2$D$_3$ caused the cells to acquire
a monocyte-like phenotype. These results indicate that the PMA-
resistant HL-525 and HL-534 cells have not lost their ability to
differentiate but were specifically resistant to differentiation
induced by PMA. In contrast, cells from the PMA-resistant
HL-402 variant were also resistant to the induction of cell
differentiation by 1,25(OH)$_2$D$_3$ (Table 1).

Analysis of the subcellular distribution of the activity of
protein kinase C revealed that about 90% of the activity was
detected in the soluble fraction of the various cell types
(Fig. 5). Incubation of the differentiation-susceptible HL-205
cells with PMA resulted in a time-dependent reduction in the
activity of protein kinase C in the cytosolic fraction. This
activity began to decrease within 2 min after the beginning of
PMA treatment and reached its lowest level (40% of control
level) 5-10 min after treatment. The decrease in the cytosolic
kinase C activity after 5 min of treatment with 1.6 to 160 nM PMA
was dose dependent. In contrast, PMA caused little or no decrease in the cytosolic kinase C activity in the PMA-resistant
HL-525, HL-534, and HL-402 cells (Fig. 5).

Concomitant with the decrease in the cytosolic protein
kinase C activity in the PMA-treated differentiation-susceptible
cells, we observed a significant increase in this activity in
the membrane fraction. Treatment of HL-205 cells with 160 nM
PMA for 5 min resulted in a more than 15-fold increase in protein kinase C activity in the membrane fraction, which was also
time and dose dependent. In contrast, no significant increase
in PMA-induced membrane-associated protein kinase C was observed
in the three cell variants (HL-525, HL-534, or HL-402 cells)
that are resistant to PMA-induced cell differentiation (Fig. 5).

These experiments, as well as those reported by others
(23,24), indicate that after PMA interacts with the receptor, it
induces a rapid translocation of protein kinase C activity from
the cytosol to the membrane fraction in cells susceptible to
PMA-induced cell differentiation but not in cells resistant to
such an induction. On the basis of these results, we believe
that induction of differentiation by tumor-promoting phorbol
diesters and related agents is initiated after they bind to
their receptor, protein kinase C. This binding results in a
translocation of the kinase from the cytosol to the phospho-
lipid-rich membrane fraction, thus causing the activation of
protein kinase C. The activated protein kinase, which is either
located in the vicinity of the nucleus or migrates to the
nuclear region, phosphorylates different nuclear proteins,

TABLE 1. Induction of differentiation markers in HL-60 cell variants at 6 days after treatment with either PMA or $1,25-(OH)_2D_3$

Inducer	HL-205	HL-525	HL-534	HL-402
	Cells reacting with OKM1 antibody (%)			
Control	8	≤5	≤5	≤5
PMA	≥95[a]	≤5	≤5	≤5
$1,25-(OH)_2D_3$	≥95	82	90	≤5
	Morphological differentiated cells (%)			
Control	<10	<10	<10	<10
PMA	88	<10	<10	<10
$1,25-(OH)_2D_3$	≥95	≥95	≥95	<10
	Cells stained for nonspecific esterase (%)			
Control	12	≤5	≤5	≤5
PMA	≥95	≤5	≤5	≤5
$1,25-(OH)_2D_3$	≥95	76	62	≤5

[a]Positive results are underlined. (From Ref. 13.) The concentration of PMA was 3 nM and of $1,25-(OH)_2D_3$ was 0.3 μM.

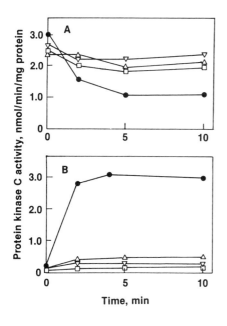

FIG. 5. Protein kinase C activity in the cytosol (A) and the membrane (B) fractions of control cells (● , 205) and HL-60 variant cells (▲ , 525; ▽ , 534; ◻ , 402) treated with 160 nM PMA.

including those required to initiate the sequence of gene expression that results in terminal cell differentiation in normal cells and partial maturation and continuous cell growth in cells initiated by carcinogens, as suggested in the working hypothesis.

In brief, I suggest that tumor formation may, in principle, result from continuous expression of growth facilitating genes that, as a result of irreversible changes during the initiation step, are placed under the control of genes that are expressed during normal differentiation. Thus, to understand carcinogenesis we must decipher the processes that lead to the acquisition of a mature phenotype in both normal and tumor cells and characterize the growth dependency of tumor cells to inducers of cell differentiation. Furthermore, the growth of a variety of tumors may be controlled through the use of inducers of maturation that activate genes that are located beyond the gene that is altered during tumor initiation.

ACKNOWLEDGMENT

Special thanks goes to Susan H. Barr for her editorial assistance. This work is supported by the U.S. Department of Energy under contract No. W-31-109-ENG-38.

REFERENCES

1. Aldaz, C. M., Conti, C. J., Klein-Szanto, A. J. P., and
    Slaga, T. J. (1987): Proc. Natl. Acad. Sci. USA,
    84:2029-2032.

2. Anderson, N. L., Gemmell, M. A., Coussens, P. M.,
    Murao, S.-I., and Huberman, E. (1985): Cancer Res.,
    45:4955-4962.

3. Ashendel, C. L., Staller, J. M., and Boutwell, R. K.
    (1983): Cancer Res., 43:4333-4337.

4. Bishop, J. M. (1987): Science, 235:305-311.

5. Castagna, M., Takai, Y., Kaibuchi, K., Sano, K.,
    Kikkawa, U., and Nishizuka, Y. (1982): J. Biol. Chem.,
    257:7847-7851.

6. Cohen, S., and Carpenter, G. (1975): Proc. Natl. Acad.
    Sci. USA, 72:1317-1322.

7. Collins, S. F., Rusetti, F. W., Gallagher, R. E., and
    Gallo, R. C. (1978): Proc. Natl. Acad. Sci. USA,
    75:2458-2462.

8. Driedger, P. E., and Blumberg, P. M. (1980): Proc. Natl.
    Acad. Sci. USA, 77:576-581.

9. Foon, K. A., Schroff, R. W., and Gale, R. P. (1982):
    Blood, 60:1-19.

10. Fujiki, H., Hecker, E., Moore, R. E., Sugimura, T., and
    Weinstein B. I., editors (1984): Cellular Interactions
    by Environmental Tumor Promoters. Japan Scientific
    Societies Press, Tokyo, Japan.

11. Furth, J. (1982): In: Cancer, A Comprehensive Treatise,
    Vol. 1, edited by F. F. Becker, pp. 89-137. Plenum
    Press, New York.

12. Hennings, H., Shores, R., Wenk, M. L., Spangler, E. F.,
    Tarone, R., and Yuspa, S. H. (1983): Nature,
    304:67-69.

13. Homma, Y, Henning-Chubb, C. B., and Huberman E. (1986):
    Proc. Natl. Acad. Sci., USA, 83:7316-7319.

14. Horowitz, A. D., Greenbaum, E., and Weinstein, I. B.
    (1981): Proc. Natl. Acad. Sci. USA, 78:2315-2319.

15. Huberman, E., and Barr, S. H., editors (1986):
    Carcinogenesis - A Comprehensive Survey: The Role of
    Chemicals and Radiation in the Ethiology of Cancer,
    Vol. 10. Raven Press, New York.

16. Huberman, E., Braslawsky, G. R., Callaham, M. F., and
    Fujiki, H. (1982): Carcinogenesis, 3:111-114.

17. Huberman, E., and Callaham, M. F. (1979): Proc. Natl.
    Acad. Sci. USA, 76:1293-1297.

18. Huberman, E., Heckman, C., and Langenbach, R. (1979):
    Cancer Res., 39:2618-2624.

19. Klein, G., and Klein, E. (1985): Nature, 315:190-195.

20. Knudson, A. G. (1985): Cancer Res., 45:1437-1442.

21. Knutson, J. C., and Poland, A. (1984): J. Cell Physiol.,
    121:143-151.

22. Koeffler, H. P., Bar-Eli, M., and Territo, M. C. (1981):
    Cancer Res., 41:919-926.
23. Kraft, A. S., and Anders, W. B. (1983): Nature,
    301:621-623.

24. Kraft, A. S., Anderson, W. B., Cooper, H. L. K., and
    Sando, J. J. (1982): J. Biol. Chem., 258:13193-13196.

25. Lotem, J., and Sachs, L. (1979): Proc. Natl. Acad. Sci.
    USA, 76:5158-5162.

26. Metcalf, D. (1985): Science, 299:16-22.

27. Murao, S.-I., Gemmell, M. A., Callaham, M. F.,
    Anderson, N. L., and Huberman E. (1983): Cancer Res.,
    43:4989-4996

28. Murphee, A. L., and Benedict, W. F. (1984): Science,
    223:1028-1033.

29. Niedel, J. E., Kuhn, L., and Vanderbark, G. R. (1983):
    Proc. Natl. Acad. Sci., USA, 80:36-40.

30. Nishizuka, Y. (1984): Nature, 308:693-698.

31. Peraino, C., Richards, W. L., and Stevens, F. J. (1983):
    In: Mechanisms of Tumor Promotion, Vol. 1, Tumor
    Promotion in Internal Organs, T. J. Slaga, ed.,
    CRC Press, Boca Raton, FL, pp. 1-53.

32. Pitot, H. C., Groso, L., and Dunn, T. (1984): In: <u>Genes and Cancer</u>, J. M. Bishop, J. D. Rowley, and M. Greaves, eds., Alan R. Liss, Inc., NY, pp. 81-98.

33. Rovera, G., O'Brien, T. G., and Diamond, L. (1979): <u>Science</u>, 204:868-870.

34. Ryffel, B., Henning, C. B., and Huberman, E. (1982): <u>Proc. Natl. Acad. Sci. USA</u>, 79:7336-7340.

35. Sachs, L., and Lotem, J. (1984): <u>Nature</u>, 312:407-412.

36. Sager, R. (1986): <u>Cancer Res.</u>, 46:1573-1580.

37. Solanki, V., Slaga, T. J., Callaham, M., and Huberman E. (1981): <u>Proc. Natl. Acad. Sci. USA</u>, 78:1722-1725.

38. Stanbridge, E. J. (1976): <u>Nature</u>, 260:17-20.

39. Totterman, T. H., Nilsson, K., and Sundstrom, C. (1980): <u>Nature</u>, 288:176-178.

40. Vanderbark, G. R., and Niedel, J. (1984): <u>J. Natl Cancer Inst.</u>, 73:1013-1019.

41. Weissman, B. E., Saxon, P. J., Pasquale, S. R., Jones, G. R., Geiser, A. G., and Stanbridge, E. J. (1987): <u>Science</u>, 236:175-180.

42. Yam, L. T., Li, C. Y., and Crosby, W. H. (1971): <u>Amer. J. Clin. Path.</u>, 55:283-290.

Tumor Promoters: Biological Approaches for
Mechanistic Studies and Assay Systems,
edited by Robert Langenbach et al.
Raven Press, New York © 1988.

SPONTANEOUS AND PHORBOL ESTER INDUCED CHROMOSOMAL ALTERATIONS IN NORMAL AND TRANSFORMED MOUSE KERATINOCYTES IN CULTURE

Norbert E. Fusenig, R.T. Petrusevska, and N. Pohlmann

Division of Differentiation and Carcinogenesis in vitro,
Institute of Biochemistry, German Cancer Research Center,
Im Neuenheimer Feld 280, 6900 Heidelberg, FRG

INTRODUCTION

Carcinogenesis is a progressive, multistep process which has been operationally defined as initiation, promotion and progression (for review see 35). Tumor promotion in mouse skin could be further subdivided into at least two stages (19, 51). First stage or complete tumor promoters, such as the phorbol ester TPA, are effective, after a limited number or even single treatments, in converting target cells into a state in which they are sensitive to further promotion to tumors by second stage, or incomplete, promoters, such as RPA (21).

The biologic effects exerted by a single application of TPA to mouse skin, which "conditioned" the epidermal target cells to further promotion, was long lasting with a "half-life" (in tumor realization) of 10 to 12 weeks (22). Moreover, this action of TPA was initiation-independent and effective whether the promoter was applied weeks before or after the initiator. These long-lasting carcinogen-independent effects of a complete promoter could no longer be explained by pure epigenetic mechanisms or interpreted as clonal expansion of carcinogen-initiated cells, but rather pointed to the involvement of genetic mechanisms.

Although TPA was not mutagenic in different test systems (42, 52), effects at the DNA and chromosomal level have been reported in different cell systems (for review see 13). In particular, DNA single strand breaks have been observed in human leukocytes (6) and mouse keratinocytes (12, 34). Moreover, TPA-induced numerical and/or structural chromosomal alterations in yeast (45), human leukocytes (9, 15) human fibroblast cultures (33, 39) have been reported. In addition, TPA caused congenital kidney defects and increased embryo mortality in CD-1 mice (37).

These findings were mostly derived from cells or tissues which can not be considered target organs for the tumor promoting activity of phorbol esters and thus, their relevance for the process of tumor promotion was questioned. Using epidermal target cells, however, we could recently demonstrate that TPA significantly enhances structural chromosomal alterations in mouse skin keratinocytes in primary and in permanent cultures (13, 14, 27).

Moreover, quite recently it has been reported that papillomas induced in mouse skin by the two stage carcinogenesis regimen, with DMBA as initiator and TPA as promoter had a substantial percentage of aneuploid cells which steadily increased with the promotion period (10). Malignant keratinocyte cell lines derived from DMBA- and TPA-induced mouse skin carcinomas had aneuploid karyotypes with characteristic, cell-line specific, structural chromosomal alterations (marker chromosomes) (1, 30, 31).

In general, numerical and structural chromosomal alterations are characteristic of virtually every malignant cell population. Specific non-random karyotypic changes found in a variety of animal and human tumors led to the recognition that chromosomal mutations may play a major role in the emergence of malignant neoplasms (49, 50, 55). The chromosomal changes were interpreted as the result of direct interactions of carcinogenic agents with the DNA of target cells and these processes were believed to be the crucial steps in carcinogenesis (8).

We here report that the complete tumor promoter TPA, although not mutagenic, induces both numerical and structural chromosomal alterations in normal and transformed mouse keratinocyte cultures. The alterations are observed after single treatments and within two cell cycles, but they increase after multiple treatments and are stable over several cell cycles. Non-promoting phorbol esters are ineffective and the incomplete or second stage promoter RPA exerts only slight effects at the chromosomal level. The cytogenetic alterations are obviously related to tumor promoting activity, since inhibitors of tumor promotion in vivo, inhibit, to a large extent, the induction of the chromosomal alterations. The cytogenetic aberrations observed within a few days of treatment with the tumor promoter are very similar to those occurring slowly during long term culture of normal keratinocytes and during the process of spontaneous immortalization and malignant conversion in vitro (31). Thus, the cytogenetic alterations induced rapidly by TPA may be of causal relevance, not only for the first stage of tumor promotion in mouse skin, but, in general, for the process of malignant cell transformation.

MATERIAL AND METHODS

Two permanent tumorigenic C_3H mouse keratinocyte cell lines (HEL-30 and HEL-37) with well defined morphological, biochemical and cytogenetic characteristics and known sensitivity to pleiotropic effects of phorbol esters were used (7, 20, 26, 30, 44). Cells were plated at a density of 1 to 2 x 10^5 cells per 60 mm Petri dish and treated for 1, 2 or 3 cell cycles when subconfluent.

Primary cultures of skin keratinocytes from newborn C_3H mice were prepared as described (24, 32). Cultures were washed 24 h after plating and treated with promoter the next day for 2 cell cycles, either once or three times at two-day intervals. All cells were grown in plastic Petri dishes (Falcon) in a modified

MEM (4 x MEM) (24) with 15 % FCS, at 30°C or 37°C in humidified
incubators with 5 % CO_2 in air. Alternatively, primary cultures
were grown in 4 x MEM with a reduced Ca^{++}-concentration of
0.08 mM (low Ca^{++} medium) as described by Hennings et al. (36).

The cell cycles were determined after BrdU (10^{-5}M) treatment
by the differential staining of the chromosomes. By simultaneous
treatment with BrdU and phorbol esters their effects on cell
cycle traverse were analyzed (see 14).

The phorbol esters 12-0-tetradecanoyl-phorbol-13-acetate (TPA),
12-0-retinoylphorbol-13-acetate (RPA), 4-0-methyl-TPA (4-0-MeTPA)
and 4-α-phorbol-didecanoate (4-α-PDD) were dissolved in acetone,
mixed with culture medium and applied at final concentrations of
10^{-8}M (and 10^{-6}M, respectively). Acetone at a final concentration
of 0.05 % was used as a control. The cyclooxygenase and lipoxy-
genase-inhibitor eicosatetraynoic acid (ETYA) was used at a
concentration of 10^{-6}M while the protease inhibitor antipain
(dissolved in PBS) was applied at a dose of 100 μg/ml.

Cell harvesting, banding of chromosomes and description of the
breakpoints were performed as reported previously (14). For
determination of numerical chromosomal alterations, an average of
100 metaphases were screened per experiment, and a minimum of 50
G-banded metaphases analyzed for the identification of specific
numerical aberrations and of structural chromosomal aberrations.

RESULTS

Structural chromosomal alterations induced by TPA in HEL-cell lines

The two spontaneously developed mouse keratinocyte cell lines
(HEL-37 is a subline of HEL-30) have maintained epidermal characteristics and are tumorigenic in appropriate hosts. While HEL-30
cells have maintained their differentiation capacity to a high
degree, this is to a large extent lost in HEL-37 cells (7, 26,
30). HEL-30 cells bind TPA by specific receptors (44), are sensitive to TPA effects on differentiation (26) and to TPA-induced
stimulation of cell proliferation and of the arachidonic cascade
(20).

TPA at doses of 10^{-6}M and 10^{-8}M did not significantly alter
the cell cycle traverse of both cell lines but led to a substantial increase in structural chromosomal aberrations (see
14). The effects were similarly expressed in HEL-30 and HEL-37
cells both at low and high passage levels. Alterations were visible as early as after one cell cycle and after doses as low as
10^{-9}M TPA but were largely independent of the TPA doses applied
(10^{-9}M - 10^{-6}M). The frequency of metaphases with additional
structural aberrations increased several fold after a single treatment but was further enhanced by multiple treatments (up to 5,
for each of two cell cycles) yielding more than 60 % of metapha-

ses with aberrations. The TPA-induced changes remained stable over at least 6 cell cycles after removal of the phorbol ester.

The chromosomal changes included gaps, chromatid and isochromatid breaks but also intra- and interchromosomal exchanges with formation of ring chromosomes as well as tri- and quadriradial exchange figures, alterations which were virtually absent in the untreated cell lines. More interestingly, different chromosomes were non-randomly affected by breaks, similar to the findings with primary epidermal cultures, and chromosomes no. 1 and 2 were mostly involved. In addition to the clastogenic effects of TPA, the frequency of metaphases carrying double minute (DM) chromosomes, the cytogenetic equivalent of gene amplification, increased 2 to 3-fold after TPA treatment.

In contrast, the non-promoting phorbol esters 4-O-MeTPA and 4-α-PDD even when applied at a concentration of 10^{-6}M did not produce any chromosomal alterations in HEL-cells.

Cytogenetic characteristics of normal skin keratinocytes in primary culture

The HEL-cell lines may not be considered the correct target cells for studying the cytogenetic effects of tumor promoters, since they are already transformed and have an altered karyotype. In particular, their aneuploidy did not allow analysis of numerical changes in the chromosome complement. We therefore extended these studies to primary cultures of mouse skin keratinocytes. The known instability of the mouse genome was reflected in the early appearance of numerical and structural chromosomal alterations which increased with culture time (Tab. 1). Depending on the culture conditions (normal and low Ca^{++} medium), the number of metaphases carrying numerical and structural chromosomal alterations increased at different rates over extended culture periods of up to 2 months. While in normal medium the number of tetraploid metaphases doubled within this period, their frequency reached 50 % in low Ca^{++} medium. During the same period, the number of diploid metaphases decreased while the fractions of hypo- and hyperdiploid cells increased, again to a higher level in low Ca^{++} cultures.

Concomitant with the spontaneous numerical changes structural aberrations showed a steady rise reaching 36 % and 47 % in normal and in low Ca^{++} medium, respectively, after 2 months. These changes included simple aberrations such as gaps, breaks and fragments but also inter- and intrachromatid exchanges, while double minutes were very rare, even in 2 month old cultures. Interestingly, the frequency of Robertsonian translocations, which was high (10 %) even in 2 day old cultures, nearly further doubled within the observation period (17 % and 20 %).

Tab. 1
Numerical and structural chromosomal alterations in mouse skin keratinocytes in primary culture[1]

Culture time (days)	Culture medium	Polyploid metaph.[2] (%)	near diploid metaph. (%)[3]			metaph.[3] with struct. aberrations (%)	Roberts.[3] transloc. (%)
			(40)	(34–39)	(41–43)		
1–4	4 x MEM+	10	94	6	0	2	10
	low Ca	11	94	6	0	4	12
5–10	4 x MEM+	15	88	10	2	3	10
	low Ca	17	85	12	3	15	11
11–30	4 x MEM+	18	82	14	4	17	14
	low Ca	20	79	16	5	27	15
31–60	4 x MEM+	20	79	15	6	36	17
	low Ca	54	60	31	9	47	26

1) Cells were cultured at 30°C at high density without passaging
2) Screened in at least 100 metaphases
3) Analyzed in at least 50 G-banded metaphases per experiment

At later culture stages, when cells usually become immortal (6 months in 4 x MEM and 3 months in low Ca^{++} medium) the majority of cells were in a near tetraploid state with an even higher percentage of metaphases with structural aberrations (47). As soon as the cells could be repeatedly passaged, they had a near tetraploid chromosomal complement with specific structural chromosomal alterations (marker chromosomes) (see 31). The chromosomal alterations always proceeded the spontaneous development of immortalized and eventually tumorigenic cell lines and are considered causal for this process.

Enhancement of numerical and structural chromosomal alterations by phorbol esters in normal mouse keratincytes in primary culture
As shown earlier, TPA (10^{-6} to 10^{-9}M) transiently inhibited proliferation of mouse skin keratinocytes followed by increased proliferation (25). The analysis of the cell cycle traverse by BrdU incorporation indicated, however, no substantial changes after TPA and RPA treatment at doses of 10^{-8}M each, while TPA at 10^{-6}M slightly accelerated the proliferation rate (see 46).

Following a single TPA-treatment (for two cell cycles) with 10^{-8}M the number of tetraploid metaphases remained unchanged while the percentage of hypo- and particularly hyperdiploid cells increased (Tab. 2). This was even more pronounced after 3 consecutive treatments when analyzed in 9 day old cultures. Similarly, the percentage of structural alterations increased 10 to 20 fold after one and three TPA applications, respectively. This was paralleled by a comparable increase in the frequency of metaphases with Robertsonian translocations. When the TPA dose was raised to 10^{-6}M, a single treatment further increased the numerical and structural alterations, although no clear cut dose dependency was observed (46).

On the other hand, the incomplete promoter RPA, at 10^{-8}M (and 10^{-6}M, not shown here), did not cause any significant alterations in the numerical chromosome content and only a slight increase in the percentage of metaphases carrying structural aberrations and Robertsonian translocations. While the structural changes after RPA were mostly breaks and centromeric splitting, TPA also induced, in addition to a higher number of breaks, complex changes such as ring chromosomes, tri- and quadriradial exchange figures and other chromosomal rearrangements (see Fig. 1). Comparable with the earlier observations in HEL cells the breaks were not randomly distributed in the genome but chromosomes no. 1, 2, 5, and 18 were more frequently involved (Petrusevska et al. in preparation).

The non-tumor promoting phorbolesters 4-O-MeTPA and 4-α-PDD did not induce substantial numerical or structural chromosomal alterations, except for an increase in the number of tetraploid metaphases by 4-O-MeTPA and of Robertsonian translocations by 4-α-PDD.

In order to get some information about the possible mechanism involved in the TPA-induced chromosomal alterations and to demon-

Tab. 2
Numerical and structural chromosomal aberrations induced by different phorbolesters in primary mouse keratinocyte cultures[1]

Phorbol ester[2] (10^-8 M)	No. of Expts.	Polyploid metaph.[3] (%)	near diploid metaph. (%)[4]			metaph.[4] with struct. aberrations (%)	Roberts.[4] transloc. (%)
			(40)	(36-39)	(41-44)		
Acetone	5	15	98	2	0	3	3
TPA(1x)	5	13	87	8	5	33	13
TPA(3x)	2	26	81	12	7	70	28
RPA	5	16	96	3	1	7	12
4-O-MeTPA	1	21	100	0	0	3	2
4-α-PDD	2	12	96	4	0	0	16

1) Cells were cultured at 37°C and treated for 2 cell cycles (54 h) starting 2 days after plating
2) applied 1 or 3 times respectively
3) Screened in at least 100 metaphases per experiment
4) Analyzed in at least 50 G-banded metaphases per experiment

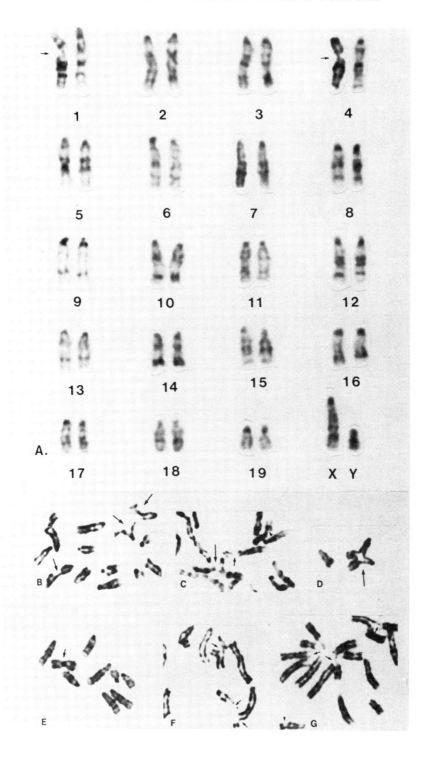

strate the relevance of these changes for tumor promotion in vivo, the effect of two inhibitors of tumor promotion were studied
at the chromosomal level in these cells (Tab. 3). On simultaneous
treatment with TPA both antipromoters were able to reduce the
frequency of metaphases with structural aberrations to a level,
close to that of the controls. ETYA itself had a slight effect on
structural chromosomal changes causing breaks and centromeric
splitting, comparable to those observed after RPA. Only the number of metaphases with Robertsonian translocations was not altered. On the other hand, ETYA had no effect on the induction of
hypo- or hyperdiploid metaphases, while the number of polyploid
metaphases was reduced. The effect of antipain on the induction
of numerical aberrations by TPA was insignificant.

DISCUSSION

Chromosomal abnormalities (numerical and structural) are consistently associated with malignant tumors, but the role of karyotypic changes and their causal relationship with distinct stages
in the process of carcinogenesis are not fully elucidated. Loss
of chromosomal stability due to chromosomal mutations, leading to
genomic rearrangements and altered gene expression, has been
suggested as an important step in the mechanism of cell transformation (5, 40, 41). It was hypothesized (38) that malignant cell
transformation might require at least two specific chromosomal
events which must coincide within a single target cell: i) induction of genetic changes, possibly mutations, that are recessive
and therefore latent in diploid somatic cells and ii) numerical
or structural chromosomal changes that could convert the heterozygous cell, created by the first process, into a homozygous or
hemizygous one. While the first process can be caused by a single
application of the carcinogen (most of them are mutagens) during
initiation, the second mechanism should occur during tumor promotion and progression.

Recent studies on the role of oncogenes in tumor development
have demonstrated that one way of protooncogene activation is by
point mutations at specific sites (48, 54, 56). Quite recently,

←——————————————————————

Fig. 1. Structural chromosomal alterations in mouse keratinocytes induced by TPA.
A). Karyogram of a 4 day old primary culture of mouse skin keratinocytes after 54 h treatment by 10^{-8}M TPA with isochromatid and
chromatid breaks (arrows). B). Multiple isochromatid breaks
(arrows). C). Triradial chromosome configuration (large arrows),
isochromatid break (small arrow) and chromatid gap (arrowhead).
D). Quadriradial chromosome configuration (arrow). E). Robertsonian translocation (arrow). F). Multiple isochromatid breaks
(arrows). G). Chromatid grap (arrowhead) and centromeric splitting with chromosomal associations (arrows).

Tab. 3

Effects of the inhibitors of tumor promotion ETYA and antipain on TPA induced chromosomal alterations in mouse keratinocytes

Treatment schedule[1]	No. of Expts.	Polyploid metaph.[2] (%)	near diploid metaph. (%)[3] (40)	(36-39)	(41-44)	metaph. with struct. aberrations[3] (%)	Roberts. transloc.[3] (%)
Acetone	5	15	98	2	0	3	3
TPA 10^{-8}M	5	13	87	8	5	33	13
ETYA 10^{-6}M	1	4	95	4	1	7	15
ETYA + TPA	2	6	88	7	5	10	13
Antipain 100 µg/ml + TPA 10^{-8}M	3	12	94	6	0	8[4]	22

[1] Single treatment with TPA and simultaneous treatment with inhibitors

[2] Screened from at least 100 metaphases per experiment

[3] Analyzed from at least 50 metaphases per experiment

[4] Including 6 % simple chromosomal aberrations (centromeric splitting)

Balmain and coworkers have demonstrated that mouse skin carcinomas contain activated Harvey ras oncogenes and that even papillomas induced in two-stage carcinogenesis (involving DMBA and TPA) already contain the activated ras-oncogene, mutated at codon 61, a typical site for DMBA induced mutation (3, 4). However, while the mutation could be demonstrated in one allele only in papillomas (being thus in a heterozygous state), the activated oncogene was either homozygous or amplified in fully developed carcinomas. It is reasonable to assume that these later changes are brought about by numerical and/or structural chromosomal changes during the development of papillomas and their malignant conversion.

So far, it had been difficult to determine the role and onset of karyotypic alterations during tumorigenesis, since only late tumor stages were commonly studied. Furthermore, the heterogeneous cell populations in solid tumors and the technical difficulties involved in getting reliable cytogenetic data, were serious limitations to the elucidation of the significance of chromosomal changes during the carcinogenesis process. Very recently, Conti and coworkers demonstrated that aneuploid cell populations were already present in very early papillomas and that these cell fractions increased with the promotion period and subsequently replaced the diploid stem lines before histologically visible carcinomas had developed (10). The increasing aneuploidy in papillomas was visible as discrete hyperdiploidy, i.e. by the gain of a few additional chromosomes, probably due to non-disjunction and unequal chromosome distribution in mitosis. The actual rate of aneuploidy is expected to be even higher since the authors did not count and consider hypodiploid metaphases, which should be expected to occur in a similar frequency. The carcinomas which developed eventually were all aneuploid with a hyperdiploid mode and variable fractions of near tetraploid cells (1, 2, 10).

These findings confirmed our earlier studies on mouse skin as well as on human skin-derived squamous cell carcinoma cell lines which were all aneuploid and developed during culture period into near tetraploid cell lines (31, 53). Similarly, during spontaneous or induced epithelial cell transformation in vitro aneuploidy was usually the first visible indication of early transformation stages, e.g. when cells were immortalized (11, 28, 31).

In this report, we have shown that rather numerical and structural chromosomal alterations, which accumulate during the latency period occur early during the spontaneous transformation process of mouse keratinocytes. These changes are obviously dependent on culture time and culture conditions and start to occur immediately after plating (13, 28, 29, 30). Most interestingly, chromosomal loss and gain was not random but specific chromosomes such as no. 5 were mostly overrepresented while others such as no. 7 and 14 were more often underrepresented. These very same chromosomes were also over- and underrepresented in the established cell lines, transformed either spontaneously, after DMBA treatment in vitro, or derived from carcinomas of mouse skin (31, 47).

While the development of these cytogenetic changes occurred slowly over several months spontaneously in keratinocytes in primary culture (depending on the culture conditions), similar changes were induced to occur rapidly after TPA treatment. Although multiple treatments led to a dramatic increase in the number of metaphases with numerical and/or structural chromosomal aberrations, one single application was sufficient to enhance the number of cells with a structurally and numerically altered karyotype by a factor of 10. The changes were not lethal to cells but were stably maintained over several cell cycles (14).

Thus, the studies have demonstrated that TPA caused various effects at the chromosomal level which could all contribute to disturbances in the genome to produce hemi- or homozygosity of already altered genes, their activation by gene rearrangement, and amplification. Moreover, preliminary data from recent experiments indicate that TPA induces similar changes in keratinocytes in vivo when the promoter is applied to mouse skin (unpublished data). The significance of the chromosomal effects of TPA on tumor promotion in vivo is further evidenced by the inhibition exerted by ETYA and antipain, since both are effective in reducing the efficiency of tumor promotion on mouse skin in vivo and transformation of cells in vitro (18, 23, 38).

At present we can only speculate about the mechanism by which tumor promoters act at the chromosomal level. From our data we can not infer whether the cytogenetic effects are mediated by oxygen radicals or via the arachidonic acid cascade as postulated by Cerutti (9, 16, 17). The effects exerted by the inhibitor ETYA indicate that these mechanisms may be involved.

It is, however, interesting to note that, not only had the non-tumor promoting phorbolesters no effect at the chromosomal level but also that the incomplete or second stage tumor promoter RPA is obviously not, or only very weakly, clastogenic and has no effect on the ploidy level. Similar results were obtained when the dose of RPA was raised to 10^{-6}M and repeated applications were used (46). Thus, this represents the first biologic assay system showing qualitative differences in the effects of first and second stage tumor promoters. This discrepancy in the biologic activity at the chromosomal level could explain why the convertogenic activity of TPA is i) achieved by one single treatment; ii) initiator independent (since it is active at the genetic level), and iii) long-lasting with a half-life of several months in mouse skin. The fact, that the chromosomal changes are obviously not completely irreversible at the tissue level (the skin) could be explained by the turnover of the proliferative cells in the epidermis. Following mitosis the proliferative cells are consecutively pushed into differentiation and lost as keratinized horn scales. The only persistent cell population, the putative stem cells, are commonly believed to cycle very slowly (43), so that the probability of these cells occurring in the mitotic cell compartment (and being analyzed cytogenetically) is rather low. Thus, although the cytogenetic alterations can be irreversible at the single cell level, their biological consequences can be reversible at the tissue level due to the elimination of the affected cells during turnover of the whole tissue.

From these data we hypothesize, that complete tumor promoters exert their initiator-independent, long-lasting effects on mouse skin by their actions at the chromosomal level: i.e. by creating aneuploidy, by their clastogenic as well as recombinogenic potency and by their capacity to amplify genes. The long-lasting effects of these genetic alteraltions might be crucial events in converting the heterozygous carcinogen-induced mutations into a hemi- or homozygous or amplified state. The interference with control mechanisms of neighbouring cells may be the specific role of second stage promoters in providing the conditions for clonal expansion of the benign tumor cells.

ACKNOWLEDGEMENTS

The technical assistance of Charlotte Rausch and Monika Blum is gratefully acknowledged. We thank Monika Matejka for typing and Dr. Cathy Ryle for stylistically correcting the manuscript. This work was supported by the Deutsche Forschungsgemeinschaft, Sonderforschungsbereich SFB 136, Heidelberg.

REFERENCES

1. Aldaz, C.M., Conti, C.J., O'Connell, J., Yuspa, S.H., Klein-Szanto, A.J.P., and Slaga, T.J. (1986): Cancer Res. 46:3565-3568
2. Aldaz, C.M., Conti, C.J., Klein-Szanto, A., and Slaga, T.J. (1986): Cancer Genet. Cytogenet. 20:223-229
3. Balmain, A. and Pragnell, I.B. (1983): Nature 303:72-74
4. Balmain,A., Ramsden, M., Bowden, G.T., and Smith, J. (1984): Nature 307:658-660
5. Barrett, J.C., Thomassen, D.G., and Hesterberg, T.W. (1983): Ann. N.Y. Acad. SCi. 407:291-300
6. Birnboim, H.C. (1982): Science 211:1247-1249
7. Breitkreutz, D.., Boukamp, P., Lueder, M., and Fusenig, N.E. (1981): Front. Matrix Biol. 9:57-82
8. Cairns, J. (1981): Nature 289:353-357
9. Cerutti, P., Amstad, P., and Emerit, I. (1983): In: Radioprotectors and anticarcinogens, edited by O.F. Nygaard and M.G. Simic, pp. 527-538, Raven Press, New York
10. Conti, C.J., Aldaz, C.M., O'Connell, J., Klein-Szanto, A.J.P., and Slaga, T.J. (1986): Carcinogenesis 7: 1845-1848
11. Cowell, J.K. and Wigley, C.B. (1982): J. Natl. Cancer Inst. 69:425-433
12. Dutton, D. and Bowden, G.T. (1985): Carcinogenesis

        6:1279-1284
13. Dzarlieva, R.T. and Fusenig, N.E. (1982): Cancer Lett. 16:7-17
14. Dzarlieva-Petrusevska, R.T. and Fusenig, N.E. (1985):
        Carcinogenesis 6:1447-1456
15. Emerit, I. and Cerutti, P.A. (1982): Proc. Natl. Acad. Sci.
        USA 79:7509-7513
16. Emerit, I. and Cerutti, P. (1983): Carcinogenesis 4:1313-1316
17. Emerit, I., Levy, A., and Cerutti, P. (1983): Mutat. Res.
        110:327-335
18. Fischer, S.M., Mills, G.D., and Slaga, T.J. (1983): In:
        Advances in Prostaglandin, Thromboxane and Leukotriene
        Research, Vol. 12, edited by B. Samuelsson, R. Paoletti,
        and P. Ramwell, pp. 309-312. Raven Press, New York.
19. Fürstenberger, G., Berry, D.L., Sorg, B., and Marks, F.
        (1981a): Proc. Natl. Acad. Sci. 78:7722-7726
20. Fürstenberger, G., Richter, H., Fusenig, N.E., and Marks, F.
        (1981): Cancer Lett. 11:191-198
21. Fürstenberger, G., Sorg, B., and Marks, F. (1983): Science
        220:89-91
22. Fürstenberger, G., Kinzel, V., Schwarz, M., and Marks, F.
        (1985a): Science 230:76-78
23. Fürstenberger, G. and Marks, F. (1985): In: Arachidonic Acid
        Metabolism and Tumor Promotion, edited by S.M. Fischer and
        T.J. Slaga, pp. 49-72, Martinus Nijhoff Publishing, Boston
24. Fusenig, N.E. and Worst, P.K.M. (1975): Exp. Cell Res.
        93:443-457
25. Fusenig, N.E. and Samsel, W. (1978): In: Carcinogenesis - A
        Comprehensive Survey, Vol. 2, Mechanisms of Tumor
        Promotion and Cocarcinogenesis, edited by T.J. Slaga et
        al., pp. 203-220, Raven Press, New York
26. Fusenig, N.E., Breitkreutz, D., Boukamp, P., Lueder, M.,
        Irmscher, G., and Worst, P.K.M. (1979): In: Neoplastic
        Transformation in Differentiated Epitelial Cell Systems
        in vitro, edited by L.M. Franks et al., pp. 37-87
27. Fusenig, N.E. and Dzarlieva, R.T. (1982): In: Carcinogenesis
        - A Comprehensive Survey, Vol. 7, edited by E. Hecker,
        N.E. Fusenig, W. Kunz, F. Marks, and H.W. Thielmann, pp.
        201-216. Raven Press, New York
28. Fusenig, N.E., Breitkreutz, D., Dzarlieva, R.T., Boukamp, P.,
        Herzmann, E., Bohnert, A., Pöhlmann, J., Rausch, C.,
        Schütz, S., and Hornung, J. (1982): Cancer Forum 6:209-240
29. Fusenig, N.E. (1983): In: Biology of Cancer, pp. 91-104,
        Alan R. Liss, Inc.
30. Fusenig, N.E., Breitkreutz, D., Dzarlieva, R.T., Boukamp, P.,
        Bohnert, A., and Tilgen, W. (1983): J. Invest. Dermatol.
        81:168s-175s
31. Fusenig, N.E., Dzarlieva-Petrusevska, R.T., and Breitkreutz,
        D. (1985): In: Carcinogenesis, edited by J.C. Barrett and
        R.W. Tennant, Vol. 9, pp. 293-326, Raven Press, New York
32. Fusenig, N.E. (1986): In: Biology of the Integument, Vol. 2
        Vertebrates, edited by J. Bereiter-Hahn, A.G. Matoltsy,

K.S. Richards, pp. 409-442, Springer Verlag
33. Gainer, H.S. and Kinsella, A.R. (1983): Int. J. Cancer
    32:449-453
34. Hartley, J.A., Gibson, N.W., Zwelling, L.A., and Yuspa, S.H.
    (1985): Cancer Res. 45:4864-4870
35. Hecker, E., Fusenig, N.E., Kunz, W., Marks, F., and
    Biological Effects of Tumor promoters. Carcinogenesis -
    A Comprehensive Survey, Vol. 7, Raven Press, New York.
36. Hennings, H., Michael, D., Cheng, C., Steinert, P., Holbrook,
    K., and Yuspa, S.H. (1980): Cell 19:245-254
37. Huber, E. and Brown, N.A. (1985): Res. Commun. Pathol.
    Pharmacol. 49:17-34
38. Kinsella, A.R. and Radman, M. (1980): Proc. Natl. Acad. Sci.
    USA 77:3544-3547
39. Kinsella, A.R., Gainer, H.S., and Butler, J. (1983):
    Carcinogenesis 4:717-719
40. Kraemer, P.M., Travis, G.L., Ray, R.F., and Cram, L.S.
    (1983): Cancer Res. 43:4822-4827
41. Krontiris, T.G. (1983): New Engl. J. Med. 309:404-409
42. Lankas, G.R., Baxter, C.S., and Christian, R.T. (1977):
    Mutat. Res. 45:153-156
43. Lavker, R.M. and Sun, T.-T. (1983): J. Invest. Dermatol. 81:
    121s-127s
44. Murray, A.W. and Fusenig, N.E. (1979): Cancer Lett. 7:71-77
45. Parry, J.M, Parry, E.M., and Barrett, J.C. (1981): Nature
    294:263-265
46. Petrusevska, R.T., Pohlmann, N., and Fusenig, N.E. (1987):
    In: Accomplishments in Oncology, edited by H. zur Hausen
    and J. Schlehofer, J.B. Lippincott, Philadelphia, in press
47. Pohlmann, N. (1986): Ph.D. Thesis, University of
    Kaiserslautern
48. Reddy, E.P., Reynolds, E., Santos, E., and Barbacid, M.
    (1982): Nature 300:149-152
49. Sandberg, A.A. (1983): Cancer Genet. Cytogenet. 8:277-285
50. Sasaki, M. (1982): Cancer Genet. Cytogenet. 5:153-172
51. Slaga, T.J., Fischer, S.M., Nelson, K., Gleason, G.L. (1980):
    P.N.A.S. 77:3659-3663
52. Thompson, L.M., Baker, R.M., Corrano, A.V., and Brookman,
    K.W. (1980): Cancer Res. 40:3245-3251
53. Tilgen, W., Boukamp, P., Breitkreutz, D., Dzarlieva, R.T.,
    Engstner, M., Haag, D., and Fusenig, N.E. (1983): Cancer
    Res. 43:5995-6011
54. Yuasa, Y., Srivatstava, S.K., Dunn, C.Y., Rhim, J.S., Reddy,
    E.P., and Aaronson, S.A. (1983): Nature 303:775-779
55. Yunis, J.J. (1983): Science 221:227-236
56. Zarbl, H., Sukumar, S., Arthur, A.V., Martin-Zanka, D., and
    Barbacid, M. (1985): Nature 315:382-385

Tumor Promoters: Biological Approaches for Mechanistic Studies and Assay Systems,
edited by Robert Langenbach et al.
Raven Press, New York © 1988.

HUMAN LUNG CELLS: IN VITRO MODELS FOR STUDYING CARCINOGENS

John F. Lechner, Tohru Masui, Masao Miyashita, James C. Willey,
Roger Reddel, Moira A. LaVeck, Yang Ke, George H. Yoakum,
Paul Amstad, Brenda I. Gerwin, and Curtis C. Harris

Laboratory of Human Carcinogenesis,
Division of Cancer Etiology, National Cancer Institute,
Bethesda, MD 20892

Lung cancer is now the most common form of malignancy facing the American population. Studies of animal models have yielded a substantial amount of knowledge about the pathogenesis of lung cancer. However, animal models have a number of limitations. For example, differential efficiencies of metabolism of chemical carcinogens are known to occur among different animal species and even between inbred strains of the same species. (1) Further, animal cells are chromosomally less stable than human cells,(2) and finally, compared to human cells, chemical and/or viral transformation of animal fibroblastic cells occurs at higher frequency.(2)

In an attempt to overcome some of these shortcomings, we embarked several years ago on a project to develop defined (serum-free) methods for establishing replicative cultures of normal human lung epithelial cells. We have now accomplished this goal for both mesothelial cells,(3-6) the target cell type of asbestos-induced human mesothelioma and for large airway epithelium,(3, 7-13) the presumed target cell type of human bronchogenic cancers. However, space permits only the latter model, the bronchial epithelial cell system to be discussed in this overview.

When we initially elected to expand our carcinogenesis model systems to include bronchial epithelial cells as well as bronchial epithelium, methods for establishing replicative cultures of this type of human epithelial cell were unavailable. However, by adapting the feeder-cell technique of Rheinwald and Green(14) to the requirements of normal human bronchial epithelial (NHBE) cells, we ascertained that replicative cultures of these cells were efficacious and further, single cells could be grown into colonies.(8) Nonetheless, it had always been our goal to develop a defined method to culture these cells since it is impossible to eliminate the role of the

feeder-cells when measuring the responses of the bronchial
epithelial cells to mitogens, differentiation inducing agents
or carcinogens.   It was our good fortune at this time that
Drs. Peehl & Ham were developing a feeder-cell-free method for
culturing human keratinocytes.(15) We quickly discovered that a
slightly modified serum-free version of their formula would
support the clonal growth of NHBE cells.(9)

Several different media have been used for growing the cells.
The primary reason for this is that the formula evolved as our
understanding of the requirements improved.   Further, we have
discovered that no one formula is optimal for all experiments.
The nutrient base is a modified form of Peehl and Ham's MCDB 152
keratinocyte medium.(15)   The changes we found to be efficacious
for NHBE cells were: to increase the calcium concentration
threefold to 110 µM; to double the concentration of the
essential amino acids; and to lower the mOsmols from 345 to
280 mOs/kg by reducing the concentrations of NaCl, HEPES and
Na-bicarbonate 18% along with the CO_2 partial pressure of the
atmosphere in the incubator.   Another major deviation from the
procedures published by Peehl and Ham was to develop a substrate
coating solution consisting of collagen, FN and BSA, which
significantly enhances the attachment of the cells to the
culture dish surface.(9)

After thus having established that NHBE cells could be
propagated without feeder-cells or serum, we turned our
attention to characterizing the cells.(11,13)   The salient
epithelial cell markers are keratin-tonofilaments and
desmosomes.   The cells also have two commonly accepted markers
of normalcy, i.e., the normal human giemsa-banded karyotype and
a finite culture life span.   The karyotype remains normal
throughout their culture life span which averages 35 population
doublings or 4 to 5 passages.   Further, the cells will grow as
colonies, although the colony forming efficiency is low.
However, the maximal clonal growth rate when measured in our
most optimized medium averages 1.1 population doublings per day.
Finally, the cells will metabolically activate procarcinogens
such as benzo[a]pyrene to the proximal forms.(16)

After developing this culture system it became possible to
initiate investigations focused upon dissecting the physiological controls operating in normal human lung epithelial cells
without the confounding effects of serum or feeder-cells. For
our first experiments we elected to ascertain the role of
ornithine decarboxylase (ODC) activity and cAMP cellular
concentration as a function of epidermal growth factor (EGF),
epinephrine (EPI) and bovine pituitary extract (BPE).   We chose
to evaluate these biochemical parameters because two of the
early changes repeatedly noted upon mitogenic stimulation of
fibroblastic and transformed cells are increased intracellular
concentrations of polyamines, the synthesis of which are
controlled by ODC and cAMP levels.(17)

TABLE 1

EPIDERMAL GROWTH FACTOR, EPINEPHRINE AND PITUITARY EXTRACT INTERACTIONS: RELATIONSHIP OF ORNITHINE DECARBOXYLASE ACTIVITY, cAMP LEVEL AND THE CLONAL GROWTH RATE OF NHBE CELLS

Additive	Ornithine Decarboxylase*	cAMP**	Population Doublings/Day
LHC-O	100	100	0.45
+ Pituitary Extract	115	140	0.45
+ Epinephrine	220	500	0.45
+ Epidermal Growth Factor	300	130	0.67
+ Pituitary Extract and Epinephrine	240	−NT	0.45
+ Epidermal Growth Factor and Epinephrine	660	670	0.67
+ Epidermal Growth Factor and Pituitary Extract	440	115	0.91
+ All Three	515	1200	1.24

*Ornithine Decarboxylase = 0.65 ($\pm$0.2) U/mg protein
**cAMP = 0.35 ($\pm$0.05) pMoles/10^6 cells.

We measured these two parameters six hours after the cells were exposed to the medium additives because preliminary experiments showed that both had attained plateau levels by that time. As can be seen in Table 1, EPI did not increase the rate at which the cells multiplied even though the concentration of ODC doubled and the level of cAMP increased five fold. On the other hand, EGF which did increase the clonal growth rate increased only the ornithine decarboxylase activity. We further evaluated this finding by testing the effect of α-difluoromethyl ornithine, a noncompetitive inhibitor of ODC, and found that this compound inhibited the mitogenic activity of EGF in a dose-response manner. In addition, we discovered that exogenously added putrescine would overcome the effects of α-difluoromethyl ornithine.

Of the dual combinations, only EGF and BPE caused a greater rate of cell multiplication, and again, the pattern was a markedly enhanced activity without a significant increase in the level of cAMP (Table 1). In contrast, the combination of EGF and EPI caused great increases in both ODC activity and the level of cAMP, but the growth rate of the cells was equal to that of EGF alone. Finally, the combination of all three additives further enhanced both the growth rate of the cells and the intracellular level of cAMP. We further found that the B-adrenergic receptor antagonist propranolol abolished the increase in growth rate caused by adding EPI to media containing EGF and BPE.

FIGURE 1

SQUAMOUS DIFFERENTIATION PATHWAYS OF NORMAL HUMAN BRONCHIAL
EPITHELIAL CELLS

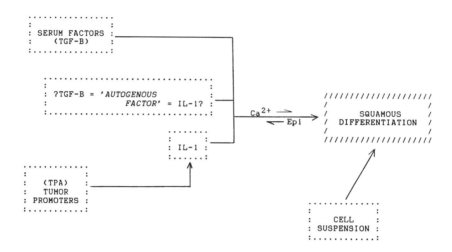

We concluded from these experiments that increased ODC activity is necessary but not sufficient for NHBE cell division to occur because EPI alone will significantly increase ODC activity without altering the growth rate. We also concluded that a high level of cAMP is not correlated with rapid growth unless pathways controlled by undefined factors in BPE are also operative.

Establishing the interactions that control normal cell multiplication and how these processes differ in cancer cells is central for understanding carcinogenesis. However, it is also important to remember that epithelial cancers likely arise as a consequence of aberrations in tissue renewal processes, resulting in cells expressing partially differentiated phenotypes that have uncontrolled and unlimited proliferative capacities.(18) Therefore, it is of equal importance to determine the role medium constituents play in controlling normal cellular differentiation. Bronchial epithelial cells undergo several types of differentiation including cilia and mucin secretion, but we have focused primarily on squamous differentiation because: 1) Squamous metaplasia of bronchial epithelium is universally present in the airways of smokers as a consequence of chemical wounding of the tissue and 2) 40% of human lung cancers are squamous cell carcinomas. Therefore, we have concentrated our initial efforts on defining the pathways that control NHBE cell squamous differentiation (see Fig. 1).

However, before initiating these investigations, we determined the markers of squamous differentiation for NHBE cells: (a) cell division and DNA synthesis cease irreversibly; (b) the cells acquire a squamous morphology; (c) they increase the release of plasminogen activator; and (d) they form cross-linked envelopes as measured by resistance to SDS treatment.

By far, the most surprising medium additive that will induce NHBE cells to undergo squamous differentiation is serum.(9,11) Our first approach towards identifying the active factor(s) in serum responsible for inducing squamous differentiation was to compare the activity of whole blood serum against serum formed by the clotting of plasma.(19) We found that plasma- derived serum did not induce squamous differentiation nor was plasma mitogenic. Since plasma did not induce squamous differentiation, we began testing lysed formed-element extracts and discovered that lysed platelet extracts were potent inducers of squamous differentiation. Therefore, we tested highly purified platelet derived growth factor (obtained from H. Antoniades at Harvard). Although this highly purified platelet derived growth factor preparation was mitogenic for normal human bronchial fibroblastic cells, it had no effect, either mitogenic or squamous differentiation inducing, on NHBE cells.

Subsequently, we focused on another major constituent of platelets, transforming growth factor beta (TGF-B) and determined that this peptide is indeed the primary serum squamous differentiation inducing factor.(20) TGF-B induces all of the markers associated with NHBE cells undergoing squamous differentiation. In addition, the IgG fraction of rabbit anti-TGF-B antiserum neutralizes the inhibition of DNA synthesis caused by either TGF-B or serum in a dose-dependent manner and also prevents squamous differentiation of NHBE cells in the presence of TGF-B or serum. The conclusion from these data is that TGF-B is playing a necessary and primary role in the differentiation induction process caused by serum.

The fact that serum, and more specifically, transforming growth factor beta are potent inducers of squamous differentiation of NHBE cells is in marked contrast to the well known results of Hennings and Yuspa (21) whose data suggest that the primary trigger of squamous differentiation of murine epidermal keratinocytes is a medium concentration of Ca^{2+} ions greater than 300 uM. Their experiments, however, differed from ours in three significant ways: (1) Their cells were cultured at high cell densities, whereas, the NHBE cells were cultured at clonal cell density. (2) They used serum-containing media, whereas, we used serum-free conditions. (3) They studied epidermal keratinocytes as opposed to our investigations with NHBE cells. Nonetheless, their Ca^{2+} observations stimulated us to investigate the effects of medium Ca^{2+} levels on NHBE cells and to ascertain if serum and/or cell density could explain the differences between our results and Hennings' and Yuspa's results.(9,10,12).

Calcium dose-response experiments carried out at clonal (100 cells/cm^2) and high (2500 cells/cm^2) cell densities in the absence of serum showed that calcium has no effect on the growth or differentiation of NHBE cells inoculated at clonal densities whereas, and in marked contrast, rapid induction of squamous differentiation occurs when the cells are inoculated at high cell density in medium calcium concentrations greater than 0.3 mM. On the other hand, when the density calcium dose-response experiments were conducted at clonal cell density with medium containing a low concentration of serum (1.25%; an amount less than that required to induce squamous differentiation), the percent of squamous NHBE cells increased directly as a function of the calcium concentration.

Our preliminary interpretation of these differences between high and low cell density cultures suggest that: NHBE cells elaborate an autocrine squamous differentiation inducing factor that only rises to an effective concentration in high density cell cultures because a larger number of cells are secreting the factor and Ca^{2+} potentiates factor release and/or serves as a co-factor to activate the released factor. Because TGF-B has been identified as an endogenous growth inhibitory and differentiation inducer, NHBE cell-conditioned medium was tested for the amount and form of TGF-B. NHBE cells secrete considerable amounts of TGF-B in a latent form.(22) Although the activation process of latent TGF-B is not known and considered an important controlling point in vivo, it is feasible that TGF-B has a differentiation controlling role for NHBE cells. Recently, however, a second peptide (interleukin-1; IL-1) has been identified as a possible autocrine inducing agent.(23) This factor is produced by murine keratinocytes when induced to undergo squamous differentiation (24) and when added to cultures of NHBE cells these cells cease DNA synthesis and become squamous. Preliminary northern blotting experiments have shown that IL-1 mRNAs are synthesized by NHBE cells. Thus, additional experiments are planned to investigate the potential roles of both TGF-B and IL-1 as autocrine squamous differentiating signals for NHBE cells.

Endogenous (and/or autocrine) agents are not the only stimuli that will induce NHBE cells to undergo squamous differentiation. A second condition is cell suspension. Rheinwald first reported this phenomenon and showed that normal keratinocytes are rapidly induced to undergo terminal squamous differentiation when incubated in suspension.(14) We know very little about how suspension induces the NHBE cells to undergo squamous differentiation except that the process is time dependent and it is very efficient. Finally, exogenous agents such as the phorbol ester 12-0-tetradecanol-phorbol-13-acetate (TPA), the indole alkaloid teleocidin B, aplysiatoxin, and certain aldehydes and peroxides can induce terminal squamous differentiation of NHBE cells in vitro.(25,26,27) Most of these latter agents are classified as tumor promoters according to the mouse skin two-stage carcinogenesis model.

A key to understanding the pathways of squamous differentiation is to find metabolic inhibitors. We have found that excess amino acids and retinoic acid will decrease the rate by which the putative autogenous factor induces squamous differentiation.(13) However, potentially more interesting are our observations that epinephrine and other cAMP enhancers are potent antagonists of squamous differentiation inducers.(20,22) Epinephrine and TGF-B are mutually antagonistic; epinephrine neutralizes the inhibition on DNA synthesis and inhibits the induction of squamous differentiation caused by TGF-B, whereas TGF-B inhibits the growth enhancement caused by epinephrine. We have measured the cAMP levels in NHBE cells exposed to TGF-B and epinephrine. As expected, epinephrine causes increased levels of cAMP. On the other hand, TGF-B cancels the growth enhancement caused by epinephrine and induces differentiation of NHBE cells without altering the cAMP levels in the cells. Therefore, epinephrine and TGF-B appear to affect different intracellular pathways that control growth and differentiation processes of NHBE cells, and that the differentiation-inducing effect of TPA is partially antagonized by epinephrine.(22) This latter observation supports the suggestion that TGF-B and TPA may share common steps and that epinephrine may cause certain effects that are antagonistic to differentiation induction. In summary (see also Fig. 1), both endogenous and exogenous inducers of terminal squamous differentiation of NHBE cells cultured in vitro have been identified and cAMP enhancers antagonize the activity of these agents.

We have characterized several lung carcinoma cell lines from the perspective of comparing the multiplication and differentiation control processes operating in these cells against the mechanisms already determined for the normal cells. Three significant differences between the NHBE and established lines of lung carcinoma cells have become apparent.(19) First, none of the carcinomas are induced by serum to undergo squamous differentiation, i.e., they all grow in 8% serum supplemented medium. Second and surprisingly, the carcinomas are more fastidious than are the normal cells, i.e., all of the carcinoma cells grow slowly or not at all when incubated at clonal cell density in serum-free media optimized for rapid growth of NHBE cells. Third, only the carcinoma cells exhibit the ability to respond to serum-borne mitogens. (We have observed similar results with primary lung tumors. Specifically for 9 of 9 primary explants of lung tumor tissue obtained from different donors the same serum differential effect was noted, e.g., cell outgrowth occurred only from explants incubated in LHC medium supplemented with 2% FBS, unpublished.) We have also determined that neither confluence nor cell suspension cause the carcinoma cells to undergo squamous differentiation. Finally, the carcinoma cells are relatively resistant to induction of squamous differentiation caused by tumor promoters.(26,27) Thus, aberrations of both multiplication and differentiation control mechanisms occur as a consequence of carcinogenesis. These significant differences between normal and carcinoma cells provide the framework to identify premalignant and malignant cells after bronchial epithelial cells have been exposed to initiating or promoting agents, transfected with oncogenes or subjected to the combination of agent exposure and oncogene transfection.

Initially, we determined the long-term effect of cultured NHBE cells exposed to Ni_2SO_4.(28) The cells were continuously exposed to a dose (5-20 ug/ml) of Ni_2SO_4 that reduced their colony-forming efficiency 30-80%. After 40 days of incubation, the cultures consisted of large squamous cells, and mitotic cells were not observed. The cells were then maintained in medium without Ni_2SO_4. After 40-75 total days of incubation, colonies of mitotic cells appeared at a rate of one colony per 100,000 cells originally at risk. On the other hand, no colonies appeared in control cultures or in cultures exposed to $5ugNi_2SO_4$/ml for 90 days. Twelve Ni_2SO_4-altered cell cultures isolated from five experiments have been expanded into mass cultures. Most of the cell populations recovered have an increased population-doubling potential. Some exhibit aberrations in the terminal squamous differentiation process whereas others have lost the requirement for EGF for clonal growth. Aneuploidy and marker chromosomes have also been noted. However, none of these Ni_2SO_4-altered cell cultures was anchorage -independent nor produced tumors upon injection into athymic nude mice. Therefore, in contrast to the reported results with rodent cells (29), we found that the long-term exposure of NHBE cells to Ni_2SO_4 did not result in malignantly transformed cells. Instead, we have found that the cells, after prolonged exposure to Ni_2SO_4-altered cultures, have reduced growth factor requirements and an extended culture population-doubling potential, reduced responsiveness to differentiation inducers, i.e., serum and TPA, and chromosomal abnormalities. Although these properties are found in carcinoma cells, the altered cells have also retained normal cell characteristics, i.e., they do not recognize FBS factors as mitogens, are anchorage-dependent, and are not tumorigenic.

Recently we have initiated investigations similar in design to those described above for Ni_2SO_4 with cigarette smoke condensate (CSC).(30,31) Initially, we ascertained the effect of whole CSC and some fractions (two basic fractions (B_{Ia}, B_{Ib}) of CSC, the ethanol extracted weakly acidic fraction (WA_e) and the methanol-extracted neutral fraction (N_{meoh}) on the clonal growth rate, (PA) activity, (CLE) formation, (ODC) activity, EGF binding, thiol levels, and DNA single strand breaks (SSB). Neither CSC nor any of the fractions were mitogenic over the range 0.01-100 ug/ml; all were growth inhibitory at higher concentrations. The 50% growth inhibitory concentration (IC_{50})

for CSC, B_{Ia}, B_{Ib}, WA_w, and N_{meoh} were 10, 10, 10, 3, and 1 ug/ml, respectively. Effects of CLE formation, morphology, PA, and ODC activities, EGF binding, and thiol levels were evaluated using IC_{50} concentrations. We found that CSC and all fractions caused an increased formation of CLEs; from a baseline of 0.5% in the untreated cells to a maximum increase of 25% induced by N_{meoh}. A squamous morphological change was observed within one hour after exposure to N_{meoh}, WA_e, and CSC. The B_{Ia} and B_{Ib} fractions had little effect. Only N_{meoh}, increased PA significantly, from 2.5 +/- 0.4 to 5.1 +/- 0.3 units/mg cellular protein. CSC and the WA_e and N_{meoh} fractions caused a decrease in EGF binding, in each case reaching a maximum effect after a 10-12 hour incubation. This effect on EGF binding was further characterized in the case of N_{meoh}. In untreated NHBE cells, by Scatchard analysis the K_d was 2.0 nM and there were 1.2×10^5 receptors per cell. In cells incubated in medium containing N_{meoh} (3 ug/ml) the k_d was 3.2 nM and there were 1.1×10^5 receptors per cell. Thus, inhibition of EGF binding by N_{meoh} was due primarily to a decrease in the affinity. At the IC_{50} neither CSC nor any of the fractions significantly affected intracellular thiol levels. While a 3 hour incubation in medium containing CSC caused significant DNA SSB only at a concentration of 100 ug/ml, N_{meoh} caused a marked effect at 5 ug/ml. Neither CSC nor any of the fractions had an effect on ODC activity.

Due to the effects of the N_{meoh} fraction on growth, morphology, EGF binding, PA activity, and formation of SSB, we considered it likely that this portion of CSC contained compounds with actions similar to those of indole alkaloid and polyacetate tumor promoters. Therefore, we investigated the inhibition of phorbol dibutyrate (PDBU) binding by both whole CSC and subfractions. Both whole condensate and the N_{meoh} fraction caused a significant inhibition of PDBU binding. However, the degree of inhibition is relatively small. Whole CSC and the N_{meoh} fraction reduced this binding from 100% of the control value to 86 +/- 13% and 81 +/- 11%, respectively; the basic and acidic fractions had no effect. Thus, the TPA-like component(s) appears to be a minor portion of the tumor promoting activity of whole CSC.

Another mechanism by which whole CSC and its fractions might have a selective effect on NHBE cells is through induction of terminal differentiation. This possibility is supported by the morphologic data that whole CSC and the N_{meoh} fraction changed NHBE cells to be more squamous in appearance with a marked increase in cell surface area. In contrast, none of the tested carcinoma cell lines exhibited marked morphological changes when exposed to CSC or its fractions. A second possible promoter mechanism is differential cytotoxicity. CSC contains a number of compounds known to have cytotoxic effects.(32) Support for this hypothesis derives from our recent observations that for all of the carcinoma lines tested, the cells continued to multiply at concentrations of whole CSC or its fractions that were cytotoxic to the NHBE cells. Thus, neoplastic cells may have selective clonal expansion advantage due to their decreased sensitivity to the differentiation inducing and cytotoxic agents in tobacco smoke.

Certain oncogenes have been shown to readily transform fibroblastic cells, i.e., NIH 3T3 cells, and oncogene expression plays a role in carcinogenesis.(33) To date three families of oncogenes, ras, myc, and raf, have been associated with human lung carcinomas. Initially, NHBE cells were transfected by v-Ha-ras oncogene by protoplast fusion (34) and selected in the presence of serum in the medium, since previous studies had shown that lung carcinoma cells are relatively resistant to differentiation induction and grow better in the presence of serum. Transformed foci resulted and one cell line (TBE-1) has been studied extensively. The v-Ha-ras-transfected cells are not induced to differentiate terminally by either 2% BDS or 100 nM TPA. TBE-1 cells also rarely grow in semisolid medium. When they are xenotransplanted into athymic nude mice, TBE-1 cells initially produce small, regressing tumors, and after 7 to 10 months these tumors reappeared in only a few mice. In contrast, cells isolated from colonies of TBE-1 cells growing in agar (i.e., TBE-SA) have a higher activity of type IV collagenase and produce progressively growing tumors with a latency period of approximately 2 months. These tumor cells (i.e., TBE-1SAT) have been shown to be of human origin on the basis of their isoenzyme patterns and the chromosomal analysis of the cultured cells. When TBE-1SAT cells are injected into athymic nude mice, they again display their tumorigenic properties. When analyzed by immunoperoxidase staining, these anaplastic tumors contain small amounts of keratin; they also produce B human chorionic gonadotropin. The mechanism by which the v-Ha-ras p21 initiates this multistage process is unknown. The possibility that a secondary alteration causing increased expression of a non-ras oncogene might have occurred was tested by extracting total RNA and screening by "dot-blot" hybridization with probes specific for H-ras, N-myc, c-myc, and raf. In no case was increased expression of these oncogenes observed.

We have also transfected NHBE cells with three other oncogenes, c-raf-1 (22), Bmyc (22) and SV40-T-antigen gene (35). C-raf-1 is expressed routinely in neural crest-derived cells and cells of hematopoietic origin. As these cells differentiate the level of raf-1 mRNA decreases. In addition, for all SCLC cells examined to date, both cell lines (12, including classic and variant phenotypes) and fresh metastatic tissues, express elevated levels of c-raf-1 RNA compared with NHBE cells and normal lung tissues. However, in contrast to the above described results following the introduction of the v-Ha ras gene into NHBE cells, the transfection of the c-raf-1 oncogene into the cells is without observable consequence.

It has been reported that the introduction of v-myc into U-937 cells, a human monoblast cell line, leads to inhibition of differentiation induced by TPA. Thus, we have transfected NHBE cells with Bmyc using the protoplast fusion method (22); pSV_2 neo was transfected as a control since the Burkitt's myc gene had been subcloned into pSV_2 neo. After serum (4%) or TPA (10nM) selection for three weeks, resistant colonies were stained and counted. $Bmyc/pSV_2$ neo transfected cultures of NHBE cells show a five fold increase in the frequency of differentiation resistant colonies compared to the control. However, the cells populating the resistant colonies proved not to be immortal.

NHBE cells have also been transformed by transfection with a recombinant plasmid containing the SV40 large T-antigen gene, or by infection with either SV40 virus or adenovirus-12 SV40 hybrid virus.(35) Several colonies of transformed cells derived by each of these means have been cultured and characterized. These cells have colony forming efficiencies 3- to 6-fold greater than NHBE cells and a culture lifespan that is significantly greater (70 population doublings [PD]) than NHBE cells (ca. 30 PD), and growth rates ranging from normal (0.7 PD/day in medium without epinephrine) to 1.5 times normal. All of these cells have keratin and SV40 T-antigen as detected by indirect immuno-fluorescence, and retain electron microscopic features of epithelial cells. All are aneuploid, and most are polyploid. Cells injected into nude mice have so far formed no tumors after periods ranging from 2 to 8 months. Unlike bronchial carcinoma cell lines but, significantly, like NHBE cells, many of these cultures undergo terminal squamous differentiation in response to serum, while a few are relatively resistant to serum.

Experiments are in progress to study multistage carcinogenesis of these cells using carcinogens and transfected oncogenes and to determine the relationship, if any, between the loss of the ability of these cells to respond to squamous differentiating signals and the onset of tumorigenicity. In addition, the SV40T-antigen gene has been transfected into the Ni_2SO_4 phenotypically-altered (see above) cells. Although their characterization is not yet completed, these "two step" cells do express several different growth control properties. The reverse experiment (T-antigen transfection followed by continuous exposure to Ni_2SO_4) is in progress.

CONCLUSIONS

A highly reproducible and well-characterized, serum-free in vitro model system is now available for studying the processes of growth, differentiation and carcinogenesis of normal human bronchial epithelial cells. When these cells are incubated in defined media, epinephrine increases the intracellular cAMP but the growth rate is not affected unless pathways controlled by as yet undefined pituitary factors are also operating. Serum (platelet) factors, calcium, cell density-suggested factors, certain tumor promoters, and cell suspension induce the cells to undergo squamous differentiation and epinephrine and cholera toxin antagonize these inducers of squamous differentiation. Finally, both multiplication and differentiation aberrations are associated with transformation of human bronchial epithelial cells.

Recently, several laboratories have pointed to the importance of aberrant differentiation as an important step in carcinogenesis (36,37). This hypothesis is especially well suited to living epithelial cells. Continuous multiplication is considered to be the primary steady state for these cells and the cessation of multiplication is a restriction imposed upon the system through cellular differentiation. Any event that produces a heritable block in the cell's natural terminal differentiation processes will _ipso_ _facto_ result in continuous cell multiplication. We have shown that some activated or introduced oncogenes can alter a cell's ability to recognize/process natural differentiation inducing signals and thus, impede normal differentiation patterns, including squamous differentiation and programmed cell death "mortality." Thus, it is not unreasonable to regard growth factor/receptor oncogenes through "agents" that prevent the cell from exiting from the cycle of DNA synthesis. The immediate consequence of this point of view of carcinogenesis from the treatment perspective is that, if valid, the prospects for finding agents that can discriminate the multiplication control processes of malignant cells from their normal homologues is remote. On the other hand, the search for physiologically tolerable agents that can induce malignant cells to terminally differentiate should be encouraged.

REFERENCES

1. Autrup, H., Harris, C.C. (1983): In: Human Carcinogenesis, edited by C.C. Harris, and H.N. Autrup, pp 169-194. Academic Press, New York.
2. DiPaolo, J.A. (1983): J. Natl. Cancer Inst., 70:3-8.
3. Lechner, J.F., Haugen, A., Trump, B.F., Tokiwa, T., and Harris, C.C. (1983): In: Human Carcinogenesis, edited by C.C. Harris, and H.N. Autrup, pp 561-585. Academic Press, New York.
4. Lechner, J.F., Tokiwa, T., Yeager, Jr., H., and Harris, C.E. (1985): In: In Vitro Effects of Mineral Dusts, edited by E.G. Beck and J. Bignon, pp 197-200, Springer-Verlag, Berlin.
5. Lechner, J.F., Tokiwa, T., LaVeck, M., Benedict, W.F., Banks-Schlegal, S., Yeager, Jr., H., Banerjoe, A., and Harris, C.C. (1985): Proc. Natl. Acad. Sci., 82:3884-3888.

6. Gabrielson, E.W., Lechner, J.F., Gerwin, B., Sporn, M.B., Wakefield, L.M., Roberts, A.B., and Harris (1986): J. Cell. Biochem. Sup., 10C:179.

7. Stoner, G.D., Katoh, Y., Foidart, J., Myers, G.A., and Harris, C.C. (1980): Meth. Cell Biol., 21A:15–35.

8. Lechner, J.F., Haugen, A., Autrup, H., McClendon, I.A., Trump, B.F., and Harris, C.C. (1981): Cancer Res., 41:2294–2304.

9. Lechner, J.F., Haugen, A., McClendon, I.A., and Pettis, E.W. (1982): In Vitro, 18:633–642.

10. Lechner, J.F., Haugen, A., McClendon, I.A., and Shamsuddin, A. (1984): Differentiation, 25:229–237.

11. Lechner, J.F. (1984): In Vitro Monog., 5:80–83.

12. Lechner, J.F., and LaVeck, M.A. (1985): J. Tissue Culture Meth., 9:43–48.

13. Lechner, J.F., Stone, G.D., Yoakum, G.H., Willey, J.C., Grafstrom, R.C., Masui, T., LaVeck, M.A., and Harris, C.C. (1986): In: In Vitro Models of Respiratory Epithelium, edited by L.J. Schiff, pp 143–159. CRC Press, Boca Raton.

14. Rhienwald, J.G. (1980): Methods Cell Biol., 21A:229–254.

15. Peehl, D.M., and Ham, R.C. (1980): In Vitro, 16:526–538.

16. Autrup, H., Lechner, J.F., and Harris, C.C. (1983): In: Safety Evaluation and Regulation of Chemicals, edited by F. Homburger, pp. 151–159. S. Karger AG, Basel.

17. Willey, J.C., McClendon, I.A., LaVeck, M.A., and Lechner, J.F. (1985): J. Cell Physiol., 124:207–212.

18. Pierce, G.B. (1970): Fed. Proc., 19:1248–1254.

19. Lechner, J.F., McClendon, I.A., LaVeck, M.A., Shamsuddin, A.K., and Harris, C.C. (1983): Cancer Res., 43:5915–5929.

20. Masui, T., Wakefield, L.M., Lechner, J.F., LaVeck, M.A., Sporn, M.B., and Harris, C.C. (1986): Proc. Natl. Acad. Sci., 83:2438–2442.

21. Hennings, H., Michaels, D., Cheng, C., Steinert, P., Holbrook, K., and Yuspa, S.H. (1980): Cell, 19:245–254.

22. Masui, T., Lechner, J.F., Mark, G.E. III, Pfiefer, A.M.A., Miyashita, M., Yoakum, G.H., Willey, J.C., Mann, D.L., and Harris, C.C. (in press): J. Cell. Biochem.

23. Lechner, J.F., LaVeck, M.A., Gerwin, B., and Harris, C.C. (unpublished).

24. Lugar, T.A., Stadler, B.M., Katz, S.I., and Oppenheim, J.J. (1981): J. Immunol., 127:1493–1498.

25. Harris, C.C., Yoakum, G.H., Lechner, J.F., Willey, J.C., Gerwin, B., Banks-Schlegel, S., Masui, T., and Mark, G. (1986): In: Biochemical and Molecular Epidemiology of Cancer, edited by C.C. Harris, pp. 213–226. Alan R. Liss, New York.

26. Willey, J.C., Saladino, A.J., Ozanne, C., Lechner, J.F., and Harris, C.C. (1984): Carcinogenesis, 5:209–215.

27. Willey, J.C., Moser, C.E., Lechner, J.F., and Harris, C.C. (1984): Cancer Res., 44:5124–5126.

28. Lechner, J.F., Tokiwa, T., McClendon, I.A., and Haugen, A. (1984): Carcinogenesis, 5:1697-1703.
29. DiPaolo, J.A., and Castro, B.C. (1979): Cancer Res., 39:1008-1013.
30. Willey, J.C., Grafstrom, R.C., Moser, Jr., C.E., Ozanne, C., Sundqvist, K., and Harris, C.C. (in press): Cancer Res.
31. Miyashita, M., Willey, J.C., Sasajima, K., Lechner, J.F., and Harris, C.C. (submitted): Cancer Res.
32. Harris, C.C., Willey, J.C., Saladino, A.J., and Grafstrom (1985): In: Carcinogenesis, Vol. 8, edited by J. Mass, et.al., pp 159-171. Raven Press, New York.
33. Land, H., Parada, L.F., and Weinberg, R.A. (1983): Science, 222:771-775.
34. Yoakum, G.H., Korba, B.F., Lechner, J.F., Tokiwa, T., Gazdar, A.F., Secky, T., Siegel, M., Leeman, L., Autrup, H., and Harris, C.C. (1983): Science, 222:385-389.
35. Ke, Y., Reddel, R.R., Lechner, J.F., Su, R., Park, J.B., Rhim, J.S., and Harris, C.C. (1986): J. Cell Biol. Abs., in press.
36. Harris, H. (1986): J. Cell Sci. Suppl., 4:431-444.
37. Muller, R. (1985): Trends Biochem. Sci., 11:129-132.

Tumor Promoters: Biological Approaches for
Mechanistic Studies and Assay Systems,
edited by Robert Langenbach et al.
Raven Press, New York © 1988.

EFFECTS OF A TUMOR PROMOTER ON CULTURES OF NORMAL

AND CARCINOGEN-TREATED HUMAN ENDOMETRIAL STROMAL CELLS:

EVIDENCE FOR DICHOTOMOUS SELECTION

David G. Kaufman and Jill M. Siegfried[*]

Department of Pathology and Cancer Research Center,
University of North Carolina, Chapel Hill, NC 27514
and [*]Carcinogenesis Section, Environmental Health Research
and Testing, Inc., Research Triangle Park, NC 27709

ABSTRACT

The tumor promoter 12-0-tetradecanoylphorbol 13-acetate (TPA)
was found to enhance the expression of alterations induced by
N-methyl-N'-nitro-N-nitrosoguanidine (MNNG) in stromal cells
derived from normal human endometrium. Cells "initiated" by MNNG
exposure were exposed to TPA continuously over several months.
Alterations in growth parameters and expression of gamma-glutamyl-
transpeptidase (GGT) were enhanced when these cells were compared
to cells exposed to MNNG followed by ethanol, the vehicle for TPA
treatments. In cells that had not been treated with MNNG, TPA
appeared to inhibit alterations in growth parameters or GGT. This
suggests that the promoter exerted different effects on normal and
carcinogen-altered cells: a dichotomous selection.

INTRODUCTION

Development of malignancies is known to occur in progressive
stages in both human cancer (2,11,17,20) and in animal models of

carcinogenesis (4,5,19,21). Not only have progressive histologic changes been documented in vivo, but in cell culture models, progressive alterations in growth properties have been identified after carcinogen treatment (3,14). Tumor promoting agents, such as phorbol esters and hormones, are known to enhance progression toward malignancy in vivo (1,12,18,25) and in vitro (9,15,24,26). Cell culture studies have largely utilized cells of rodent origin to demonstrate tumor promotion.

We studied whether a process resembling promotion could be documented in cells of human origin and examined whether tumor promoters could induce selective growth of cells that had been treated with a carcinogen. These studies were done with cultures of stromal cell derived from normal human endometrial tissue. In this report, we describe the properties of these cells in culture, the effects of treatments with MNNG in vitro, and the results of treatments of these cells with the tumor promoter TPA.

BIOLOGY OF THE HUMAN ENDOMETRIUM

The endometrium is a complicated tissue both because of its organization and because of the hormone-induced changes that occur in it during the menstrual cycle. The endometrium is entirely derived from mesoderm and composed primarily of two cell types. Epithelial cells compose the surface of the endometrial cavity and also line endometrial glands. Stromal cells are the most numerous cells of the tissue and they form a spongy framework surrounding glands and blood vessels. Stromal cells are a specific cell type and are different from the fibroblasts that form the stroma of most other organs. Endometrial stromal cells, like endometrial epithelial cells, have steroid hormone receptors and are hormonally responsive. Stromal cells are metabolically active, and respond to changes in the hormonal environment by undergoing morphologic and biochemical changes during the menstrual cycle (6,27).

The menstrual cycle is characterized by changes in ovarian follicles, serum hormone levels and endometrial morphology. During theproliferative phase of the menstrual cycle, the endometrium is characterized by a low columnar epithelium lining glands and the tissue surface. The stromal cells are bipolar and resemble fibroblasts. Both populations undergo cell division and contribute to the formation of an enlarged uterine lining. During the secretory phase, epithelial cells become higher and form tortuous glands. The stromal cells become larger and rounder and assume an epithelioid, pavement-like configuration at sites of predecidual differentiation (10). During pregnancy they become the decidual cells at the placental implantation site, a change to a more differentiated state of stromal cells.

CULTURE OF HUMAN ENDOMETRIAL CELLS

When endometrial tissue is subjected to brief enzymatic digestion with collagenase and then placed into primary culture, two major types of cells are established as cultures on the plates. One type forms compact colonies of swirling, tadpole-shaped cells; these cells are incapable of surviving repetitive subculture under conditions used in our laboratory to the present. The other cell type is readily subcultured. They have a polygonal shape and are arranged in a pavement-like pattern when grown in CMRL-1066 medium but they are bipolar and appear similar to fibro-blasts when grown in Dulbecco's minimal essential medium (DMEM). The cell of origin for these two types of cell cultures was deter-mined based on histochemical and immunochemical studies (7). The staining properties of endometrial tissue in frozen sections was compared with the staining properties of the different types of cells in culture. For example, alkaline phosphatase is a good marker for epithelial cells in glands in the intact tissue and also stains the colonies with swirling, tadpole shaped cells. Similarly, fibronectin proved to be a good marker for stromal cells in frozen sections and the subculturable cells were shown to react positively by immunochemical staining. Because stromal cells could be maintained in cell culture, they were used in subsequent studies.

Endometrial stromal cells in culture display many of the characteristics of stromal cells in vivo. They have enzyme activities, such as leucine aminopeptidase (7), which are found in the endometrial stroma. They express predecidual morphology and produce glycogen in response to hormonal priming with estrogen followed by treatment with progesterone in simulated menstrual cycles in vitro (8,23). Stromal cells have been maintained in culture for more than a year through 50 passages, but they still have a finite lifespan. In DMEM, stromal cells maintain a bipolar fibroblastic pattern, while in CMRL medium, stromal cells take on a polygonal appearance. The stromal cells can be induced to take on the appearance of pseudodecidual cells by programmed hormonal treatment. These steps of differentiation are reversible and are dependent on the conditions of culture. Thus the endo-metrial cell cultures demonstrate the pathway of differentiation of human endometrial stromal cells as deduced from observations of the intact tissue. The whole range of differentiation can be reproduced in culture by adjustments of the culture medium.

CARCINOGEN-INDUCED TRANSFORMATION OF HUMAN STROMAL CELLS

The initial goal of this study was to develop a cell culture system in which normal diploid human cells could be transformed in a multi-step process as occurs in vivo. Such a system might be used to discover the biologic nature of these individual steps and achieve a detailed mechanistic insight. It was our thought that this system should use cells which have a high growth capacity in primary culture and which had not been preselected for growth or exposed to any other extreme conditions of cell culture. Furthermore, we used repetitive carcinogen treatments that caused little toxicity. This was thought to better approximate the conditions of human exposures in vivo than single large doses that produce high levels of cell toxicity. A system for chemical carcinogenesis in vitro with these properties (TABLE 1) was established using human endometrial stromal cells.

TABLE 1. Specifications for cell transformation system in vitro

---

    1. Start with Normal, Diploid, Adult Human Cells
    2. Cells Not Strongly Selected by Growth Conditions
    3. Carcinogen Treatments with Low Toxicity
    4. Multiple, Repetitive Carcinogen Treatments
    5. Multiple Step Process of Transformation In Vitro

TABLE 2 shows the protocol for carcinogen treatments with MNNG. Carcinogen treatments were multiple and repetitive. Exposures to 0.5 or 1.0 µg/ml MNNG in acetone vehicle, which were used most commonly, produced little toxicity in the cultures. Control cells were treated with equal volumes of the acetone vehicle. The progress of the treatment protocol was noted as the number of individual treatments or by specifying the cumulative carcinogen exposure that the cells had received.

TABLE 2. Experimental plan for MNNG treatments

MNNG TREATMENTS: 1 2 3 4 5 6 7 8 9 10
                    ↓ ↓ ↓ ↓ ↓ ↓ ↓ ↓ ↓ ↓
            CARCINOGEN-TREATED EXPERIMENTAL CELLS

            ACETONE-TREATED VEHICLE CONTROL CELLS

Our studies have demonstrated that upon repetitive treatment with the methylating agent MNNG, stromal cells in culture undergo a series of progressive changes which are reminiscent of cell transformation (TABLE 3). With increasing numbers of MNNG treatments, the stromal cells show progressive morphologic alterations. Cells develop a higher plating efficiency and saturation density, they grow with a shorter doubling time, and they become anchorage independent (23). They acquire the ability to form colonies in restrictivemedia (13,22) and express the enzyme gamma glutamyltranspeptidase (23). In contrast, after 50 weeks of culture, normal untreated stromal cells are not changed to an appreciable extent. Even after a single carcinogen treatment the morphology of the treated cells is not greatly altered either soon after the treatment or after a year of subsequent maintenance in culture.

TABLE 3. Sequence of appearance of MNNG-induced alterations

Number of Treatments		Carcinogen-Induced Alteration
1 -		
2 -	E	Resist Carcinogen-Induced Toxicity
	A	
3 -	R	Slight Morphologic Changes
	L	Plating Efficiency Increases
4 -	Y	Saturation Density Increases
		Pronounced Morphologic Change
5 -	M	
	I	Growth Rate Double that of Normals
6 -	D	Anchorage-Independent Growth
	D	
7 -	L	Appearance of GGT Positive Cells
	E	Cloning in Restrictive Media
8 -		
	L	Severe Morphologic Abnormalities
9 -	A	Growth of Cells in Suspension
	T	Colonies form Macroscopic Foci
10 -	E	Expression of Abnormal LDH Isoenzymes

STUDIES OF A "PROMOTION-LIKE" PROCESS IN CULTURED STROMAL CELLS

Next, we undertook to determine whether the prototype strong tumor promoter, TPA, could produce a "promotion-like" process in this system in vitro. Since the expression of carcinogen-induced phenotypic changes in this system was primarily dependent on total carcinogen exposure (8), cultures could be obtained at different stages by varying the total number treatments or the cumulative quantity of exposures to MNNG (TABLE 4).

TABLE 4. Experimental plan for MNNG treatments

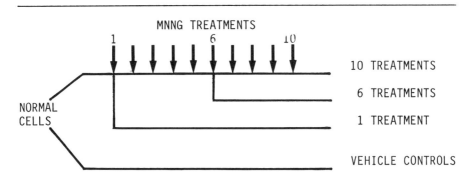

Expression of further alterations was then monitored period-ically after chronic TPA treatment. Our approach to studying "promotion-like" phenomena in cell culture again was formulated with a view of the conditions of the process of tumor promotion in vivo. In particular, we chose to examine the influence of promoters on cultured cells after prolonged continuous exposures lasting from three to six months.

TABLE 5. Experimental plan for TPA treatments

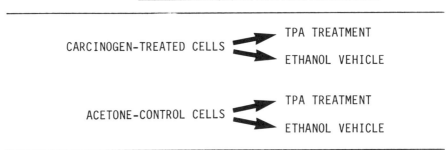

The general plan for these studies (TABLE 5) was to compare the effects of the promoter to the effect of its vehicle (ethanol). These comparisons were to be made between cells previously-treated with MNNG and their vehicle controls (acetone). TABLE 6 illustrates the experimental plan for these studies in a more comprehensive manner. It shows that cells with different cumulative exposures to carcinogen were also compared.

TABLE 6. Experimental plan for MNNG and promoter treatments

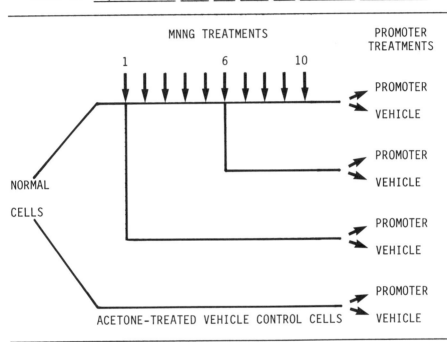

In these studies we considered the effects of TPA treatment in terms of changes in cell culture morphology, cloning efficiency in medium permissive for cloning (DMEM), cloning efficiency in media restrictive for cloning, including CMRL and DMEM with low calcium, and the development of an additional abnormal phenotypic change (gamma glutamyltranspeptidase expression) (TABLE 7).

In control cultures, TPA produced a morphologic change that reverted to normal within 24 hours. In contrast, MNNG-treated cultures exposed to TPA developed a profound change in morphology which reverted to normal only after 48-72 hours. Also, "initiated" cultures did not become refractory to this change as did controls. Such differences were noted after only three exposures to MNNG or after culturing cells for six months after one MNNG exposure.

TABLE 7. <u>End-points of studies with tumor promoters</u>

Morphologic Changes

Plating Efficiency in Permissive Medium

Plating Efficiency in Restrictive Media

Acquisition of Further Phenotypic Abnormalities

Normal stromal cells cultured in DMEM medium have a less-differentiated, bipolar shape. When exposed to TPA chronically for 3 months in culture, they have a regular polygonal pattern like more differentiated stromal cells maintained in CMRL medium (22). Endometrial stromal cells that had been treated once with MNNG, and then maintained for 3 months without promoter treatment, preserved a regular pattern of growth and the bipolar shape of untreated controls. A single treatment with MNNG followed by 3 months of exposure to TPA caused the development of foci of small round cells with poorly defined boundaries. This is the type of change that had been seen with greater numbers of MNNG treatments or a larger cumulative exposure. These findings suggest that the TPA treatment causes the morphologic differentiation of normal stromal cells. In cells that had been treated previously with MNNG, this same TPA treatment appears to impede differentiation and causes progressive changes in these cells that resemble the alterations found following more extensive carcinogen treatment.

In order to examine the effect of promoter treatment on phenotypic changes which occur late in the sequence of events after repetitive carcinogen exposure, stromal cells were treated three times with MNNG (1 µg/ml) to obtain multiply-treated cells.

TABLE 8. <u>Effect of chronic TPA treatment on saturation density</u>

Number of MNNG exposures	TPA	Months of Continuous TPA Treatment			
		1	2	3	4
0	-	2.04	2.04	1.78	1.81
	+	2.04	2.80	0.89	1.60
3	-	1.53	1.99	2.04	1.91
	+	2.54	2.93	3.44	4.97

Thereafter, cultures were exposed to TPA (0.01 µg/ml) chronically over a period of months and were evaluated periodically (22). Over four months, a progressive increase in saturation density was observed in cultures receiving MNNG and TPA treatment, but not in control groups (TABLE 8). This effect was only discernable in cultures which had received three or fewer MNNG exposures; in cultures that had been more extensively treated with MNNG, saturation density had already increased as the result of carcinogen alone.

Stromal cells that had been treated with MNNG and maintained in TPA continuously for 6 months were tested for their ability to form colonies in permissive medium (TABLE 9). Colony-forming ability was measured in DMEM with normal calcium, in which stromal cells usually demonstrate a colony-forming efficiency of 10-15%. Colony-forming efficiency in the presence and absence of TPA was compared and expressed as a ratio. The results show that TPA inhibited colony formation cells not treated with MNNG but potentiated colony formation by cells that had been treated with MNNG.

TABLE 9. Effect of TPA on colony-formation in permissive medium

Number of MNNG exposures (1 µg/ml)	TPA 0.01 µg/ml	Colony-forming efficiency	Ratio
0	-	12.5 + 0.01	0.07
	+	0.9 + 0.20	
1	-	18.3 + 1.00	0.70
	+	12.8 + 0.01	
6	-	7.1 + 0.70	1.14
	+	8.1 + 0.60	
10	-	17.1 + 0.40	1.65
	+	28.3 + 2.30	

TPA treatment also increased the number of cells which were capable of clonal growth in two restrictive media (TABLE 10). Human endometrial stromal cells normally have a high dependence on calcium for cell growth, and in certain media such as CMRL, undergo predecidual differentiation similar to that seen at the end of the menstrual cycle in vivo. Repeated carcinogen treatment resulted in cultures capable of forming colonies in low calcium medium and in CMRL (18). TPA exposure enhanced colony forming ability in both restrictive media, and this enhancement showed a general dependence on the total MNNG exposure used for initiation. In CMRL medium, TPA treatment caused an increase in the number of uninitiated cells which could form colonies. This may relate to the ability of TPA to alter differentiation in cell populations.

TABLE 10.   Effect of TPA on colony formation in restrictive media

Cumulative dose of MNNG (μg/ml)	TPA 0.1 μg/ml	Mean number of colonies per 500 cells plated	
		CMRL 1066	DMEM with 1 μg Ca^{++}/ml
0	−	0.40 + 0.35	0.0 + 0.0
0	+	4.77 + 2.69	0.0 + 0.0
2.0	−	1.80 + 0.20	0.0 + 0.0
2.0	+	4.30 + 0.45	0.1 + 0.1
3.5	−	1.16 + 0.39	0.0 + 0.0
3.5	+	9.01 + 1.00	0.35 + 0.30
5.0	−	1.08 + 0.20	0.13 + 0.01
5.0	+	18.3 + 0.25	2.60 + 0.50

TABLE 11.   Effect of TPA on gamma glutamyltranspeptidase activity

Number of MNNG exposures (1 μg/ml)	TPA 0.01 μg/ml	Percentage of GGT positive cells
0	−	2.0 + 1.0
	+	3.1 + 1.0
1	−	2.8 + 1.0
	+	11.0 + 3.0
6	−	3.4 + 1.0
	+	32.4 + 3.4
10	−	47.0 + 3.0
	+	44.0 + 6.0

Gamma glutamyltranspeptidase (GGT) was demonstrated histochemically in cultures subjected to chronic TPA exposure (TABLE 11). Chronic exposure to TPA for three months was compare to chronic exposure to the ethanol vehicle alone with regard to effects on GGT expression in cultures. Control cells which had not been treated with MNNG showed no change in GGT expression when exposed to TPA or ethanol vehicle alone. Cells initiated with one exposure to MNNG showed a 3.5-fold increase in the number of GGT-positive cells. After six exposures to MNNG, TPA treatment caused a 10.4-fold increase. Both of these increases were statistically significant ($p < 0.05$). In cultures that had been treated with MNNG 10 times, a maximal expression of GGT had been achieved and exposure to TPA produced no further enhancement.

DISCUSSION AND CONCLUSIONS

The development of several alterations of growth properties and phenotypic changes associated with transformation has been enhanced in human cells derived from human endometrium following their exposure to TPA in culture (TABLE 12). Marked changes were observed only in cultures that had been treated with a carcinogen, MNNG, prior to exposure to TPA. These results suggest that a process that resembles tumor promotion occurs and can be measured in human cells.

TABLE 12. Effects of TPA on endometrial stromal cells

CARCINOGEN-TREATED CELLS:

    Morphologic Changes Like More Extensive Treatment
    Increased Colony Forming Efficiency in Permissive Medium
    Increased Colony Forming Efficiency in Restrictive Media
    Acquisition of More Abnormal Phenotype

"NORMAL" (VEHICLE CONTROL) CELLS:

    Morphologic Changes Like Differentiation
    Reduced Colony Forming Efficiency in Permissive Medium
    Little or No Colony Formation in Permissive Media
    No Significant Progressive Changes in Phenotype

Moolgavkar and Knudson (16) have suggested that tumor promotion may be viewed as expansion of an altered stem cell population which leads to an increased probability of further genetic change and tumor expression. Yuspa and Morgan (28) have also documented the ability of TPA to induce differentiation of normal, but not initiated, epidermal epithelial cells from mouse skin. Based on these findings, we postulated that TPA may cause promotion in endometrial stromal cells by allowing altered cells to proliferate, while impeding growth of normal cells.

To test this hypothesis, we determined the fraction of cells capable of clonal growth in nonrestrictive medium in initiated and control cultures at various times after chronic TPA exposure. Over a period of six months, we observed a progressive decline in the number of control cells exposed to TPA which were capable of clonal growth, while the number of MNNG-initiated cells exposed to TPA which were capable of clonal growth increased (TABLE 9). The effect was most apparent after six months. This effect was not due to differences in attachment, nor to acute effects of TPA; it depended on the "initiated" state of the cells. It is possible that this type of response to tumor promoters may provide a means for detecting cells which have been "initiated", but are otherwise indistinguishable from controls.

This observation and the other results of this study address a fundamental question concerning tumor promoters. The issue is whether tumor promoters act directly by causing further genetic alteration in cells damaged by carcinogen treatment, or whether promoters act indirectly by allowing expansion of the "initiated" population in preference to normal cells. In this study, cells not previously exposed to MNNG did not show progressive changes even following chronic TPA treatment. If TPA can cause genetic changes directly, it does so with vastly less efficiency than does an agent like MNNG. These results suggest that TPA acts largely as the result of selective effects on the population of carcinogen-initiated cells in this system. These effects enhance progressive changes associated with transformation in the initiated cells, but do not have this effect on normal cells.

TABLE 13 illustrates a concept of the action of promoters based on these observations. It is hypothesized that promoters have different - dichotomous - effects on cells which depend on the prior history of the cells with regard to exposure to carcinogens. Cells previously exposed to carcinogens, "initiated" cells in the accepted jargon, are facilitated in their growth and their progressive acquisition of altered phenotypic properties, as a result of secondary exposure to a promoter like TPA. Quite in contrast, normal cells or cells treated only with vehicle are inhibited with regard to growth, appear to undergo differentiation, and do not acquire futher changes in phenotype. As a consequence, in a mixed cell population like in an intact tissue, the promoter might act to facilitate the emergence of the initiated population, while at the same time it surpresses the growth of the normal cells.

TABLE 13. Dichotomous effects of a promoter on stromal cells

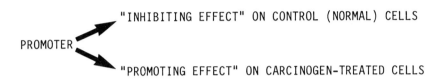

One cannot ignore the limitations of this type of system for studying the mechanisms of promotion. It is an in vitro system and the effects of a single promoter are reported. Still, these results could be viewed as providing another type of evidence for the tangibility of the concept of promotion. In this case the promoter appears to do something that is somewhat different than what a complete carcinogen would do in this system. Since this system utilizes human cell cultures, the results suggest that promotion can occur in human cells in vitro, and if this is the case, then perhaps it also occurs in humans in vivo.

ACKNOWLEDGEMENT

This work was done in collaboration with Dr. Karen G. Nelson and Ms. Jane L. Martin. The work was supported by grant CA31733 from the National Cancer Institute.

REFERENCES

1. Armuth, V. and Berenblum, I. (1972): Cancer Res., 32: 2259-2262.

2. Auerbach, O., Stout, A.P., Hammond, E.C., and Garfinkel, L. (1961): N. Eng. J. Med., 265: 253-267.

3. Barrett, J.C. (1979): Progr. Exp. Tumor Biol., 24: 17-27.

4. Boutwell, R.K. (1964): Progr. Exp. Tumor Res., 4: 207-250.

5. Cohen, S.M. Arai, M., Jacobs, J., and Friedell, G.H. (1979): Cancer Res., 39: 1207-1217.

6. Dallenbach-Hellweg, G. (1975): Histopathology of the Endometrium. Springer-Verlag, New York, pp. 22-82.

7. Dorman, B.H., Varma, V.A., Siegfried, J.M., Melin, S.A., Adamec, T.A., Norton, C.R., and Kaufman, D.G. (1982): In Vitro 18: 919-928.

8. Dorman, B.H., Siegfried, J.M., and Kaufman, D.G. (1983): Cancer Res., 43: 3348-3357.

9. Driedger, P.E., and Blumberg, P.M. (1977): Cancer Res., 37: 3257-3265.

10. Finn, C.A. (1977): In: Biology of the uterus, edited by R.M. Wynn, pp. 245-308. Plenum Publishing Co., New York.

11. Green, G.H. and Donovan, J.W. (1970): J. Obstet. Gynec. Brit. Cwlth, 77: 1-9.

12. Hicks, R.M., Wakefield, J.St.J., and Chowaniec, J. (1975): Chem.-Biol. Interact., 11: 225-233.

13. Kaufman, D.G., Siegfried, J.M., Dorman, B.H., Nelson, K.G., and Walton, L.A. (1983): In: Human Carcinogenesis, edited by C.C. Harris and E. H. Autrup, E.H., pp. 469-508. Academic Press, New York.

14. Knowles, M.A. and Franks, L.M. (1977): Cancer Res., 37: 3917-3924.

15. Lasne, C., Gentil, A., and Chouroulinkov, I. (1974): Nature, 247: 490-491.

16. Moolgavkar, S.H. and Knudson, A.G. (1981): J. Natl. Cancer Inst., 66: 1037-1052,.

17. Muto, J., Bussey, H.J.R., and Morson, B.C. (1975): Cancer, 36: 2251-2270 .

18. Narsawa, T., Magadia, N.E., Weisburger, J.H., and Wynder, E.L. (1974): J. Natl. Cancer Inst., 53: 1093-1097.

19. Peraino, C., Fry, R.J.M., Saffeldt, E., and Kisieleski, W.E. (1973): Cancer Res., 33: 2701-2704.

20. Saccomanno, G., Archer, V.E., Auerbach, O., Saunders, R.P., and Brennan, L. (1974): Cancer, 33: 256-270.

21. Schreiber, H., Saccomanno, G., Martin, D.H., and Brennan, L. (1974): Cancer Res., 34: 689-698.

22. Siegfried, J.M. and Kaufman, D.G. (1983): Int. J. Cancer 32: 423-429.

23. Siegfried, J.M., Nelson, K.G., Martin, J.L., and Kaufman, D.G. (1984) In Vitro 20: 25-32.

24. Steele, V.E., Marchok, A.C., and Netteshein, P. (1980): Int. J. Cancer, 26: 343-348.

25. Terzaghi, M., Klein-Szanto, A., and Netteshein, P. (1983): Cancer Res., 43: 1461-1466.

26. Traul, K.A., Hink, R.J., Kachevsky, V., and Wolff, J.S. (1981): J. Nat. Cancer Inst., 66: 171-175.

27. Wynn, R.M. (1977): In: Biology of the Uterus edited by R.M. Wynn, pp. 341-376. Plenum Press, New York.

28. Yuspa, S.H. and Morgan, D.L. (1981): Nature, 293: 72-74.

Tumor Promoters: Biological Approaches for
Mechanistic Studies and Assay Systems,
edited by Robert Langenbach et al.
Raven Press, New York © 1988.

ALTERATIONS IN CELLULAR ONCOGENES DURING NEOPLASTIC

TRANSFORMATION OF RAT TRACHEAL EPITHELIAL CELLS

Cheryl Walker, Tona Gilmer, and Paul Nettesheim

Laboratory of Pulmonary Pathobiology
National Institute of Environmental Health Sciences
P.O. Box 12233
Research Triangle Park, North Carolina 27709

The molecular mechanisms underlying carcinogen induced neoplastic transformation of normal cells are not yet well understood. It has been demonstrated in a number of cell systems that
neoplastic transformation occurs in discrete stages, which can be
recognized by sequential phenotypic changes such as acquisition
of unlimited growth capacity (immortalization), anchorage independence, and tumorigenicity. The molecular mechanisms involved
and which, if any, of the known cellular oncogenes are instru-
mental in bringing about these different phenotypic alterations
are not known.

In order to study how cellular oncogenes participate in airway epithelial cell carcinogenesis, we have begun to study the
expression of cellular oncogenes in primary rat tracheal epithelial (RTE) cells transformed by carcinogens in vitro. In this
system normal diploid tracheal epithelial cells can be transformed by carcinogens such as N-methyl-N-nitro-N-nitrosoguanidine
(MNNG), and the transformants progress with repeated subculture
to become immortal and ultimately neoplastic (14), closely
paralleling the events which occur during tracheal carcinogenesis
in vivo (22). Tumors produced by these neoplastic transformants
can be explanted into tissue culture allowing the isolation of
tumor derived cell lines. As end-stage transformants these
tumor derived lines would be expected to express a spectrum of
cellular oncogenes which become activated during the neoplastic
progression of the transformed cells and, thus, may be useful in
identifying those cellular oncogenes which play a role in the
neoplastic process. In addition, the level of expression of the
relevant oncogenes can be quantitated in these lines relative to
normal RTE cells.

The most frequently used assay to detect activated oncogenes
following carcinogen exposure is the NIH 3T3 transfection assay.

TABLE 1. In Vivo Activation of Cellular Oncogenes by Chemical Carcinogens

Species	Carcinogen	Lesion	Cellular Oncogene	Ref.
Rat	NMU (N-nitroso-N-methyl urea)	Mammary carcinoma	H-ras	27
		Schwannoma	neu	1
	DMBA (dimethylbenz(a)anthracene)	Mammary carcinoma	H-ras	27
	ENU (N-ethyl-N-nitrosourea)	Neuro/Glioblastoma	neu	2
	DMN-OME [methyl(methoxymethyl)nitrosomine]	Renal carcinoma	K-ras,N-ras	21
	MMS (methyl-methane-sulfonate)	Nasal carcinoma	non-ras	11
	DMCC (dimethyl-carbamyl chloride)	Nasal carcinoma	negative	11
Mouse	DMBA	Skin carcinoma	H-ras	17
	DB(c,h)ACR (dibenz(c,h)acridine)	Skin carcinoma	H-ras	4
	B(a)P [benzo(a)pyrene]	Skin carcinoma	negative	4
	NMU	Thymic lymphoma	N-ras	13
	MCA (3-methyl-cholanthrene)	Fibrosarcoma	K-ras	9
	MCA	Thymic lymphoma	K-ras	10
	MNNG (N-methyl-N-nitro-N-nitrosoguanidine)	Skin carcinoma	negative	17
	BPL (β-propriolactone)	Skin carcinoma	H-ras	11
	DMCC	Skin carcinoma	negative	11

TABLE 1. Continued

Species	Carcinogen	Lesion	Cellular Uncogene	Ref.
	Furfural	Hepatoma	H-, K-ras, non-ras	18
	Furan	Hepatoma	H-, K-ras, non-ras	18
	N-HO-AAF (N-hydroxy-2-acetylaminofluorene)	Hepatoma	H-ras	25
	VC (vinylcarbamate)	Hepatoma	H-ras	25
	HO-DHE(1-hydroxy-2-3-dehydroestraqole)	Hepatoma	H-, K-ras	25
Guinea Pig	MNNG	Transformed fetal cells	N-ras	20
	DEN (diethyl-nitrosamine)	Transformed fetal cells	N-ras	20

This assay tests the ability of donor DNA to morphologically transform recipient 3T3 cells, and it appears to be particularly selective for activated oncogenes of the ras family. Therefore, it is not surprising that activated ras oncogenes have been the most common oncogenic lesions detected in chemically transformed cells (Tables 1 & 2). However, oncogene expression and/or activation in many cases appear to be dependent on both the specific carcinogen and the transformation system itself. It has been shown using in vivo models of chemical carcinogenesis that the same carcinogen can activate different oncogenes in different systems. For example, N-nitroso-N-methylurea (NMU) activates H-ras in rat mammary carcinomas (27), N-ras in mouse thymic lymphomas (13) and c-neu in rat schwannomas (1). In mouse skin, where papillomas and carcinomas can be induced by topical application of a wide range of chemicals, activation of specific oncogenes such as H-ras also appears to be a function of the carcinogen used. Dimethylbenz(a)anthracene (DMBA) induces a high frequency of papillomas and carcinomas in which H-ras is activated by an AT→TA transversion at the second position of the 61st codon (17). In contrast, carcinomas induced by MNNG do not contain this activating mutation (17), and DNA from dimethyl carbamyl chloride (DMCC) induced mouse skin carcinomas also lacks detectable transforming activity in the NIH 3T3 focus assay (11).

It is notable that MNNG in particular has not been shown to result in the direct activation of cellular oncogenes detectable by the 3T3 assay. N-ras activation has been observed in MNNG transformed guinea pig cell lines (20), but this appears to be a late event because early passages of these MNNG transformants are negative in the 3T3 assay (20).

To further investigate the role of cellular oncogenes in chemical carcinogenesis, specifically transformation induced by MNNG, we have assayed for the presence of activated cellular oncogenes in 4 MNNG transformed cell lines using the NIH 3T3 assay. The cell lines chosen for this analysis were derived from tumors produced after inoculation of nude mice with 4 cell lines derived from MNNG transformed primary rat tracheal epithelial (RTE) cells (19). DNAs from the 4 tumor derived lines, EGV_4T, EGV_5T, EGV_6T and $EGV_{10}T$, were tested in 3-5 independent assays. Whereas T24 DNA which contains an activated H-ras oncogene (12) yielded transformed foci with a frequency of 0.417 foci/μg DNA, DNAs from all 4 EGV-T lines were negative for the presence of activated cellular oncogenes detectable by the 3T3 assay.

The absence of detectable 3T3 transforming activity suggested that these cells may have been transformed by an alternative mechanism such as alteration in the level of expression of specific cellular oncogenes. In contrast to the numerous studies on qualitative alterations in cellular oncogenes during chemical carcinogenesis, studies to date on quantitative alterations in cellular oncogene expression have been very limited. These types of changes have been analyzed in detail in mouse skin (23,16)

TABLE 2. In vitro activation of cellular oncogenes
by chemical carcinogens

Species	Carcinogen	Cells	Cellular oncogene	Ref.
Guinea Pig	MNNG	Day 43 fetal cells	N-ras	20
	B(a)P	Day 43 fetal cells	N-ras	20
	MCA	Day 48 fetal skin	N-ras	20
	MNNG	Passage 90 cell line	negative	20
Mouse	DMBA	DI/UCD mammmary cell line	H-ras	8
	MCA	C3H IOT1/2 and Balb 3T3 cell lines	K-ras	15
Human	MNNG	SV40 immortalized keratinocytes	negative	19

during liver hepatocarcinogenesis (3,6,7,26) and in a carcinogen-
induced mouse thymoma (5). In these systems, a small subset of
cellular oncogenes (ras, myc, myb, abl) have been observed to
display alterations in levels of expression. Results from these
studies are difficult to interpret in terms of identifying carcinogen-induced alterations. An example is mouse skin which
appears to undergo a transient elevation in K-ras expression
during papilloma development (16), but this does not appear to
persist, or occurs variably among carcinomas (23,16). An additional complication in interpreting increased expression of oncogenes such as myc is the difficulty in separating elevated
expression due to direct carcinogen interaction from increased
expression which occurs as a consequence of increased proliferation due to loss of growth control. It is therefore sometimes
difficult to choose the correct "normal" control against which
to measure c-onc expression in transformed cells. For example,
to examine c-onc expression in mouse thymomas, normal thymus in
which the cells are quiescent and thus may express only low
levels of c-onc such as myc may not be an appropriate control.
Finally it is notable that to date no data on quantitative
alterations in c-onc expression during in vitro transformation
is currently available.

To quantitate oncogene expression in transformed RTE cells,
tumor derived cell lines were screened with a panel of 15
cellular oncogenes (Table 3). Slot-blot analyses were performed using cytoplasmic total RNA from these lines, and the
level of expression of various c-onc was quantitated relative to
their level of expression in normal 1° RTE cells. As shown in
Table 3, erb-B, abl, N-myc, fes, myb, ros, sis, and kit were not
detectably expressed in normal or transformed cells. H-ras was
slightly (3-fold) but significantly elevated relative to normal

TABLE 3. Quantitation of c-onc Expression in EGV-T Cell Lines

	fms	H-ras	K-ras	raf	fos	L-myc	c-myc	N-myc, abl, erb-B, fes, myb, ros, sis, kit
Normal rat tracheal epithelial (RTE) cells	1	1	1	1	1	1	1	No detectable expression
EGV4T	5*	3*	2	2	<1	<1	<1	
EGV5T	5*	3*	2	2	<1	<1	<1	
EGV6T	19*	3*	<1	2	<1	<1	<1	
EGV10T	<1	<1	<1	<1	ND	<1	ND	

*significant $p < .05$
ND = not determined

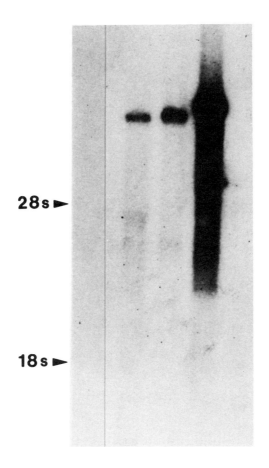

FIG. 1. Northern analysis. Samples (5 μg) of poly A+ cytoplasmic RNA from rat embryo fibroblasts (REF) or EGV-T cell lines were separated by electrophoresis in formaldehyde/agarose gels, transferred to nitrocellulose, and hybridized to 3'v-fms probe.

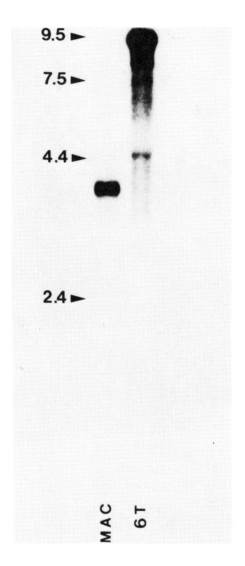

FIG. 2.   Northern analysis. Samples (5 μg) of poly A+
         cytoplasmic RNA from EGV₆T and normal rat aveolar
         macrophages (MAC) were separated by electrophoresis
         in formaldehyde/agarose gels, transferred to nitro-
         cellulose, and hybridized to 3' v-fms probe.

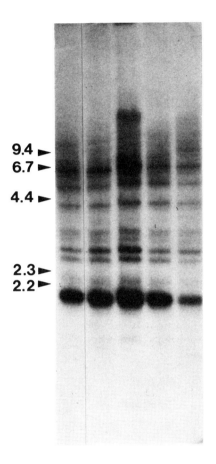

9.4 ►
6.7 ►
4.4 ►
2.3 ►
2.2 ►

REF 4T 5T 6T 10T

FIG. 3. Southern blot analysis of genomic DNA from normal rat
embryo fibroblasts (REF) and EGV-T cell lines. DNA
samples digested with HindIII and hybridized to
3'v-fms probe. The amount of DNA loaded per slot was
monitored by ethidium bromide staining and U.V. illumination of the agarose gel before DNA transfer onto
nitrocellulose. After normalization for variations in
DNA loading, no amplification of fms sequences could
be detected in any of the EGV-T lines.

EGV-T cells in 3 of the 4 cell lines, (EGV$_4$T, EGV$_5$T, and EGV$_6$T), but the biological relevance of this marginal increase in expression is questionable. Expression of one oncogene, fms, was elevated 5-19 fold in the EGV$_4$T, EGV$_5$T, and EGV$_6$T cell lines. The c-fms oncogene is related and possibly identical to the gene for the receptor for the macrophage growth factor CSF-1 and has not previously been reported to be expressed in chemically trans- formed epithelial cells.

Northern analysis was performed on the EGV-T cell lines to determine the size of the fms mRNA expressed. This analysis confirmed the presence of a fms-related transcript in EGV$_4$T, EGV$_5$T, and EGV$_6$T which was absent in normal rat embryo fibro- blasts (Figure 1). However, this transcript was determined to be 9.5 kb in contrast to the 4.0 kb fms mRNA size pre- viously reported in human and mouse cells (24). Northern analysis of RNA isolated from rat alveolar macrophages, which normally express the fms/CSF-1 receptor, indicated that the fms/CSF-1 receptor mRNA was expressed as a 3.8 kb transcript in these cells (Figure 2), suggesting that the presence of the 9.5 kb transcript is not a result of species specific difference in fms/CSF-1 receptor expression. Southern analysis of DNA from the EGV-T cell lines revealed neither amplification of fms sequences in EGV-T cells which express the 9.5 kb transcript (Figure 3) nor any detectable gene rearrangement. We conclude from these results that the MNNG-induced RTE tumor derived lines are expressing a novel gene related to, but distinct from, the CSF-1 receptor/fms cellular oncogene.

We are presently investigating when during the multi-stage transformation process this fms related gene is first expressed. Preliminary results suggest that this occurs during the transi- tion from the preneoplastic to neoplastic stage. This would suggest that the expression of this gene is temporally removed from the initial MNNG exposure and not a direct consequence of interaction with the carcinogen. Studies are under way to characterize this gene and to determine whether it also codes a receptor which we speculate may be specific for another, as yet undetermined, hematopoietic growth factor.

References

1. Barbacid, M. (1986): Carcinogenesis, 7:1037-1042.
2. Bargmann, C.I., Hung, M., and Weinberg, R.A. (1986): Cell, 45:649-657.
3. Beer, D.G., Schware, M., Sawada, N., and Pitot, H.C. (1986): Cancer Res., 46:2435-2441.
4. Bizub, D., Wood, A.W., Skalka, A.M. (1986): Proc. Natl. Acad. Sci. USA, 83:6048-6052.
5. Chinsky, J., Lilly, F., Childs, G. (1985): Proc. Natl. Aad. Sci. USA, 82:565-569.

6. Corcos, D., Defer, N., Raymondjean, M., Paris, B., Corral, M., Tichonisky, L., and Kruh, J. (1984): Biochem. Biophys. Res. Comm., 122:259-264.
7. Cote, G.J., Lastra, B.A., Cook, J.R., Huang, D., and Chiu, J. (1985): Cancer Lett., 26:121-127.
8. Dandekar, S., Sukumar, S., Zarbl, H., Young, L.J.T., and Cardiff, R.D. (1986): Mol. Cell. Biol., 6:4104-4108.
9. Eva, A., and Aaronson, S.A. (1983): Science, 220:955-956.
10. Eva, A., and Trimmer, R.W. (1986): Carcinogenesis, 7:1931-1933.
11. Garte, S.J., Hood, A.T., Hochwalt, A.E., Eustachio, P.D., Synder, C.A., Segal, A., and Albert, R.E. (1985): Carcinogenesis, 6:1709-1712.
12. Goldfarb, M., Shimizu, K., Perucho, M., and Wigler, M. (1982): Nature, 296:404-409.
13. Guerrero, I., Villasante, A., Corces, V., and Pellicer, A. (1985): Proc. Natl. Acad. Sci. USA, 82:7810-7814.
14. Nettesheim, P., and Barrett, J.C. (1984): in: Critical Reviews in Toxicology, edited by Goldberg,L., Vol. 12, pp. 222-225. CRC Press, Boca Raton.
15. Parada, L.F., and Weinberg, R.A. (1983): Mol. Cell. Biol., 3:2298-2301.
16. Pelling, J.C., Ernst, S.M., Strawhecker, J.M., Johnson, J.A., Nairn, R.S., and Slaga, T.J. (1986): Carcinogenesis, 7:1599-1602.
17. Quintanilla, M., Brown, K., Ramsden, M., and Balmain, A. (1986): Nature, 322:78-80.
18. Reynolds, S.H. personal communication.
19. Rhim, J.S., Fujita, J., Arnstein, P., and Aaronson, S.A. (1986): Science, 232:385-388.
20. Sukumar, S., Pulciani, S., Doniger, J., DiPaolo, J.A., Evans, C.H., Zbar, B., and Barbacid, M. (1984): Science, 223:1197-1199.
21. Sukumar, S., Peratoni, A., Reed, C., Rice, J.M., and Wenk, M.L. (1986): Mol. Cell. Biol., 6:2716-2720.
22. Terzaghi, M., and Nettesheim, P. (1979): Cancer Res., 39:4003-4010.
23. Toftgard, R., Roop, D.R., and Yuspa, S.H. (1985): Carcinogenesis, 6:655-657.
24. Walker, C., Nettesheim, P., Barrett, J.C., and Gilmer, T.M. (1987): Proc. Natl. Acad. Sci. USA, in press.
25. Wiseman, R.W., Stowers, S.J., Miller, E.C., Anderson, M.W., and Miller, J.A. (1986): Proc. Natl. Acad. Sci. USA, 83:5825-5829.
26. Yaswen, P., Goyette, M., Shank, P.R., and Fausto, N. (1985): Mol. Cell. Biol., 5:780-786.
27. Zarbl, H., Sukumar, S., Author, A.V., Martin-Zanca, D., and Barbacid, M. (1985): Nature, 315:382-385.

Tumor Promoters: Biological Approaches for Mechanistic Studies and Assay Systems, edited by Robert Langenbach et al. Raven Press, New York © 1988.

MULTISTEP CARCINOGENESIS:

STUDIES WITH PRIMARY FIBROBLASTS AND KERATINOCYTES

Gian Paolo Dotto, Michael Z. Gilman, and Robert A. Weinberg

The Whitehead Institute, Nine Cambridge Center
Cambridge, Massachusetts 02142

STUDIES WITH PRIMARY FIBROBLASTS

An important problem in multistep carcinogenesis is to understand how the several steps required for tumor formation in vivo relate to the activation and interaction of oncogenes. In this paper we present our attempts to address this problem by using two different model systems, involving primary cells of either fibroblastic or epithelial origin in culture as models for multistep carcinogenesis in vivo.

For our studies, we have chosen as a point of reference the mouse skin system, which represents one of the best in vivo models for multistep carcinogenesis (Hecker et al.,1982). In this system, the several steps necessary for tumor formation - initiation, promotion and tumor progression - seem to involve a minimum of two genetic lesions (Hennings et al., 1983). This establishes an apparent parallel with the observation that introduction of two genetic elements, such as an activated ras and myc oncogenes, into primary fibroblasts in culture is necessary to elicit a fully transformed phenotype (Land et al., 1983a). We wondered therefore whether activation of either a ras or a myc oncogene alone would be sufficient for the first step of this process.

Initiated cells are an elusive entity and can be detected only in an indirect way. For this reason, we chose to define operationally an initiated cell as a cell that is present among the normal cell population but enjoys a specific growth advantage in the presence of a tumor promoter. We reasoned that we could mimic this situation in culture by introducing into a fraction of normal cells either a ras or a myc oncogene and then ask whether the growth of the oncogene-bearing cells was modified and enhanced, relative to the surrounding normal cell population, by the presence of a tumor promoter. Although primary keratinocytes are the natural target for in vivo carcinogenesis and should have been the cells of choice for these studies, their complex growth requirements did not allow the kind of quantitative analysis that we wanted to perform. Therefore, as a first approximation, we used the primary rat embryo fibroblasts (REFs), the same cells used by H. Land in his ras-myc cooperation studies (Land et al.,1983b).

In previous work with REFs, oncogenes had been introduced into cells via DNA transfection. However, the efficiency of gene transfer by that method is low and the number of transfected cells hard to control. For that reason, we decided to introduce the activated oncogenes into cells by infection with retroviral vectors that carry the oncogene of interest in addition to a second gene that confers resistance to the antibiotic G418 and serves as an independent selectable marker (Cepko et al.,1984; Dotto et al.,1985). The recombinant viruses were produced by $\psi 2$ cells (Mann et al.,1983) as a high titer stock, free of helper, so that no further spread of virus would occur following the initial infection. In this way, the number of infected cells in a dish could be carefully calibrated by simply varying the multiplicity of infection. This was important since, as mentioned before, we wanted to create a mixed population of cells in which only a minor fraction would carry an oncogene of interest. Three viruses were used: ras-zip 6, carrying the ras oncogene from the HaSV virus; VM, carrying the myc oncogene from the MC29 virus; and SVX, a control virus with no oncogenes. Details of the construction of these viruses have been presented elsewhere (Cepko et al., 1984; Dotto et al., 1985).

TPA-induced focus formation of ras-bearing fibroblasts.

Tertiary cultures of rat embryo fibroblasts (REFs) were exposed to virus at low multiplicity so that only about 1% of the cell population was infected. Cells were split 2 days after infection into either normal medium, medium with TPA (10 ng/ml) or medium with G418 (0.5 mg/ml). Dishes were scored 7-10 days later for focus or colony formation. No foci could be detected in the monolayers in the presence of normal medium, irrespective of the oncogene introduced into cells (fig.1a). In the presence of TPA, however, ras-bearing cells formed a large number of foci, while no foci could again be detected with the myc or the control cells. The number of foci obtained with the ras-bearing cells was very similar to the number of G418-resistant colonies obtained from the same population when plated on selective medium (fig.1a). Thus, almost every cell that expressed the G418 resistance gene of the viral ras chimera was also able to form a focus in the presence of TPA. This ability of TPA to affect all the ras cells present in the monolayer conforms to epigenetic effects associated with tumor promoters and contrasts with the rarely occurring genetic alterations associated with initiating agents. As we have reported elsewhere (Dotto et al.,1985), effects similar to the ones observed with TPA were observed with cells treated with second stage tumor promoters such as mezerein and RPA (12-O-retinoylphorbol-13-acetate) (Slaga et al., 1980; Furstenberger et al., 1981) but not with biologically inactive phorbol esters such as 4α-PDD (4-α-phorbol-12,13-didecanoate).

Microscopically, cells in the ras-induced foci exhibited a classical ras-transformed morphology, while the myc-infected cells underwent more subtle morphological alteration which did not result in macroscopically observable foci (fig. 1b).

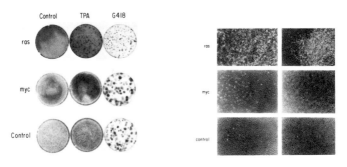

Fig. 1a   Fig. 1b

Fig. 1.   Effects of TPA on focus formation of oncogene-bearing REFs in monolayer. Tertiary rat embryo fibroblasts ($7x10^5$ cells/10 cm dish) were infected with the SVX, ras- or myc-virus. After 48 hours, cells were split 1:10 into either normal medium (DME; 10% Fetal Bovine Serum) or medium plus TPA (10 ng/ml) or medium plus G418 (0.5 mg/ml). Cells were photographed (Fig. 1b) and dishes were fixed and stained (Fig. 1a) 10 days later.

Specificity of TPA effects for ras- but not myc-bearing fibroblasts.

To better quantify these results and to address the question of the specificity of action of TPA on ras- or myc-bearing cells, we decided to measure directly the number of ras or myc-bearing cells grown in the presence or the absence of TPA. This was possible, since the viral vectors used to introduce the oncogenes also contain the G418 resistance gene. Therefore, the cells could be split at various time intervals after growth in the presence or absence of TPA and plated in G418. The number of G418 resistant colonies provided a measurement of the proportion of ras- or myc-bearing cells in the population, irrespective of any focus-formation assay. It is clear from fig. 2 that the proportion of myc or control cells was not significantly affected by the presence of TPA, while the proportion of ras cells was much greater (20 fold higher by 7 days) in the presence of the tumor promoter. This confirms that growth of ras-bearing fibroblasts in the monolayer is strongly stimulated by TPA and shows that this effect is specific for cells harboring the ras oncogene.

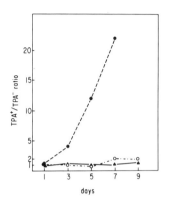

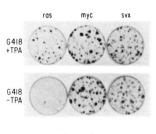

Fig. 3

Fig. 2

Fig. 2.   Effects of TPA on the growth of oncogene-bearing REFs in monolayer. REFs were infected the same as described in Fig.1. After 48 hours cells were split 1:10 into either normal or TPA containing media and separate dishes were withdrawn at various times after that. Cells were trypsinized, counted and replated at a density of 1 and 5×10^5 cells/10 cm dish in G418-containing medium (0.5 mg/ml, Gibco). Colonies were counted 2 weeks later and the ratio between the number of colonies from cells grown with and without TPA was calculated. Two independent dishes were counted for each experimental point. Values are given for cells infected with the ras- (   ), myc- (   ) and SVX (   ) virus.

Fig. 3.   Effects of TPA on the growth of oncogene-bearing REFs in the absence of surrounding normal cells. Cells were infected as described in Fig.1 and after 48 hours were split 1:10 into G418-containing medium (0.5 mg/ml), with or without TPA (10 ng/ml). Dishes were stained 1 week later.

Direct growth stimulatory effects of TPA on ras-bearing cells.

     Tumor promoters might exert their effects in the presently described experimental system through two possible mechanisms : 1) direct growth stimulation of the "ras-initiated cells"; 2) suppression of growth inhibition of the "ras cells" by the surrounding normal cell population. As a preliminary attempt to distinguish between these two possibilities, cells were infected with the various viruses as in the preceding experiments and split 2 days later in either medium with G418 alone or medium with G418 plus TPA. In this way all the adjacent normal cells were killed off and one could study the direct effects of TPA on the oncogene-bearing cells alone. As it is clear from Fig. 3, there was a strong effect of TPA on the size, but not the number or the morphology, of the "ras cell" colonies. When the cells were trypsinized and counted there were 10 times more cells in the presence of TPA then in its absence. No such difference could be detected with the myc or the control cells.

In conclusion, we have shown that introduction of an activated ras oncogene into primary fibroblasts is sufficient to confer upon these cells an initiated phenotype, since, in the presence of a tumor promoter such as TPA, they enjoy a strong and specific growth advantage relative to the surrounding normal cell population. The direct and specific growth stimulatory effect of TPA on the ras bearing fibroblasts could explain at least in part this phenomenon.

STUDIES WITH PRIMARY KERATINOCYTES

The results presented above with the primary embryo fibroblasts and the results of others obtained with the C3H10T1/2 and rat6 fibroblast lines (Hsiao et al., 1984; 1986), point to a possible involvment of ras in initiation of carcinogenesis. Nevertheless, the general validity of this conclusion is seriously limited by the fact that it is based on the study of cells of fibroblastic origin, while the natural target for in vivo carcinogenesis are epithelial cells, keratinocytes in the case of the mouse skin. Since the growth properties of the two kinds of cells are profoundly different, what is learned from one system might not necessarily apply to the other.

The same conclusion, about involvment of ras in initiation of carcinogenesis, is however now strongly supported by alternative kind of evidence, derived from systems closer to the in vivo situation (Yuspa et al., 1985; Sukumar et al.,1983; Zarbl et al., 1985; Balmain et al.,1983,1984; Brown et al. 1986). In all of these cases, however, the notion that ras activation might be sufficient for initiation of in vivo carcinogenesis remains still to be verified. A direct approach to this problem would be to grow keratinocyte in culture and again try to assess which oncogene, if any, could confer upon these cells initiated properties.

In this sense, the "low-high calcium" culture system for mouse keratinocytes developed by H. Hennings and S. Yuspa (Hennings et al.,1980) is very attractive and we decided to reproduce it in our own laboratory. In this system, cells are grown in low calcium (0.05mM) medium and can then be induced to terminally differentiate by addition of 2mM calcium to the medium. Initiating treatment with carcinogens, both in vivo or in vitro, results in a considerable increase in the number of calcium-resistant clones that one can recover from the primary keratinocytes following selection for growth in high calcium medium (Yuspa and Morgan,1981; Kilkenny et al.,1985). From this it would be tempting to equate resistance to calcium in the keratinocytes with acquisition of an initiated phenotype. This is also suggested by the fact that cells that are resistant to calcium-induced differentiation are resistant to a differentiating effect that TPA has on normal keratinocytes (Yuspa et al.,1983a; Table I and our own unpublished observations).

Table I

Differentiation parameters of primary and RBK cells.

		DNA Synthesis (% of the control)		Cornified Envelopes (%of the total cell number)	
		Balb/c;	RBK	Balb/c,	RBK
High calcium	24 hrs	2%	>100%	3%	<1%
" "	5 days	0.2%	100%	20%	3%
TPA	24 hrs	20%	100%	15%	<1%

Conditions for keratinocyte cultivation, for the isolation of the RBK line and for calcium and TPA treatment are as described elsewhere (Dotto et al., 1986). DNA synthesis was measured by ^{3}H-thymidine incorporation. Cells were pulse-labelled with ^{3}H-thymidine (1μCi/ml, 78Ci/mmol, NEN) for 1 hr, DNA was prepared by treatment with NaOH (0.2M) for 10' at 4° and TCA- precipitable counts were determined and normalized against DNA content of each sample (measured in a H33258 fluorescent assay [Labarca and Paigen, 1980]). Cornified envelopes were measured by typsinizing cells, washing in PBS and incubating at 68°C in 1% SDS, .1% β-mercaptoethanol for 10'.

As shown by Yuspa et al. (1983b; 1985), and we have observed the same in our own work, introduction of ras into primary keratinocytes leads only to rather subtle modifications of these cells and is not sufficient to induce resistance to calcium. It seems likely therefore that other events are required in these cells, in concomitance with calcium, for acquisition of the calcium and TPA resistant phenotype. As a preliminary analysis of the regulatory events underlying differentiation triggered by calcium and TPA, we have examined expression of the myc and fos protooncogenes in both primary keratinocytes and in a calcium and TPA-resistant line that we have derived from primary keratinocytes by prolonged cultivation in high calcium medium. The interest in the regulation of fos

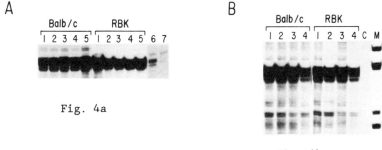

Fig. 4a

Fig. 4b

Fig.4.   myc- and fos-RNA expression in either primary
keratinocytes or calcium-resistant cells (RBK) upon increase of
calcium concentration in the medium. Same amounts of total
cellular RNA, obtained from RBK cells or primary cells kept in
culture for two weeks in low calcium (0.05 mM) medium and
switched to high calcium (2 mM) at various times, was analyzed
for   myc (4a) or myc and fos (4b) expression by SP6 ribonuclease
protection assay as described elsewhere (Dotto et al., 1986).
Control in low calcium: 1; high calcium for 30': 2; for 2 hours:
3; for 24 hours : 4; for 5 days : 5; RNA from resting Balb/c 3T3
cells serum stimulated for 1 hour : 6; RNA from quiescent Balb/c
3T3 cells : 7; tRNA control : C; size marker : M.   The RNAs
analyzed   in Fig. 1a and 1b derive from two independent
experiments.

and myc expression in these cells derived from the fact that
regulation of these genes have been found to be linked to the
control of growth and proliferation in a large variety of other
systems.

myc and fos expression in primary and calcium-resistant (RBK)
keratinocytes in response to calcium

Total cellular RNA was prepared from primary keratinocytes
and RBK cells at various times after calcium addition and
analyzed by SP6-ribonuclease protection assay (Melton et
al.,1984), using probes specific for either the myc or the fos
genes. The levels of myc mRNA found both in proliferating
keratinocytes (in low calcium medium) and in RBK cells were
significantly higher than in fibroblasts in which substantial
myc expression had been induced by a 1 hour exposure of
previously quiescent cells to serum (fig. 4a, lanes 1 and 6,7).
myc expression in the primary keratinocytes remained
substantial even after induction of differentiation. In some
experiments, it was reduced imperceptibly (fig. 4a), while in
others (fig. 4b), levels of myc decreased about 3 fold by 24
hours after calcium addition. This lower level of myc, seen in
cells where DNA synthesis is reduced to less than 5% of the

control (Table I), is still several fold higher than that seen
in fibroblasts induced to grow by serum addition (cf. fig. 4a
and 4b). Indeed, myc RNA levels remained very high even 5 days
after calcium exposure (fig. 4a, lane 5), under conditions where
DNA synthesis was completely arrested (Table I). Similarly, no
difference in myc RNA levels could be detected between freshly
isolated keratinocytes prior to plating and containing a large
fraction of differentiated cells, and actively replicating
keratinocytes kept in culture in low calcium medium for two
weeks (data not shown). The pattern of myc expression in
response to calcium was similar in primary keratinocytes and RBK
cells (fig. 4a and b).

     These findings differ from those observed with most other
cell types studied to date, which suggest some linkage between
expression of myc and cellular growth and differentiation (Kelly
et al.,1983; Campisi et al.,1984; Greenberg and Ziff, 1984). One
exception stems from tumor cells of the PC12 pheochromocytoma
line which exhibit a response related to that seen here: upon
induction of differentiation, a brief peak of myc expression is
followed by a lower level of sustained expression, long after
cell proliferation has stopped (Greenberg et al., 1985).
However, it is unclear whether this behavior reflects that of
the normal counterparts of the PC12 cells or is a consequence of
the malignant state of these cells.

     A number of cell types exhibit a sharp increase in fos
expression in response to agents that induce their
differentiation (Muller et al.,1984b; 1985; Curran and Morgan,
1985; Greenberg and Ziff, 1984; Kruijer et al.,1985; Mitchell et
al., 1985). In contrast, keratinocyte differentiation triggered
by calcium is not accompanied by induction of fos expression
(fig.1b). Instead, the low levels of fos RNA present inside the
cell undergo a slight decrease by 2 hours after exposure to
calcium (fig.4b). This pattern of fos expression was observed
with both primary and RBK cells (fig.4b). This suggests that fos
activation might not be an essential element of the mechanism
involved in triggering keratinocyte differentiation by calcium.

myc and fos expression in keratinocytes in response to TPA

     The tumor promoter TPA induces terminal differentiation in a
large proportion of primary keratinocytes in culture in a manner
similar to calcium (Yuspa et al.,1982 and 1983a; Table I). Cells
such as those of the RBK line, which have been selected for
resistance to calcium, are also found to be resistant to TPA-
induced differentiation (Yuspa et al.,1983a; Table I). This
might indicate that the two inducers act through a common
pathway.

Unexpectedly, the effects of TPA on myc and fos expression in the primary keratinocytes differed dramatically from those previously observed with calcium. Unlike the persistent expression of myc RNA seen upon addition of calcium, TPA addition led to a marked decrease (more than ten fold) in myc RNA levels within 2 hours of exposure (fig.5). This decrease in myc RNA was specific for this RNA and was not detected for other mRNAs such as tubulin mRNA (data not shown). By 24 hours after TPA addition, when DNA synthesis was diminished to less than 20% of the control (Table I), myc RNA rose again to elevated levels (fig.5). The late rise in myc expression further demonstrate that in the keratinocyte, regulation of myc expression and DNA synthesis are uncoupled.

TPA elicited a fos response quite different from that seen after application of calcium. After TPA treatment, fos RNA levels underwent a considerable (more than thirty fold) and transient increase. Maximal expression was reached by 30' after TPA addition and remained very high for at least 2 hours (fig.5). However, by 24 hours fos expression reverted to basal levels (fig. 5).

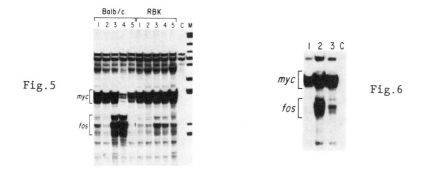

Fig.5   Fig.6

Fig. 5. fos and myc-RNA expression in either primary keratinocytes or RBK cells upon treatment with TPA (100ng/ml). RNAs were prepared and analyzed simultaneously for fos and myc as described elsewhere (Dotto et al.,1986). DMSO control (0.1%) for 30': 1; DMSO control for 2 hours: 2; TPA for 30': 3; TPA for 2 hours: 4; TPA for 24 hours: 5.

Fig. 6. Differential fos induction in RBK cells by fresh medium or TPA. Total cellular RNA from RBK cells was analyzed simultaneously for fos and myc as described in Dotto et al.,1986. Control : 1; 30' after addition of fresh medium (0.05 mM calcium) : 2; 30' after addition of TPA (100 ng/ml) : 3.

Taken together, our results with myc and fos expression suggest that calcium and TPA induce keratinocyte differentiation by two related but distinct pathways. This conclusion is supported by the different morphological changes induced by calcium and TPA (not shown) and by the uniform response of all primary keratinocytes in a culture to calcium-induced differentiation (Hennings et al.,1980), this contrasting to the incomplete response of keratinocyte populations to treatment with TPA (Yuspa et al., 1982; Parkinson et al., 1984).

The strong fos response observed with TPA and the absence of a similar response with calcium is reminiscent of that found with HL60 promyelocytic leukemia cells. There, TPA treatment triggers monocytic differentiation and causes a marked and sustained fos induction (Muller et al., 1984b, 1985; Mitchell et al., 1985), while retinoic acid and DMSO lead to granulocytic differentiation with no effect on fos expression (Mitchell et al., 1985). Thus, the nature of the fos response depends upon the inducing agent used and the type of differentiation pathway that it triggers. These, and more recent results on HL60 cells (Mitchell et al., 1986), suggest that modulation of fos expression in these myeloid cells, as well as in the presently described keratinocytes, is not tightly coupled to the differentiation programs of these cells.

The availability of RBK cells, which are resistant to calcium and TPA-induced differentiation, prompted us to examine how myc and fos expression in these cells is affected by TPA. In contrast to the TPA-induced reduction of myc in the primary cultures, myc gene expression in RBK cells was unaffected by TPA treatment (fig. 5). fos expression was similarly unresponsive; it was only slightly stimulated by TPA, in contrast to the enormous increase seen in the primary cells (fig. 5). This slight increase in fos expression persisted in the RBK cells even 24 hours after TPA addition. We conclude that as a consequence of a selection against calcium-induced differentiation the RBK cells have also acquired resistance to TPA-induced differentiation and have lost the normally observed regulation of the fos and myc genes by TPA. This situation is reminiscent of the block in fos expression recently described for some TPA-resistant variants of the HL60 cell line (Mitchell et al.,1986).

The marked decrease of fos inducibility by TPA in RBK cells led us to test whether the fos gene of these cells can still be regulated by serum, which serves as a strong fos inducer in primary keratinocytes (data not shown) as well as in fibroblasts (Greenberg and Ziff, 1984; Kruijer et al., 1984; Muller et al., 1984a). Indeed, as is seen in fig. 6, the fos gene of RBK cells remains highly responsive to serum, increasing 20 fold by 30 minutes after serum addition. This allows the additional conclusion that the fos gene in the keratinocytes can be induced through at least two distinct pathways, only one of which has been lost during the selection of the RBK cells. The second pathway would appear to be independent of the action of kinase C, the enzyme for which TPA serves as an agonist (Nishizuka, 1984).

We have shown that c-myc RNA expression in the keratinocytes is very high and remains such, irrespective of the proliferative or differentiated state of the cell. The use of primary cells and not of an established cell line allows the conclusion that this persistent mode of myc expression is a true characteristic of the keratinocyte cell type and it is not an artifact due to establishment of cells in culture. This high and persistent pattern of myc expression is drastically different from that observed in lymphocytes and fibroblasts. Thus it is difficult to envisage a role for the myc oncogene in keratinocyte transformation similar to that proposed for transformation of cells of fibroblastic or lymphocytic origin (Land et al., 1983a).

fos and myc expression in the primary keratinocytes are not significantly modulated in response to calcium while they are dramatically affected by TPA. This shows that calcium and TPA, although inducing a similar differentiation program, elicit very different molecular effects on the primary keratinocytes. Whether the modulation in protooncogene expression triggered by TPA is important for induction of differentiation by this substance is not clear. In any case, assessment of protooncogene expression in the keratinocytes provides a sensitive measure of the very early response of these cells to TPA.

In this way, it can be concluded from our study that the resistance of the RBK cells to TPA is due to an early block in the cascade of events triggered by this substance. This block might be caused by an alteration in either levels or function of protein kinase C, the cellular receptor for TPA (Nishizuka, 1984a). This possibility is suggested by the fact that the markedly reduced inducibility of fos in the RBK cells is specific for TPA and by the fact that fos induction by TPA or other mitogens is a very early event for which no protein synthesis is required (Kruijer et al., 1984; Muller et al., 1984; Greenberg et al., 1986). An elucidation of the molecular mechanism responsible for resistance to TPA could lead to an understanding of the concomitant acquisition of resistance to calcium, as it is observed in the RBK cells and in many other spontaneous or carcinogen-induced keratinocyte cell lines (Yuspa et al., 1983; Hennings et al., 1984; our unpublished observations).

Acknowledgements

G.P.D. is a fellow of the Jane Coffin Childs Memorial Fund for Cancer Research. M.Z.G. is supported by a fellowship from the U.S. Natl. Inst. of Health. R.A.W. is an American Cancer Society Research Professor. This work was supported by grant CA07353-03 from the U.S. Natl. Cancer Inst. and by a grant from the ABC Research Foundation.

REFERENCES

1. Balmain, A., and Pragnell, I.B. (1983): Nature, 303:72-74.
2. Balmain, A., Ramsden, M., Bowden, G.T., Smith, J. (1984): 307:658-660.
3. Brown, K., Quintauilla, M., Ramsden, M., Kerr, I.B., Young, S., Balmain, A. (1986): 46:447-456.
4. Campisi, J., Gray, H.E., Pardee, A.B., Dean, M., Sonenshein, G.E. (1984): Cell, 36:241-247.
5. Cepko, C.L., Roberts, B.E., Mulligan, R.C. (1984): Cell, 37:1053-1062.
6. Cochran, B.H., Zullo, J., Verman, I.M., Stiles, C.D. (1984): Science, 226:1080-1082.
7. Curran, T. and Morgan, J.I. (1985): Science, 229:1265-1268.
8. Dotto, G.P., Parada, L.F., Weinberg, R.A. (1985): Nature, 318: 472-475.
9. Dotto, G.P., Gilman, M.Z., Maruyama, M., Weinberg, R.A. (1986): Embo J., in press.
10. Endo, T. and Nadal-Ginard, B. (1986): Mol.Cell.Biol., 6:1050-1057.
11. Furstenberger, G., Berry, D.L., Sorg, B., Marks, F. (1981): Proc.Natl.Acad.Sci.USA, 78:7722-7726.
12. Greenberg, M.E. and Ziff, E.B. (1984): Nature, 311:433-438.
13. Greenberg, M.E., Greene, L.A., Ziff, E.B. (1985): Mol.Cell.Biol., 6:1050-1057.
14. Greenberg, M.E., Hermanowski, A.L. and Ziff, E.B. (1986): Mol.Cell.Biol., 6:1050-1057.
15. Hecker, H., Fusenig, N.E., Kunz, W., Marks, F., Thielman, H.W., editors (1982): Carcinogenesis. Raven Press, New York.
16. Hennings, H., Michael, D., Cheng, C., Steinert, P., Holbrook, K., Yuspa, S.H. (1980): Cell, 19:245-254.
17. Hennings, H., Shores, R., Wenk, M.L., Spangler, E.F., Tarone, R., Yuspa, S.H. (1983): Nature, 304:67-69.
18. Hennings, H., Ben, T., Yuspa, S.H. (1986): Proc.Am.Assoc.Cancer.Res., 25:146.
19. Hsiao, W-L.W., Gattoni-Celli, S., Weinstein, I.B. (1984): Science, 226:552-555.
20. Hsiao, W-L.W., Wu, T., Weinstein, I.B. (1986): Mol.Cell.Biol., 6:1943-1950.
21. Kelly, K., Cochran, B.H., Stiles, C.D., Leder, P. (1983): Cell, 35:603-610.
22. Kilkenny, A.E., Morgan, D., Spangler, E.F., Yuspa, S.H. (1985): Nature, 312:711-716.
23. Kruijer, W., Cooper, J.A., Hunter, T., Verman, I.M. (1984): Nature, 312:711-716.
24. Kruijer, W., Schubert, D., Verman, I.M. (1985): Proc.Natl. Acad.Sci.USA, 82:7330-7334.
25. Kulesz-Martin, M.F., Koehler, B., Hennings, H., Yuspa, S.H. (1980): Carcinogenesis, London, 1:995-1006.
26. Labarca, C. and Paigen, K. (1980): Analytical Biochemistry, 102:344-351.

27. Land, H., Parada, L.F., Weinberg, R.A. (1983a): Science, 222:771-778.
28. Land, H., Parada, L.F., Weinberg, R.A. (1983b): Nature, 304:596-602.
29. Mann, R., Mulligan, R.C., Baltimore, D.B. (1983): Cell, 33:153-159.
30. Melton, D.A., Krieg, P.A., Rebagliati, M.R., Maniatis, T., Zinn, K., Green, M.R. (1984): Nucleic Acids Res., 12:7035-7056.
31. Mitchell, R.L., Henning-Chubb, C., Huberman, E., Verman, I.M. (1985): Cell, 45:497-504.
32. Muller, R., Bravo, R., Burckhardt, J., Curran, T. (1984a): Nature, 312:716-720.
33. Muller, R., Muller, D., Guilbert, L. (1984b): EMBO J., 3:1887-1890.
34. Muller, T., Curran, T., Muller, D., Guilbert, L. (1985): Nature, 314:546-548.
35. Nishizuka, Y. (1984): Nature, 308:693;398.
36. Parkinson, E.K., Pera, M.F., Emmerson, A., Gorman, P.A. (1984): Carcinogenesis, 5:1071-1077.
37. Slaga, T.J., Fischer, S.M., Nelson, K., Gleason, G.L. (1980): Proc.Natl.Acad.Sci.USA, 77:3659-3663.
38. Sukumar, S., Notario, V., Martin-Zanca, D., Barbacid, M. (1983): Nature, 306:658-661.
39. Toftgard, R., Roop, D.R., Yuspa, S.H. (1985): Carcinogenesis, 6:655-657.
40. Van Beveren, C., Van Straaten, F., Curran, T., Muller, R., Verman, I.M. (1983): Cell, 32:1241-1255.
41. Yuspa, S.H. and Morgan, D.L. (1981): Nature, 293:72-74.
42. Yuspa, S.H., Ben, T., Hennings, H., Kichti, U. (1982): Cancer Res., 42:2344-2349.
43. Yuspa, S.H., Kulesz-Martin, M., Ben, T., Hennings, H. (1983a): J.Invest.Dermatol., 81:162s-168s.
44. Yuspa, S.H., Vass, W., Scolnick, E., (1983): Cancer Res. 43:6021-6030.
45. Yuspa, S.H., Kilkenny, A.E., Stanley, J., Kichti, U. (1985): Nature, 314:459-462.
46. Zarbl, H., Sukumar, S., Arthur, A.V., Martin-Zanca, D., Barbacid, M. (1983): Cancer Res., 43:6021-6030.

Tumor Promoters: Biological Approaches for
Mechanistic Studies and Assay Systems,
edited by Robert Langenbach et al.
Raven Press, New York © 1988.

PROTEIN PHOSPHORYLATION AND SIGNAL TRANSDUCTION IN TUMOR PROMOTION

Curtis L. Ashendel, Phyllis A. Baudoin, and Pamela L. Minor

*Department of Medicinal Chemistry, Purdue University
West Lafayette, Indiana 47907*

In the society of molecules that constitutes a living animal cell, it appears that the control of the cell is largely endowed in but a few molecules that carry out the general process that has recently come to be referred to as signal transduction. Understanding in molecular detail how the signal transduction system exerts this control over the growth, differentiation, and function of cells is central to understanding carcinogenesis. This is because this general regulatory system appears to be the direct or indirect target of most carcinogens, tumor promoters, and oncogenic viruses. This presentation will discuss recent data and present alternative hypothetical models concerning the role of signal transduction, and specifically protein phosphorylation, in tumor promotion.

SIGNAL TRANSDUCTION

The process by which extracellular information is received by and ultimately impacts on the functioning of cells represents a broad definition of signal transduction. However, in this presentation this term will be used only in reference to cases where information transfers across the cell membrane independently of the transfer of the signal molecules into the cells. Many distinct signal transducing systems exist in cells and the following description of their similar components represents an oversimplification of these processes. In each case the transduction of a signal must begin with an extracellular signal, be it a soluble factor or a non-diffusible entity such as substratum or a neighboring cell. This interacts specifically with a recognition site on the cell surface that in all known cases is a transmembrane receptor protein. When activated by binding the signal, the intracellular domain of the receptor activates an intracellular membrane-bound coupling protein ("G protein"), that, in the presence of guanine nucleotides, activates another intracellular membrane bound protein. Except in cases of neuronal membrane depolarization, the latter protein then produces, on the inside of the cell, low molecular weight second messenger molecules that then allosterically activate intracellular "effector" proteins. These effector proteins have numerous effects in cells that culminate in altered cell behavior.

PROTEIN PHOSPHORYLATION

Although the phosphorylation of proteins was first recognized as a significant response to hormonal stimulation 30 years ago (29,40), the general importance of this process in signal transduction has become understood only recently. Each of the four known second messengers activates a protein kinase and many cell surface receptor proteins contain tyrosyl-specific protein kinase activity. Thus, all the known signal transduction pathways involve protein kinases that appear to mediate the extracellular signals' effects on cells. Unfortunately it is technically very difficult to identify biologically significant phosphate-accepting substrates for protein kinases. Although these protein kinases exhibit some specificity for particular amino acid sequences (25), and possibly additional structural features (20), they do not generally display the high degree of specificity that might limit one protein kinase to a small number of substrates. With the exception of a few proteins already known to be involved in signal transduction pathways, few, if any, significant substrates for signal transduction-related protein kinases have been identified and characterized. However, it is generally assumed that either the receptor-linked tyrosyl kinases or the second messenger-dependent protein kinases, or both, mediate the effects of extracellular signals on cellular behavior.

A large number of distinct signal molecules may impact on the surface of any given cell, and several, perhaps dozens, will specifically bind to receptors. These result in the intracellular production of only four known second messengers -- cyclic-AMP, cyclic-GMP, calcium, and diacylglycerol -- each of which activates a single distinct protein kinase. Although each of these kinases catalyzes the phosphorylation of many different polypeptides, they have effects on cells that are limited to only a few different outcomes: cell division, differentiation, and transient functional responses (e.g., secretion, motility, mechanical functions, and membrane transport). There is no simple relationship among the biological outcomes and the changes in the concentration of a single second messenger. Thus, if protein phosphorylation ultimately regulates cellular function, then a more complex model must be postulated, perhaps including patterns of second messengers, feedback regulation, or second messenger-independent phosphorylation.

SIGNAL TRANSDUCTION AND CANCER

The importance of signal transduction to cancer is obvious when cancer is viewed as a disease of abnormal regulation of cell growth and differentiation. The components of signal transduction paths most closely associated with the cell membrane appear to represent a constriction point for flow of regulatory information into the cell. This is consistent with the observed or suspected functions of many oncogene-coded proteins in the membrane-associated aspects of signal transduction (6,41) where a small change in the function of a single protein would be expected to have a tremendous impact on cell behavior. Not all protein products of oncogenes have a direct role in signal transduction at the membrane level, however, with *myc*, adenovirus-*E1A*, and other oncogene products having nuclear or cytoplasmic localization (6,41). These latter oncogene products are also distinct in that they appear to affect cellular longevity (6,41).

The results of a separate line of investigation also implicate alterations in signal transduction as causal to induction of neoplasia: Tumor-promoting phorbol esters specifically interact with and alter the function of signal-transducing protein kinase C (PKC). The signal-transduction pathway leading to activation of PKC has been discovered over the last few years (21,35). Many signal molecules, via interaction with transmembrane receptor proteins, stimulate the production of diacylglycerol and inositol tris-phosphate. This appears to involve a calcium- and guanine nucleotide-dependent activation of a plasma membrane-localized phospholipase C that is specific for diphospho-phosphatidyl inositol (21). The inositol tris-phosphate leads to the release of calcium from the endoplasmic reticulum into the cytosol, where it, along with membrane-localized diacylglycerol, activates PKC. Phorbol esters, and functionally related compounds such as mezerein, teleocidin B, and aplysiatoxin activate PKC in a manner similar to but not quite the same as diacylglycerol (1).

This is the current extent of the substantial knowledge of the role of PKC in signal transduction because of the very limited data available on the phosphate-accepting substrates for protein kinases. PKC is known to preferentially phosphorylate proteins on seryl or threonyl hydroxyls that are two residues towards the amino terminus from a basic amino acid, although one or more basic amino acids within three residues on either side of the phosphorylation site is sufficient (25). Purified PKC will catalyze the phosphorylation of several dozen to a few hundred polypeptides upon its activation in the presence of crude extracts of cells (unpublished results). A list of 45 proteins of known function that can be phosphorylated by PKC appeared in a recent review (34). Yet the phosphorylation of one, some, or all of these proteins cannot explain the effects of phorbol esters on cells.

Despite the difficulty of proving that a protein of known identity is phosphorylated by PKC in cells as well as in cell-free systems, the only other experimental approach is even more difficult: High-resolution separation of phosphoproteins and analysis of how their levels change when PKC is activated by phorbol esters or by natural extracellular factors. Such studies observe only the large changes in the most abundant phosphoproteins in cells. The amount of effort required to identify such phosphoproteins is large, requiring years to successfully accomplish. Without some basis to choose which of those phosphoproteins to identify there is only a low chance of identification of critical substrates. The use of phorbol esters to activate PKC will be an extremely useful tool to identify relevant phosphoproteins if knowledge of the normal regulation of PKC and its perturbation by phorbol esters is employed in such a search.

ABNORMAL REGULATION OF PROTEIN KINASE C
BY PHORBOL ESTERS

Phorbol esters may exert their pleotypic effects (7) simply by mimicking the activation of PKC by diacylglycerol, as suggested by a number of indirect studies (1,34). Yet it seems that when examined at the molecular level and the level of tumor promotion, the effects of phorbol esters on PKC are rather distinct from those of diacylglycerol. Investigation of these differences may provide clues to understanding the mechanism of tumor promotion by phorbol esters. The first difference to be recognized was the one thousand-fold greater potency of phorbol esters for activation of PKC (10,43). The lower-affinity interaction of diacylglycerides probably results from the reduced number of points of interaction with PKC due to their structural simplicity compared to phorbol esters. Furthermore, the higher energetics of binding of phorbol esters to PKC appears to reduce the need for participation of calcium ions to a negligible level (3). Together these differences result in a much greater stability of the complex of PKC with phospholipid in the presence of phorbol esters than in the presence of diacylglycerol when divalent-cation chelators are used to prevent the participation of calcium. Thus, when cells treated with phorbol esters such as 12-O-tetradecanoylphorbol-13-acetate (TPA) are lysed in the presence of EDTA, the PKC remains complexed with phospholipid in the cell membranes to a greater extent than in untreated cells, as was first observed by Kraft, *et al.* (28).

This phenomenon of subcellular redistribution of PKC has become known as phorbol ester-induced translocation. From the above discussion it is clear that the three-step mechanism shown in Fig. 1 is consistent with the observations of PKC activation and translocation. This model postulates an equilibrium binding of PKC to membrane phospholipids that results in only a small fraction of PKC activity being associated with the membrane. This membrane-associated PKC is not active and is easily dissociated from the phospholipids with EDTA. When TPA is added, it partitions into the cell membranes. The small amount of membrane-associated PKC and the TPA are both laterally mobile and can interact to form a stable complex that is not dissociated by EDTA. This mechanism is favored over the alternative in which PKC forms a complex with phorbol esters without any phospholipid involvement because such a complex has never been detected. In addition it is consistent with the complexation of PKC with phospholipid that was observed in the absence of phorbol esters but with appropriate concentrations of calcium and magnesium (3). The mechanism in Fig. 1 explains how phorbol esters redistribute PKC to the membrane without having to attract PKC from the cytosol.

Translocation of PKC was not observed after treatment of cells with mitogens (3), growth factors (19,39,46), or phospholipase C (3) that should have resulted in the production of diacylglycerol. In contrast, interleukens 2 and 3 induce translocation of PKC (16,17). Although the difference in ability to translocate PKC might have been suspected to be

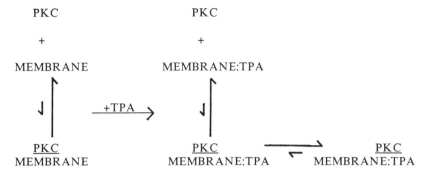

FIG 1. Proposed mechanism for the translocation of PKC by the phorbol ester 12-O-tetradecanoylphorbol-13-acetate (TPA).

related to the functional differences between diacylglycerol and phorbol esters, upon closer inspection the difference appears to depend upon the use of EDTA in the extraction of the cells. Activation of PKC by diacylglycerol is just as dependent on phospholipid as activation by phorbol esters (3,26) and so is just as likely to occur at the cell membrane. This should result in a translocation of PKC to the cell membrane, but observation of such a redistribution of PKC most likely is obscured by the instability of the complex of PKC with the membrane phospholipid and diacylglycerol when the calcium is bound by EDTA.

Although the activated complex of PKC at the cell membrane is very similar when formed with phorbol esters or with diacylglycerol, the subcellular location of such complexes may be rather dissimilar. Both of these activators are very lipophilic and can diffuse and act throughout cellular membranes. However, diacylglycerol may be produced (as part of transducing signals) only in the plasma membrane and because of its short lifetime in cells may not diffuse far. This may result in regions of the membrane that are richer in this second messenger than other regions. In contrast, there are no known obstacles to the free diffusion of phorbol esters to all regions of all cell membranes. This as yet undocumented distinction is potentially very important to the identification of proteins that are phosphorylated by PKC, since this enzyme seems to regulated more by substrate availability than substrate specificity, as discussed above.

Another difference between the action of phorbol esters and diacylglycerol on PKC is that the lifetime of phorbol esters in cells (30,36) is forty- to four hundred-times longer than diacylglycerides (10). In addition, inositol tris-phosphate is rapidly metabolized, resulting in a quick return to the normal cytosolic concentration of calcium after its increase in response to extracellular signals. As depicted in Fig. 2A, the short biological lives of the activating second messengers (10) are thought to result in the breakdown of the active complex of PKC at the membrane. This model allows for each molecule of PKC to participate in many cycles of activation and inactivation. In contrast to this, the activation of PKC by phorbol esters is not so easily reversed because the complex of PKC with a molecule of phorbol ester is so much more stable than the corresponding complex with diacylglycerol. Unable to shut off PKC action by the normal mechanism, cells treated with phorbol esters appear to resort to the more drastic method of proteolytic degradation of PKC (4,42), as depicted in Fig. 2B.

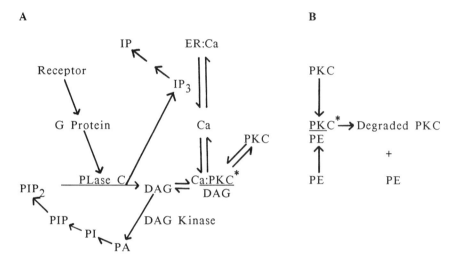

FIG 2. Reactions leading to the reversal of the activation of PKC by diacylglycerol (DAG), **A**; and by phorbol ester (PE), **B**. PIP$_2$, diphosphophosphatidyl inositol; IP$_3$, inositol trisphosphate; IP, inositol monophosphate; ER, endoplasmic reticulum; PKC*, activated PKC; PA, phosphatidic acid, PI, phosphatidyl inositol; and PIP, phosphophosphatidyl inositol.

Due to the fairly good biological stability of phorbol esters, at least in comparison to activated PKC, phorbol esters appear to enhance the degradation (down-regulation) of PKC. This enhancement would be particularly large if the proteolyzed PKC has no or low ability to bind the phorbol ester, such that each molecule of phorbol ester down-regulates several molecules of PKC, as suggested in Fig. 2B. Although fragments of PKC that retain phorbol ester-binding activity have been described (22), this has only been demonstrated in cell-free experiments. Although it is not known if down-regulation of PKC occurs in all cell types in response to treatment with phorbol esters, it has been observed in C3H 10T1/2 cells (Table 1 and 5), mouse spleen lymphocytes (5), as well as other cells (4,13,23,42). A detailed study was done of the kinetics of activation of PKC and its disappearance from cells (4,5). The results are consistent with the model shown in Fig. 2B in that activation always occurred prior to down regulation. Additionally, with greater magnitudes of activation of PKC its rate of down-regulation was higher. Although PKC can be converted to a calcium- and phospholipid-independent form by limited proteolysis *in vitro* (24) or in platelets (45) or neutrophils (32) after TPA treatment, we did not observe any increase in such activity in the EDTA-soluble fractions of C3H 10T1/2 cells treated with phorbol esters. However, several polypeptides of lower molecular weight than PKC were detected with PKC-specific antibody (5) on western blots of subcellular fractions of these cells, and the abundances of these polypeptides were changing in a time-dependent manner that was consistent with their identity as fragments of PKC.

Down-regulation of PKC does not occur in C3H 10T1/2 cells treated with the diacylglycerol dioctanoylglycerol (diC_8), as indicated by the data in Table 1. Treatment with the calcium ionophore A23187 alone or with diC_8 also did not down-regulate PKC. Although the lack of down-regulation of PKC by diC_8 may be due to the rapid metabolism of diacyl-glycerides, treatments with diC_8 every 4 h was insufficient for down-regulation of PKC. Although these data do not exclude the possibility that PKC can be down-regulated by endogenous or exogenous diacylglycer-ol, it suggests that either a continuous production of a high level of diacylglycerol may be necessary for this to occur, if it occurs at all.

TABLE 1. Down-regulation of PKC in C3H 10T1/2 cells treated for 24 h

Treatment of cells[a]	Total PKC activity[b]	Down-regulation[c]
acetone	233	0
TPA (200 nM)	13	94
diC_8 (1000 nM)	225	4
diC_8 (1000 nM, every 4 h)	212	9
A23187 (100nM) + diC_8 (1000 nM)	356	0
A23187 (100 nM)	242	0

[a]Confluent cultures of C3H 10T1/2 cells in BME medium with 10% fetal calf serum.

[b]Cells were washed once in phosphate-buffered saline, scraped from the culture flasks, homogenized by douncing in 20 mM Tris pH 7.4 buffer containing 5 mM EDTA, sedimented at 800 x *g* for 10 min, and PKC activi-ty was determined (3) in the EDTA-soluble and detergent-soluble frac-tions of the supernatant. The sum of the PKC activity in these two fractions is expressed as pmol/min/mg total protein.

[c]Indicated in percent, based upon acetone-treated cells having no down-regulation of PKC and the absence of detectable PKC defined to be 100% down-regulation.

Since incubation of cells with phorbol esters results in the nearly complete loss of PKC activity, this is likely to impare the function of PKC in signal transduction pathways in which it has a role. In the simplest model of PKC function, activation of PKC by phorbol esters mimicks the activation that would have resulted from the calcium and diacylglycerol produced in response to the extracellular signal, as described above. This model allows the prediction that down-regulation of PKC will reduce the responsiveness of cells to those natural extra-cellular signals that involve PKC.

Molecular studies of the role of PKC in signal transduction indicate that PKC phosphorylates the receptors for epidermal growth factor (11) and insulin (8). The phosphorylated EGF receptor displayed reduced ability to bind EGF with high affinity and also both the phosphorylated

EGF receptor and phosphorylated insulin receptor possessed less tyrosyl-kinase activities. At least in these cases, PKC appears to play a role in which the signal transducing system for these factors is attenuated in response to the presence of the factor outside the cell. In such cases, PKC may not have its primary role in the mediation of the intra-celluar signal, but may act to negatively modulate signal reception. The primary mediation of the signal may be done by calcium/calmodulin-dependent protein kinases or by some pathway directly linked to the tyrosyl-kinase activity of the cell surface receptors. Even if PKC is the primary signal mediator, down-regulation of PKC would be expected to reduce the negatively modulating role of PKC and *enhance* the responsive-ness of cells to extracellular signals. The synergism of phorbol esters with serum or polypeptide growth factors for mitogenesis of cells in culture (14,31) is consistent with this hypothesis, but does not distin-guish between these various models of PKC function.

DOWN-REGULATION OF PKC IN TUMOR PROMOTION

Although it remains to be established whether the normal role of PKC in signal transduction is a positive mediator, a negative modulator, or both, understanding the role of PKC in tumor promotion is also impor-tant. It is well established that tumor promotion is an effect of chronic administration of phorbol esters and that gaps in the adminis-tration of promoter, if long enough, reduce the effect of the promoting treatments (9). A similar requirement for continuous presence of phor-bol ester has been observed for promotion of cell transformation *in vitro* (18). In the C3H 10T1/2 cell transformation system the promotion of cell transformation was correlated with down-regulation of PKC in these cells when down-regulation was measured after six weeks of promo-tion (Table 2). Although this suggests that down-regulation of PKC may be necessary for tumor promotion, it may not be sufficient. This insuf-ficiency is consistent with the results of a similar experiment in which mezerein was found to be just as effective as phorbol-12,13-didecanoate (PDD) in down-regulating PKC but was much less effective than PDD in promoting cell transformation (data not shown).

TABLE 2. Correlation of PKC down-regulation with promotion of C3H 10T1/2 cell transformation.[a]

Promoter	PKC Down-regulation[b]		Transformation (foci/flask)
	at 11 d	at 42 d	
Acetone control (0.02%)	0	0	0.9
TPA (10 nM)	71	23	2.9
TPA (200 nM)	83	55	9.9
PDD (10 nM)	86	83	28.6

[a]As described previously (18) except that cells were initiatied with 100 ng/ml benzo(a)pyrene 2 d after seeding in 25 cm^2 flasks and the medium was changed every 2 d during promoter treatment.
[b]PKC activity was determined in cells that were initiated and promoted for either 11 or 42 d and expressed as percent down-regulated as in Table 2.
[c]Number of type III foci per flask of 10 flasks per treatment group.

MULTIPLE FORMS OF PHORBOL ESTER-BINDING PROTEINS

One explanation for the differences in the action of mezerein and TPA or PDD is that mezerein interacts with PKC in a manner differently than TPA or PDD. However, many studies (1) failed to show any large differences in these interactions although some subtle differences were observed (15). Recently published results of efforts to clone the cDNA of PKC (12,27,37,38) have revealed that there are several proteins with sequences very similar to PKC that are expressed in brain tissue and other cells. These proteins are likely to bind phorbol esters similarly, but may differ most in their dependence on calcium for activation. Perhaps the difference in the action of mezerein and TPA results from their interaction with sets of proteins that are largely the same but have a minor protein that is distinct. This distinct protein may only exhibit this differential interaction in cases of specific intracellular concentrations of calcium, thus rendering mezerein distinct from TPA during the first stage of promotion in SENCAR mice, yet nearly identical in the second stage (44).

TABLE 3. <u>Chromatographic resolution of two forms of PKC from rat brain.</u>[a]

Characteristic	Peak I	Peak II
Recovery of [^{3}H]TPA-binding activity[b]	55%	24%
PKC/[^{3}H]TPA-binding activity[c]	78	58
Apparent molecular weight[d]	76500,80000	76500

[a]Extracts of rat brain were separated on DEAE-cellulose (33) by elution with 25 mM PIPES (peak I) and subsequently with 120 mM NaCl (peak II).
[b][^{3}H]TPA-binding activity was determined (2) for the extract and the eluted activity peaks and expressed as percent of the activity applied to the column.
[c]pmol/min PKC activity per pmol [^{3}H]TPA bound.
[d]Determined by relative electrophoretic migration on a discontinuous sodium dodecylsulfate polyacrylamide gel, electrophoretic transfer to nitrocellulose and detection with antibody specific for PKC.

When PKC is purified from rat brain, we discovered that it could be chromatographically resolved into two fractions on DEAE-cellulose (33). The two peaks of activity were highly reproducible and also were similar in their [^{3}H]TPA-binding characteristics, protein kinase characteristics, and the ratio of phorbol ester-binding activity to protein kinase activity, as summarized in Table 3. Western blots (using PKC-specific antibodies) of these active fractions revealed that they both contain 76500 dalton polypeptides while peak I contained an additional immunoreactive polypeptide. The differences, if any, between the smaller proteins in these two fractions are currently under investigation. Although it is not known what relationship these biochemically distinguishable forms of PKC have to the PKC-related polypeptides whose sequences were deduced from cloned cDNA (12,27), the impact of the existence of multiple forms of PKC is clear. The difficulty in understanding the molecular events underlying tumor promotion and signal transduction has now been multiplied several-fold.

CONCLUSIONS

The highly specific interaction of phorbol esters with PKC makes it reasonable to assume that this interaction results in their tumor-promoting action. There is insufficient knowledge about the phosphate-accepting substrates for PKC to understand the molecular details of tumor promotion that occur subsequent to PKC. Such knowledge may be more easily obtained as the details of the regulation of PKC and the perturbation of this regulation by phorbol esters becomes more fully understood. Although the subcellular location of the activated PKC is likely to be an important component of its regulation, the translocation of PKC to cellular membranes is more of an apparent than a real difference between activation of PKC with phorbol esters and endogenous second-messenger molecules. In contrast, the down-regulation of PKC may be unique to tumor promoters that bind to PKC and may be of particular relevance to tumor promotion. At present, it remains to be determined whether the activation of PKC or the down-regulation of PKC is more significant for the chronic and acute effects of tumor promoters. In light of this, it seems premature to propose short-term assays for tumor promoting agents that are based upon only one component of the regulation of PKC, such as its activation.

The complexity of the regulation of PKC is compounded by the existence of multiple distinct forms of PKC. Furthermore, PKC's role in cellular signal transduction may be as a positive mediator, a negative modulator, or both. Yet, the apparently essential role of PKC in signal transduction indicates that tumor promoters as well as chemical carcinogens and viral oncogenes have as a common component in their mechanisms of action leading to an alteration in signal transduction. Although the details of the mechanisms of these agents differ, particularly in their reversibility, the common target suggests that these agents act in a more similar fashion than previously thought. One interpretation of this is that tumor promoters reversibly complement the actions of carcinogen-activated or viral oncogenes to lead to the development of neoplasia, similar to the complementation of multiple oncogenes or to complete chemical carcinogenesis without tumor promotion. Yet because it is likely that there are many possible ways to reversibly alter signal transduction (at least compared to the 30 or more irreversible alterations know to occur via change in the structure or expression of a particular signal transducing protein) the search for a short-term assay for tumor promoters may benefit most by focusing on general markers of perturbation of signal transduction, rather than specific alterations.

ACKNOWLEDGEMENTS

This research was supported by NIH grants CA 36262 and CA 36761 and Junior Faculty Research Award 106 from the American Cancer Society.

REFERENCES

1. Ashendel, C. L. (1985): *Biochem. Biophys. Acta*, 8:   219-242.
2. Ashendel, C. L. and Boutwell, R. K. (1981): *Biochem. Biophys. Res.*

Commun., 99: 543-549.
3. Ashendel, C. L. and Minor, P. L. (1986): *Carcinogenesis*, 7: 517-521.
4. Ballester, R. and Rosen, O. M. (1985): *J. Biol. Chem.*, 260: 15194-15199.
5. Baudoin, P. A. and Ashendel, C. L., manuscript in preparation.
6. Bishop, J. M. (1985): *Cell*, 42: 23-38.
7. Blumberg, P. M. (1980): *CRC Crit. Rev. Toxicol.*, 8: 153-234.
8. Bollag, G. E., Roth, R. A., Beaudoin, J., Mochly-Rosen, D., and Koshland, D. E. (1986): *Proc. Natl. Acad. Sci. USA*, 83: 5822-5824.
9. Boutwell, R. K. (1964): *Prog. Exp. Tumor Res.*, 4: 207-250.
10. Castagna, M., Takai, Y., Kaibuchi, K., Sano, K., Kikkawa, U., and Nishizuka, Y. (1982): *J. Biol. Chem.*, 257: 7847-7851.
11. Cochet, C., Gill, G. N., Meisenhelder, J., Cooper, J. A., and Hunter, T. (1984): *J. Biol. Chem.*, 259: 2553-2558.
12. Coussens, L., Parker, P. J., Rhee, L., Yang-Feng, T. L., Chen, E., Waterfield, M. D., Francke, U., and Ullrich, A. (1986): *Science*, 233: 859-866.
13. Darbon, J., Issandou, M., Delassus, F., and Bayard, F. (1986): *Biochem. Biophys. Res. Commun.*, 137: 1159-1166.
14. Dicker, P. and Rozengurt, E. (1978) *Nature*, 276: 723-726.
15. Dunn, J. A. and Blumberg, P. M. (1983): *Cancer Res.*, 43: 4632-4637.
16. Farrar, W. L. and Anderson, W. B. (1985) *Nature*, 315: 233-235.
17. Farrar, W. L., Thomas, T. P., and Anderson, W. B. (1985): *Nature*, 315: 235-237.
18. Frazelle, J. H., Abernethy, D. J., and Boreiko, C. J. (1983): *Carcinogenesis*, 4: 709-715.
19. Glynn, B. P., Colliton, J. W., McDermott, J. M., and Witters, L. A. (1986): *Biochem. Biophys. Res. Commun.*, 135: 1119-1125.
20. Harrison, M. L., Low, P. S., and Geahlen, R. L. (1984): *J. Biol. Chem.*, 259: 9348-9350.
21. Hokin, L. E. (1986): *Ann. Rev. Biochem.*, 54: 205-236.
22. Hoshijima, M., Kikuchi, A., Tanimoto, T., Kaibuchi, K., and Takai, Y. (1986): *Cancer Res.*, 46: 3000-3004.
23. Hovis, J. G., Stumpo, D. J., Halsey, D. L., and Blackshear, P. J. (1986): *J. Biol. Chem.*, 261: 10380-10386.
24. Inoue, M., Kishimoto, A., Takai, Y., and Nishizuka, Y. (1977): *J. Biol. Chem.*, 252: 7610-7616.
25. Kishimoto, A., Nishuyama, K., Nakanishi, H., Uratsuji, Y., Nomura, H., Takeyama, Y., and Nishizuka, Y. (1985): *J. Biol. Chem.*, 260: 12492-12499.
26. Kishimoto, A., Takai, Y., Mori, T., Kikkawa, U., and Nishizuka, Y. (1980) *J. Biol. Chem.*, 255: 2273-2276.
27. Knopf, J. L., Lee, M., Sultzman, L. A., Kriz, R. W., Loomis, C. R., Hewick, R. M., and Bell, R. M. (1986): *Cell*, 46: 491-502.
28. Kraft, A. S., Anderson, W. B., Cooper, H. L., and Sando, J. J. (1982): *J. Biol. Chem.*, 257: 13193-13196.
29. Krebs, E. G. and Fischer, E. H. (1956): *Biochem. Biophys. Acta*, 20: 150.
30. Mastro, A. M. and Popin, K. G. (1980): *Chem.-Biol. Interact.*, 30:

171-179.

31. Matrisian, L. M., Bowden, G. T., and Magun, B. E. (1981): *J. Cell. Physiol.*, 108: 417-425.
32. Melloni, E., Pontremoli, S., Michetti, M., Sacco, O., Sparatore, B., and Horecker, B. L. (1986): *J. Biol. Chem.*, 261: 4101-4105.
33. Minor, P. L. and Ashendel, C. L., manuscript in preparation.
34. Nishizuka, Y. (1986): *Science*, 233: 305-312.
35. Nishizuka, Y. (1984): *Nature*, 308: 693-698.
36. O'Brien, T. G. and Diamond, L. (1978): *Cancer Res.*, 38: 2567-2572.
37. Ono, Y., Kurokawa, T., Kawahara, K., Nishimura, O., Muramoto, R., Igarashi, K., Sugino, Y., Kikkawa, U., Ogita, K., and Nishizuka, Y. (1986): *FEBS Lett.*, 203: 111-115.
38. Parker, P. J., Coussens, L., Totty, N., Rhee, L., Young, S., Chen, E., Stabel, S., Waterfield, M. D., and Ullrich, A. (1986) *Science*, 233: 853-859.
39. Pontremoli, S., Melloni, E., Michetti, M., Salamino, F., Sparatore, B., Sacco, O., and Horecker, B. L., (1986): *Biochem. Biophys. Res. Commun.*, 136: 228-234.
40. Rall, T. W., Sutherland, E. W., and Wosilait, W. D. (1956): *J. Biol. Chem.*, 218: 483.
41. Ratner, L., Josephs, S. F., and Wong-Staal, F. (1985): *Ann. Rev. Microbiol.*, 39: 419-449.
42. Rodriguez-Pena, A. and Rozengurt, E. (1984): *Biochem. Biophys. Res. Commun.*, 120: 1053-1059.
43. Sharkey, N. A., Leach, K. L., and Blumberg, P. M. (1984): *Proc. Natl. Acad. Sci. USA*, 81: 607-610.
44. Slaga, T. J., Fischer, S. M., Nelson, K., and Gleason, G. L. (1980): *Proc. Natl. Acad. Sci. USA*, 77: 3659-3663.
45. Tapley, T. H. and Murray, A. W. (1984): *Biochem. Biophys. Res. Commun.*, 122: 158-164.
46. Vaarjes, W. J., deHaas, C. G. M., and van den Bergh, S. G. (1986): *Biochem. Biophys. Res. Commun.*, 138: 1328-1333.

Tumor Promoters: Biological Approaches for
Mechanistic Studies and Assay Systems,
edited by Robert Langenbach et al.
Raven Press, New York © 1988.

THE MECHANISM OF ACTION OF PROTEIN KINASE C: NEW INSIGHTS THROUGH THE STUDY OF INHIBITORS AND GENE CLONING

Catherine A. O'Brian, Gerard M. Housey, Mark D. Johnson,
Paul Kirschmeier, Rob M. Liskamp, and I. Bernard Weinstein

Division of Environmental Sciences, the Cancer Center
and Institute of Cancer Research, Columbia University,
701 West 168th Street, New York, N.Y. 10032.

INTRODUCTION

Tumor promoters are compounds which have no or only weak carcinogenic activity when administered alone, but markedly enhance tumor formation when administered after an initiating agent. The resulting tumors are often benign but, in some cases, may progress to become malignant (30,41). In addition to mouse skin carcinogenesis, there is evidence that cancers of the breast, colon, bladder, and liver proceed through stages of initiation and promotion (42). Since breast and colon cancers are leading causes of cancer mortality in Western industrial societies (second only to lung cancer) (12), a detailed understanding of tumor promotion could have a major impact on cancer prevention and treatment in these countries. An indepth understanding of tumor promotion requires elucidation of the mechanism(s) of this operationally defined process at the molecular level. Currently there is substantial evidence at the molecular level for a mechanism of tumor promotion that involves the activation of protein kinase C (PKC) (29,30). A mechanism that involves the generation of free radicals has also been implicated in tumor promotion (2). Recent studies suggest that these processes may actually be related, since the activation of PKC has been correlated with the production of oxygen radicals in human neutrophils (34,38). This review will focus on the evidence that PKC activation may be a critical event in tumor promotion and will discuss research which has been directed toward an understanding of the mechanism of regulation of this enzyme, through studies of PKC inhibitors and through the molecular cloning of a PKC gene and other closely related genes.

EVIDENCE FOR A ROLE OF PKC IN TUMOR PROMOTION

High-affinity receptors for tumor-promoting phorbol esters have been observed in the membranes of numerous cell types. These receptors also bind tumor-promoting polyacetates (such as aplysiatoxin) and indole alkaloids (such as teleocidin) with high affinity. However, these receptors do not specifically bind nonpromoting phorbol esters, polyacetates, or indole alkaloids (16). The high affinity binding of chemically diverse tumor promoters (but not nonpromoting structural analogues) to the same membrane receptor provides evidence that the receptor may actually be the primary target of action of these tumor promoters.

There is now convincing evidence that PKC, the Ca^{2+} - and phospholipid-dependent protein kinase, is the major membrane-associated receptor for the phorbol ester tumor promoters and related compounds. PKC and the phorbol ester receptor have been copurified to apparent homogeneity from both bovine brain and rat brain (19,37), and the relative potencies of a series of phorbol esters in tumor promotion tend to correlate with their relative potencies in PKC activation (5). In addition, tumor promoting indole alkaloids (such as teleocidin B) and polyacetates (such as aplysiatoxin) activate PKC, whereas the nonpromoting polyacetate anhydrodebromoaplysiatoxin does not activate the enzyme (3). The activation of PKC by nanomolar concentrations of chemically diverse and potent tumor promoters suggests a critical role for PKC in tumor promotion. The correlation, however, between the potencies of these agents in tumor promotion and PKC activation is not exact (3,5), and certain second stage tumor promoters, such as mezerein and 12-0-retinoyl-phorbol-13-acetate, are also potent PKC activators (3,15). In addition, certain tumor promoters, such as tetrachlorodibenzo-p-dioxin and phenobarbital, do not activate isolated PKC (8). Therefore, while PKC does appear to be of critical importance in the mediation of tumor promotion by certain tumor promoters, it is not yet clear whether PKC is, in fact, a general mediator of tumor promotion.

INHIBITORS OF PKC

Objectives of PKC Inhibitor Studies

We have been studying PKC inhibitors with three major objectives: 1) the acquisition of a more refined understanding of the mechanism of regulation of PKC, 2) the development of specific PKC inhibitors which could allow a specific, pharmacological manipulation of PKC in intact cells, and 3) the development of antiproliferative drugs. The mechanism of regulation of PKC is very complex, since the phosphotransferase reaction involves two substrates and several cofactors (phospholipid, Ca^{2+}, TPA, diacylglycerol, Mg^{2+}), and yet the enzyme is a single polypeptide chain. PKC inhibitors can perturb the activation of the enzyme, and thereby provide a new perspective from which the regulation of PKC can be analyzed.

Specific PKC inhibitors could be used as pharmacological probes
in order to identify biochemical pathways which are mediated by
the enzyme and biological properties which require the enzyme.
Thus, they could provide an important complement to tumor
promoters in the mouse skin carcinogenesis model, and they could
be used in this model to test the hypothesis that the activation
of PKC is a critical event in tumor promotion. The design of
specific PKC antagonists may be an important approach for the
development of antiproliferative drugs. Specific PKC
antagonists may be useful drugs in the control of abnormal
proliferative disease states such as psoriasis, particularly
since PKC appears to be an important mediator of growth factor
action. In addition, PKC antagonists may be useful in the
treatment of cancer. The current understanding of PKC-tumor
promoter interactions suggests that a PKC antagonist may block
tumor promotion and may even inhibit the growth of established
tumors. Site-directed PKC antagonists may be able to modulate
the function of specific membrane receptors and channels by
inhibiting their phosphorylation in intact cells by PKC.

The Inhibition of PKC by Tamoxifen and
Related Triphenylethylenes

The triphenylethylene tamoxifen is an antiestrogen, which
can effectively inhibit tumor growth in the treatment of human
breast cancer (27). 4-Hydroxytamoxifen and
N-desmethyltamoxifen, which are metabolites of tamoxifen (9),
are also antiestrogens (6,39). All three of these
triphenylethylene derivatives bind to the estrogen receptor with
apparent Kd's of less than 5 nM (39) and to the antiestrogen
receptor with apparent Kd's of less than 50 nM (25,40).
Recently it was demonstrated that micromolar concentrations of
these antiestrogens have growth inhibitory effects on cultured
human breast cancer cells, which cannot be completely reversed
by estrogen. (11,39). This finding suggests that there may be
a low affinity receptor for the antiestrogens, which mediates
those aspects of their action observed only at micromolar
concentrations of the drugs. Such a low affinity receptor could
be important in the mechanism of tamoxifen-mediated tumor
regression, since tamoxifen-treated breast cancer patients have
uM levels of tamoxifen in their plasma (1,9,10) and also high
levels (about 25 ng tamoxifen/mg protein) of the drug in their
tumor tissue (9).
We have found that PKC is a target of tamoxifen,
4-hydroxytamoxifen, N-desmethyltamoxifen, and the
fertility-stimulating drug clomiphene, at micromolar
concentrations of these drugs (31,32). Each of these drugs
inhibits PKC whether the enzyme is under the regulation of
Ca^{2+} and phospholipid or TPA and phospholipid. Thus, these

compounds form a new structural class of PKC inhibitors, since they are all cationic amphiphiles containing a triphenylethylene backbone (31,32). Phenothiazines are structurally related PKC inhibitors (28), in that they are also cationic amphiphiles. The triphenylethylene and phenothiazine PKC inhibitors are also pharmacologically related, since both classes of compounds also inhibit calmodulin-dependent enzymes (4,22,28).

We determined the potencies of tamoxifen (IC_{50}=100uM), 4-hydroxytamoxifen (IC_{50}=25uM), clomiphene (IC_{50}=25uM), and N-desmethyltamoxifen (IC_{50}=8uM) in the inhibition of the Ca^{2+} and PI(phosphatidylinositol)-dependent phosphorylation of histone III-S catalyzed by isolated rat brain PKC. N-desmethyltamoxifen, the most active compound, contains a secondary amine, suggesting that the secondary amine might be an important feature of its potency as a PKC inhibitor. The mechanism of action of these drugs appeared to be the same whether the enzyme was activated by Ca^{2+} and PI or TPA and PI, since the potency of each drug was similar in both of these reactions (31,32)

Protamine sulfate is unusual as a PKC substrate since it is phosphorylated by PKC in the absence of any allosteric cofactors, i.e., Ca^{2+}, phospholipid, DAG or TPA (19). We found no inhibition of PKC-catalyzed protamine sulfate phosphorylation by the triphenylethylenes, providing evidence that these drugs do not inhibit PKC by interacting directly with its active site (31,32).

We observed that the potency of each triphenylethylene as a PKC inhibitor was decreased as the concentration of the phospholipid cofactor was increased. The observation that increasing phospholipid concentrations overcome the inhibition of PKC by triphenylethylenes suggests that the triphenylethylene-mediated inhibition of PKC involves drug-phospholipid interactions and lends further support to our evidence that triphenylethylenes are not active site inhibitors of PKC (31,32).

Our evidence that triphenylethylenes inhibit PKC by interactions with the phospholipid cofactor suggests that their potencies could be affected by the lipid environment of the cell. Therefore, in order to estimate the potencies of these triphenylethylenes on PKC in intact cells, we determined their potencies as inhibitors of [3H]PDBu binding in intact mouse fibroblasts. N-Desmethyltamoxifen, 4-hydroxytamoxifen, tamoxifen, and clomiphene inhibited [3H]PDBu binding in intact mouse embryo C3H/10T1/2 cells with IC_{50}'s of 5,10, 5, and 6uM respectively. Thus, these drugs do appear to interact with the PKC-lipid complex at micromolar concentrations in intact cells (31,32).

The mechanism of inhibition of PKC by the triphenylethylenes is apparently similar to that of the phenothiazines. Neither the triphenylethylenes nor the phenothiazines inhibit the Ca^{2+}- and phospholipid-independent activity of PKC. In addition, the inhibition of PKC by phenothiazines, as well as by triphenylethylenes, decreases when the phospholipid concentration is increased. Thus, both classes of drugs appear to inhibit PKC by phospholipid interactions (28,31,32), although additional interactions of these drugs with PKC itself are not excluded.

Reddel et al. (39) have reported that micromolar quantities of N-desmethyltamoxifen, 4-hydroxytamoxifen, and tamoxifen are cytotoxic to MCF-7 cells and that their order of potency is N-desmethyltamoxifen>4-hydroxytamoxifen>tamoxifen. This order of potency does not correlate with estrogen receptor affinities or antiestrogen receptor affinities. In addition, this order of potency is not observed in the inhibition of calmodulin-dependent phosphodiesterase by these triphenylethylenes (4). We have found (31) however, that these drugs inhibit PKC with the same order of potency as that reported for MCF-7 cytotoxicity, which suggests that inhibition of PKC by triphenylethylenes mediates, at least in part, the estrogen-irreversible antiproliferative effects of the drugs.

The Inhibition of PKC by Rhodamine 6G

The drug rhodamine 6G is selectively toxic to carcinoma cells in vitro. Although the drug initially localizes in the mitochondria of cultured cells, it subsequently becomes dispersed through-out the cytoplasm at doses which are toxic to carcinoma cells (23). We have examined the effects of rhodamine 6G on the regulation of the phosphotransferase activity of PKC.

We have found that rhodamine 6G inhibits PKC, and that this drug falls into the same class of PKC inhibitors as triphenylethylenes and phenothiazines, since its inhibitory effect is reduced at elevated phospholipid concentrations, it does not inhibit the Ca^{2+} plus phospholipid-independent activity of the enzyme, and it is a cationic amphiphilic compound (33). We employed rhodamine 6G in order to further explore the mechanism of inhibition of PKC by this class of cationic amphiphilic drugs. We have found that rhodamine 6G can inhibit PKC whether the enzyme is activated by Ca^{2+} plus phosphatidylserine (10ug/ml) or Ca^{2+} plus arachidonic acid (10ug/ml). It is of interest that rhodamine 6G is over ten times more potent as an inhibitor of PKC when the activating cofactors are Ca^{2+} plus arachidonic acid (IC_{50}=50uM), than when the cofactors are Ca^{2+} plus phosphatidylserine (IC_{50}=800uM). We have also found that the extent of inhibition of the Ca^{2+} plus arachidonic acid-dependent protein kinase activity by rhodamine 6G is decreased when the arachidonic acid concentration is increased. In addition,

rhodamine 6G can inhibit PKC under conditions in which the only
allosteric cofactor present is arachidonic acid (i.e., in the
absence of Ca^{2+} or TPA), but the drug cannot inhibit PKC in
the absence of allosteric cofactors (33).

Our observations that the potency of rhodamine 6G-mediated
PKC inhibition is markedly affected by the structure of the
lipid cofactor (i.e. phosphatidylserine versus arachidonic
acid), that rhodamine 6G can inhibit PKC when the only
allosteric cofactor is a lipid, and that the drug cannot inhibit
PKC in the absence of allosteric cofactors, provide the first
molecular evidence that the inhibition of PKC by certain
cationic amphiphilic drugs occurs through drug-lipid
interactions. These results complement kinetic evidence that
certain cationic amphiphilic drugs inhibit PKC by drug-lipid
interactions (28,30). Our results also indicate that the lipid
microenvironments within various cell types could profoundly
affect the abilities of cationic amphiphilic drugs to inhibit
PKC in vivo.

Rhodamine 6G accumulates in the mitochondria of hepatoma
cells to concentrations of approximately 2mM (21). Dispersal
through-out the cytosol and concomitant cytotoxic effects are
observed following further drug accummulation (23). Since the
mitochondria occupy about 20% of the cytosolic volume of
hepatocytes (24), it follows that upon cytosolic dispersion of
the drug, the cytosolic concentration of rhodamine 6G could
exceed 400uM. Rhodamine 6G might, therefore, accumulate in the
cytosol of certain cells at concentrations which can inhibit PKC
activity. Thus, our results suggest that inhibition of PKC may
play a role in the mechanism of cytotoxicty of certain rhodamine
compounds. Further studies are required, however, to determine
the relevance of our in vitro studies to the in vivo cytotoxic
action of rhodamine compounds.

ISOLATION OF CDNA CLONES ENCODING PKC

Structural studies of the isolated enzyme PKC have been
limited because of the great difficulty involved in purifying mg
quantities of the enzyme to homogeneity. Studies of cDNA's
encoding PKC could provide, therefore, a valuable complement to
studies of the enzyme itself, by allowing an indirect
determination of the primary structure of PKC and by providing
the means by which to characterize structurally related cDNA's,
which could encode PKC isoenzymes or related protein kinases.
In addition, the characterization of cDNA's encoding PKC is
critical for investigations into the regulation of PKC
expression. Therefore, we have undertaken the isolation of cDNA
clones encoding PKC (17).

The Design of an Oligonucleotide Probe for cDNA's Encoding PKC

In order to design an oligonucleotide probe for cDNA's encoding PKC, sequence information was obtained from isolated rat brain PKC. PKC was partially purified to a specific activity of 120nm/min/mg. The enzyme was then labelled with ^{32}P by stimulating its autophosphorylation activity, and, following preparative polyacrylamide gel electrophoresis and autoradiography, the ^{32}P-labelled PKC was identified as a homogeneous 82 kd band. This band was then excised from the gel and the protein was recovered by electroelution. The purified enzyme was reduced, carboxymethylated, dialyzed, and cleaved with endoproteinase Lys C. Cleavage peptides were separated by reverse-phase high pressure liquid chromatography (HPLC). The sequence of one of these peptides, K-S-V-D-W-W-A-F-G-V-L-L-Y-E-M-L-A-G-Q (peptide P2), was used to design an oligonucleotide probe (17).

Isolation of cDNA Clones Homologous to a PKC Probe

Initial screening of 6 x 10^5 clones from a rat brain gt10 cDNA library identified 41 clones that hybridized under low stringency conditions to the ^{32}P-labelled oligonucleotide probe. These clones were isolated and placed into distinct groups based upon intensity of hybridization signal, restriction mapping, and high-stringency Southern blot analyses of rat genomic DNA. Thus far, we have identified five distinct groups of cDNA clones and are in the process of sequencing representatives of each group and analyzing their expression levels in various tissues. Detailed studies on two of these clones, a Group I cDNA designated RP41 and a Group II cDNA designated RP16, are described below.

Sequence Analysis of the cDNA Clone RP41

Restriction enzyme mapping of the RP41 clone indicated that it contained a 1.7 kb cDNA insert. Restriction fragments were subcloned into M13 vectors, and the complete nucleotide sequence of RP41 was determined. The sequence of the 720 base pair Pst I fragment of RP41 is shown in Fig. 1. This sequence displays a 224 amino acid open reading frame followed by a stop codon (TAG) and includes a region of 19 amino acids which is identical with the PKC peptide P2. The latter finding, coupled with findings described below, provide strong evidence that the RP41 clone encodes the carboxyterminal region and catalytic domain of rat brain PKC. It is of particular interest that this sequence also exhibits homology with several domains present in almost all of the previously characterized protein kinases (18), including the conserved amino acid residues RDL, DFG, CGT, and APE (amino

```
1-90   (CTT) GCA GAG ATT GCC ATC GGT CTT TTC TTC TTG CAG AGC AAG GGC ATC ATT TAC CGT GAC CTG AAA CTT GAC AAC GTG ATG CTG GAT TCC GAG
1-30          A   E   I   A   I   G   L   F   F   L   Q   S   K   G   I   I   Y   R   D   L   K   L   D   N   V   M   L   D   S   E
                                          10                                  *   *   *                                          30

91-180        GCG CAC ATC AAA ATC GCT GAC TTT GGC ATG TGT AAA GAG AAT ATC TGG GAT GGG GTG ACA GGG GTG GAT GGG GTG ACT CCA GAC TAC
31-60         G   H   I   K   I   A   D   F   G   M   C   K   E   N   I   W   D   G   V   T   T   K   T   F   C   G   T   P   D   Y
                                                     *   *                          50                      *   *                60

181-270       ATT GCC CCA GAG ATC GCT ATT GCT TAT CAG CCC TAC GGA AAG TCT GTG GAC TGG TGG GCG TTT GGA GTC CTG CTG TAT GAA ATG TTG GCT GGC
61-90         I   A   P   E   I   A   I   A   Y   Q   P   Y   G   K   S   V   D   W   W   A   F   G   V   L   L   Y   E   M   L   A   G
                      *   *                                      70

271-360       CAG GCA CCT TTT GAA GCG GAG GAG GAT GAG GAC CTC TTC CAG TCA ATC ATG GAG CAC AAC GTG GCG TAT CCC AAG TCC ATG TCT AAG GAA
91-120        Q   A   P   F   E   E   E   D   E   D   L   F   Q   S   I   M   E   H   N   V   A   Y   P   K   S   M   S   K   E
              ___                                          100                                 110                             120

361-450       GCT GTG GCA ATC TCC AAA ATC TGC CTA ATG ACC AAA CAC CCA CAC AAG CCC CTG GGT TGT GGG CCT GAA GGG GAA CGA GAT ATT AAG GAG CAT
121-150       A   V   A   I   S   K   I   C   L   M   T   K   H   P   H   K   P   L   G   C   G   P   E   G   E   R   D   I   K   E   H
                                                             130                 +           +   +           +               150

451-540       GCA TTT TTC CGG TAT ATC GAC TGG GAA AAG CTC GAA CGC AAA GAG ATT CAG CCA CCT TAT AAA CCA AAA GCT AGA GAC AAG CGA GAC ACC
151-180       A   F   F   R   Y   I   D   W   E   K   L   E   R   K   E   I   Q   P   P   Y   K   P   K   A   R   D   K   R   D   T
                                                         +                       +           +                           170     *

541-630       TCC AAC TTC GAC AAA GAG TTC ACT CGG CAG CCT GTT GAA CTG ACT CCC ACT GAC AAA CTC TTC ATC ATG AAC TTG GAC CAA AAT GAA TTT
181-210       S   N   F   D   K   E   F   T   R   Q   P   V   E   L   T   P   T   D   K   L   F   I   M   N   L   D   Q   N   E   F
                  *   *   *                                      190                             200                             210

631-718       GCT GGC TTC TCG TAT ACT AAC CCA GAG TTT GTC ATT AAT GTG TAG  GTGAATCCAGATTCCATCCCTGACCCTGTGTAAGG CTCCAG
211-224       A   G   F   S   Y   T   N   P   E   F   V   I   N   V   -
                                                             220
```

Figure 1

acids 18-20, 37-39, 55-57, and 62-64 in Fig. 1). Computer searches of the Protein Information Resource (PIR) database, using the coding region of RP41 shown in Fig. 1, indicated that the greatest homologies in amino acid sequence (about 40% overall identity) were with the catalytic subunit of the cyclic AMP-dependent protein kinase (PKA), and the carboxy terminal (catalytic) domain of the cyclic GMP-dependent protein kinase (PKG). These sequence homologies provide strong evidence that the carboxy terminal region of RP41 constitutes the catalytic domain of PKC (17).

Sequence Analysis of the cDNA Clone RP16

Restriction enzyme mapping of the RP16 clone indicated that it contained a 2.0 Kb cDNA insert. Appropriate restriction fragments were subcloned into the M13 vectors, and the complete nucleotide sequence of RP16 was determined. Fig. 2 shows a 720 nucleotide segment of this sequence, along with the deduced amino acid sequence, beginning 18 amino acids upstream from an ATP binding site consensus sequence: GXGXXG-(16 amino acids)-K (amino acids 18-22 and 40 in Fig. 2). As with RP41, RP16 also exhibits all of the homology domains that have been previously identified in other protein kinases (18), including the RDL, DFG, CGT, and APE clusters (amino acids 135-137, 154-156, 172-174, and 179-181, respectively, in Fig. 2). Furthermore, in the region corresponding to the PKC peptide P2 (amino acids 190-208 in Fig. 2) this clone differs from RP41 at only 4 positions. The sequence of RP16 in Figure 2 displays 65% identity with the carboxy terminal region of RP41, whereas the homology between this region of RP41 and either PKA or PKG is only about 40%.

Analysis of the Transcripts Related to RP41 and RP16.

Utilizing a ^{32}P-labelled probe prepared from the coding region of the PKC cDNA clone RP41 in Northern blot analyses, we detected very high levels of two distinct transcripts of about 9 kb and 3.5 kb in the poly A$^+$ RNA fraction of rat brain (data not shown). When the same poly A$^+$ RNA samples were hybridized

---

Figure 1. Nucleotide and Deduced Amino Acid Sequences of the cDNA clone RP41. A 720 base pair Pst I fragment encoding the 224 amino acid carboxy terminal region of rat brain PKC is displayed. Asterisks denote amino acid residues conserved among previously described protein kinases. The 19 amino acid sequence that is underlined corresponds exactly to PKC peptide P2. Amino acids which appear to constitute an ATP binding site consensus sequence are denoted with a plus (+) sign (aa 138, 140, 143, and 160).

```
1-90      CAA GGC CAG GCC AAG CGC TTG GGC CTG GAT GAG TTC AAC TTC ATC AAG GTG TTA GGC AAA GGC AGC TTT GGC AAG GTC ATG CTG GCC GAG
1-30       Q   G   Q   A   K   R   L   G   L   D   E   F   N   F   I   K   V   L   G   K   G   S   F   G   K   V   M   L   A   E
                                                10                                  +  20   +           +                      30

91-180    CTC AAG GGT AAG GAT GAA GTC TAT GCT GTG AAG GTC TTA AAG AAG GAC GTC ATC CTG CAG GAT GGA CAA CGT GGA CTG CAC GAT GAC AGA
31-60      L   K   G   K   D   E   V   Y   A   V   K   V   L   K   K   D   V   I   L   Q   D   G   Q   R   G   L   H   D   D   R
                                                40  +                                  50                                      60

181-270   GAA GAG GAT TTT GGC TCT GGC GCG GAA ACA CCC TTA TCT AAC CCA ACT CTA TTG CTG CTT CCA GAC CAA GGA CCG CCT CTT CTT CGT CAG
61-90      E   E   D   F   G   S   G   A   E   T   P   L   S   N   P   T   L   L   L   L   P   D   Q   G   P   P   L   L   R   Q
                                                70                                      80                                      90

271-360   GAA TAT GTA AAC GGT GGA GAC CTC ATG TTC CAG ATT CAG CGG TCC CGA AAA TTC GAT GAG CCT CGT TCC GGG TTC TAT GCT GCC GAG GTC
91-120     E   Y   V   N   G   G   D   L   M   F   Q   I   Q   R   S   R   K   F   D   E   P   R   S   G   F   Y   A   A   E   V
                                               100                                     110                                     120

361-450   ACA TCT GCT CTC ATG TTT CTC CAC CAA CAT GGA GTG ATC TAC AGG GAT TTG AAA CTG GAC AAC ATC CTT CTA GAT GCA GAA GGT CAC TGC
121-150    T   S   A   L   M   F   L   H   Q   H   G   V   I   Y   R   D   L   K   L   D   N   I   L   L   D   A   E   G   H   C
                                               130                  *   *   *          140                                     150

451-540   AAG CTG GCT GAC TTT GGG ATG TGC AAG GAA GGG ATT CTG AAT GGC GTG ACA ACT ACC ACC TTC TGT GGG ACT CCT GAC TAC ATA GCT CCA
151-180    K   L   A   D   F   G   M   C   K   E   G   I   L   N   G   V   T   T   T   T   F   C   G   T   P   D   Y   I   A   P
                       *   *   *               160                                     170      *   *   *                   *   *

541-630   GAG ATC CTG CAG GAG TTG GAG TAC GGC CCC TCA GTG GAC TGG TGG GCC CTG GGC GTG CTG ATG TAC GAG ATG ATG GCC GGG CAG CCC CCC
181-210    E   I   L   Q   E   L   E   Y   G   P   S   V   D   W   W   A   L   G   V   L   M   Y   E   M   M   A   G   Q   P   P
           *                                  -^-------------------------^---------------^---------------^-----------------    210

630-720   TTT GAA GCT GAC AAC GAG GAC GAC TTG TTT GAA TCC ATC CTT CAC GAT GAC GTT CTC TAC CCT GTC TGG CTT AGC AAG GAG GCT GTC AGC
211-240    F   E   A   D   N   E   D   D   L   F   E   S   I   L   H   D   D   V   L   Y   P   V   W   L   S   K   E   A   V   S
                                               220                                     230                                     240
```

Figure 2

to a ^{32}P labelled probe prepared from the PKC-related cDNA clone RP16, a single transcript that was approximately 7.5 Kb in size was detected (data not shown). The abundance of the transcripts for both RP41 and RP16 were high in brain, with moderate levels in heart and liver (17). The relative abundance of the RP41 transcript in these three tissues is consistent with published data on the levels of PKC enzymatic activities, and with the amounts of PKC determined to be present in these tissues by immunoassay (14,26).

Evidence for a PKC Multigene Family and its Implications in the Mechanism of Tumor Promotion

We have observed much greater homology between the PKC cDNA clone RP41 and the cDNA clone RP16 than between either of these cDNA sequences and the corresponding sequences of other structurally characterized protein kinases. These findings provide evidence for the existence of a PKC multigene family (17). Recently, other laboratories have also obtained evidence for a PKC multigene family. Ono et al. have isolated and partially sequenced a rat brain cDNA clone, which appears to be identical to our clone RP41, and they have obtained peptide sequence data which suggest the existence of other forms of PKC (35). Knopf et al. have also partially characterized a rat brain cDNA (designated PKC III) which is virtually identical to RP41. They have also isolated and completely sequenced cDNA's encoding two other forms of PKC, PKC I and PKC II (20). Parker et al. have reported the isolation of a cDNA encoding a bovine PKC, as well as two other closely related bovine and human cDNA sequences (7,36). The sequences of the latter clones differ appreciably from the sequences of our RP41 and RP16 clones. Thus, there is now substantial evidence for the existence of a PKC-related multigene family.

The existence of a PKC-related gene family may have considerable implications with respect to growth control and tumor promotion. The existence of multiple forms of PKC may account for the previously discussed discrepancies between the potencies of certain compounds in the activation of PKC *in vitro* and in tumor promotion *in vivo*, since various forms of PKC may have distinct sensitivities to different tumor promoters. There

---

Figure 2. Nucleotide and Deduced Amino Acid Sequence of the cDNA clone RP16. A partial sequence of RP16, a PKC-related cDNA clone, is displayed. Notations are as described in the legend to Figure 1. The 19 amino acid sequence underlined (aa 190-208) is identical to PKC peptide P2 at 15 out of 19 positions. Arrowheads denote the four amino acids that differ between P2 and the corresponding region of RP16.

is precedence for a division of labor within a protein kinase family. The cAMP-dependent protein kinases fall into two major classes, type I and type II, which differ in their mechanisms of regulation and their tissue distribution (13). It seems likely that future studies employing the recently isolated PKC cDNA clones will clarify the role of this new multigene family in signal transduction, growth control and tumor promotion.

Acknowledgements: We acknowledge the excellent secretarial assistance of Mrs. Nancy Mojica and Ms. Lintonia Sheppard. These studies were supported by NIH Grant CA 02656 and funds from the Alma Toorock Memoria for Cancer Research. G.M. Housey is supported by the Medical Scientist Training Program. We thank Janusz Wideman, Stan Stein, and May Chang for valuable assistance in obtaining the amino acid data on PKC, and Cheryl Fitzer and James Murphy for valuable technical assistance.

References

1. Adam, H.K., Douglas, E.J., and Kemp, J.O. (1979): Biochem. Pharmacol., 28: 145-147.

2. Ames, B.N. (1983): Science, 221: 1256-1264.

3. Arcoleo, J.P. and Weinstein, I.B. (1985): Carcinogenesis, 6: 213-217.

4. Barrera, G., Screpanti, I., Paradisi, L., Parola, M., Ferretti, C., Vacca, A., Farina, A., Dianzani, M.U., Frati, L., and Gulino, A. (1986): Biochem. Pharmacol., 35: 2984-2986.

5. Castagna, M., Takai, Y., Kaibuchi, K., Sano, K., Kikkawa, U., and Nishizuka, Y. (1982): J. Biol. Chem., 257: 7847-7851.

6. Coezy, E., Borgna, J.L., and Rochefort, H. (1982): Cancer Res., 42: 317-323.

7. Coussens, L., Parker, P.J., Rhee, L., Yang-Feng, T.L., Chen, E., Waterfield, M.D., Francke, U., and Ullrich, A. (1986) Science, 233: 859-866.

8. Couterier, A., Bazgar, S., and Castagna, M. (1984): Biochem. Biophys. Res. Commun., 121: 448-455.

9. Daniel, P., Gaskell, S.J., Bishop, H., Campbell, C., and Nicolson, R.I. (1981): Eur. J. Cancer Clin. Oncol., 17: 1183-1189.

10. Daniel, P., Gaskell, S.J., Bishop H., and Nicolson, R.I. (1978): J. Endocrinol., 83: 401-408.

11. Darbre, P.D., Curtis, S., and King, R.J. (1984): <u>Cancer Res.</u>, 44: 2790-2793.

12. Doll, R. and Peto, R. (1981): <u>The Causes of Cancer</u>, Oxford Univ. Press, Inc., New York.

13. Flockhart, D. and Corbin, J. (1982): <u>Crit. Rev. in Biochem.</u>, 12: 133-186.

14. Girard, P.R., Mazzei, G.J., and Kuo, J.F. (1986): <u>J. Biol. Chem.</u>, 261: 3.

15. Gschwendt, M., Horn, F., Kittstein, W., Furstenberger, G., and Marks, F. (1983): <u>FEBS Lett.</u>, 162: 147-150.

16. Horowitz, A.D., Fujiki, H., Weinstein, I.B., Jeffrey, A., Okin, E., Moore, R.E., and Sugimura, T. (1983): Cancer Res, 43: 1529-1535.

17. Housey, G.M., O'Brian, C.A., Johnson, M.D., Kirschmeier, P., Roth, J., and Weinstein, I.B. (1986): <u>J. Cell Biochem. Suppl. (Abstract)</u>, 10C: 132.

18. Hunter, T. and Cooper, J.A. (1985): Ann. Rev. Biochem., 54: 897-930.

19. Kikkawa, U., Takai, Y., Minakuchi, R., Inohara, S., and Nishizuka, Y. (1982): <u>J. Biol. Chem</u>, 257: 13341-13348.

20. Knopf, J.L., Lee, M-H., Sultzman, L.A., Kriz, R.W., Loomis, C.R., Hewick, R.M. and Bell. R.M. (1986) <u>Cell</u>, 46: 491-502.

21. Kuzela, S., Joste, V., and Nelson, B.D. (1986): <u>Eur. J. Biochem.</u> 154: 553-557.

22. Lam, H.-Y. (1984): <u>Biochem. Biophys. Res. Commun.</u>, 118: 27-32.

23. Lampidis, T.J., Hasin, Y., Weiss, M.J., and Chen, L.B.(1985): <u>Biomedicine and Pharmacotherapy</u>, 39: 220-226.

24. Loud, A.V., Barany, W.C., and Pack, B.A. (1965): <u>Laboratory Investigation</u>, 14: 996-1008.

25. Miller, M.A. and Katzenellenbogen, B.S. (1983): <u>Cancer Res.</u>, 43: 3094-3100.

26. Minakuchi, R., Takai, Y., Yu, B., and Nishizuka, Y. (1981): <u>J. Biochem.</u>, 9: 1651-1654.

27. Mouridsen, H., Palshof, T., Patterson, J., and Battersby, L. (1978): <u>Cancer Treat. Rev.</u>, 5: 131-141.

28. Nishizuka, Y. (1984): <u>Science</u>, 225: 1365-1370.

29. Nishizuka, Y (1984): <u>Nature</u>, 308: 693-698.

30. O'Brian, C.A., Liskamp, R.M., Arcoleo, J.P., Hsiao, W.-L.W., Housey, G.M., and Weinstein, I.B. (1986): In: <u>New Insights into Cell and Membrane Transport Processes</u>, edited by George Poste and Stanley T. Crooke, pp. 261-274. Plenum Publishing Co., New York.

31. O'Brian C.A., Liskamp, R.M., Solomon, D.H., and Weinstein, I.B. (1986): <u>J. Natl. Canc. Inst.</u>, 76: 1243-1246.

32. O'Brian, C.A., Liskamp, R.M., Solomon, D.H., and Weinstein, I.B. (1985): <u>Cancer Res.</u>, 45: 2462-2465.

33. O'Brian, C.A., and Weinstein, I.B. <u>Biochem. Pharmacol</u>, in press.

34. O'Flaherty, J., Schmitt, J.D., and Wykle, R.L. (1985): <u>Biochem. Biophys. Res. Commun.</u>, 127: 916-923.

35. Ono, Y., Kurokawa, T., Kawahara, K., Nishimura, O., Marumoto, R., Igarashi, K., Sugino, Y., Kikkawa, U., Ogita, K., and Nishizuka, Y. (1986): <u>FEBS Lett.</u>, 203: 111-115.

36. Parker,P.J., Coussens, L., Totty, N., Rhee, L., Young, S., Chen, E., Stable, S., Waterfield, M.D., and Ullrich, A. (1986): <u>Science</u>, <u>233</u>: 853-858.

37. Parker, P.J., Stabel, S., and Waterfield, M.D. (1984): <u>EMBO</u>, 3: 953-959.

38. Pontremoli, S., Melloni, E., Michetti, M., Sacco, I., Salamino, F., Sparatore, B., and Horecker, B.L. (1986): <u>J. Biol. Chem</u>, 261: 8309-8313.

39. Reddel, R.R., Murphy, L.C., and Sutherland, R.L. (1983): <u>Cancer Res.</u>, 43: 4618-4624.

40. Watts, C.K., Murphy, L.C., and Sutherland, R.L. (1984): <u>J. Biol. Chem.</u>, 259: 4223-4229.

41. Weinstein, I.B., Horowitz, A.D., Fisher, P., Ivanovic, V., Gattoni-Celli, S., and Kirschmeier, P. (1982): In: <u>Tumor Cell Heterogeneity</u>, edited by A.H. Owens, D.S. Coffey, and S.B. Baylin, pp 261-283. Academic Press, New York.

42. Weinstein, I.B. (1981): <u>Cell Biology of Breast Cancer</u>, edited by C.M. McGrath, M.J. Brennar, and M.A. Rich, pp 425-450. Academic Press, New York.

Tumor Promoters: Biological Approaches for
Mechanistic Studies and Assay Systems,
edited by Robert Langenbach et al.
Raven Press, New York © 1988.

PRO GENES, A NOVEL CLASS OF GENES THAT SPECIFY SENSITIVITY TO
INDUCTION OF NEOPLASTIC TRANSFORMATION BY TUMOR PROMOTERS

M.I. LERMAN[1] AND N.H. COLBURN[2]

Laboratory of Experimental Pathology[1] and Laboratory of
Viral Carcinogenesis[2], National Cancer Institute, Frederick,
Maryland 21701

ABSTRACT

The advent of molecular cloning quickly led to the suggestion
that a certain set of evolutionarily conserved genes is driving
the process of carcinogenesis. The following is a brief
discussion of how tumor promoters control the expression of some
oncogenes and the recently discovered pro genes. The cellular
system, the molecular cloning, structure and possible function
of the pro genes are presented. We speculate that a subset of
oncogenes and the pro genes, when genetically altered, provide
the network that is influenced by tumor promoters.

INTRODUCTION

That the process of tumor promotion is governed at least in
part by genetically determined events, can be deduced from two
basic observations which have been known for sometime. The
first of these is that early termination of chronic exposure to
tumor promoter in mouse skin initiation-promotion or other
rodent systems does not produce a return to an initiated state
but rather to some post-initiated state (11). This implies that
at least some transitions during tumor promotion are irreversible and therefore possibly genetically determined. The second
observation is that one can obtain from pre-existing populations
(29) or by breeding experiments (8), rodents that are relatively
sensitive or resistant to initiation-promotion schemes of
carcinogenesis. Because such animals do not vary in initiation-
related events, namely in their capacity to metabolize
carcinogens to mutagenic compounds, to form DNA adducts, or to
repair these adducts (91), it appears likely that the basis for
sensitivity is at the level of tumor promotion. Similarly there
exists a variety of genetically determined human cancer prone
disorders, some of which have been postulated to involve
increased sensitivity to tumor promotion (60).

The Use of Genetic Variants for Responses to Tumor Promoters to Elucidate Critical Regulatory Functions and Genes

The purification of the tumor promoting phorbol esters as the active components of croton oil (45,103) coupled with the discovery that phorbol esters bind to specific saturable receptors (31), made possible a classical approach to elucidating events on the biologic response pathways triggered by phorbol ester receptor interaction. Genetic variants for a number of biochemical events postulated to be on the pathways leading to growth or differentiation or tumor promotion responses to phorbol esters have been sought as have variants for the biologic responses themselves, and the results have been informative (see Table 1).

TABLE 1. Genetic variants for response to tumor promoters

Cell Line(s)	Variant Parameter	References
HL-60, human promyel- ocytic leukemia	Phorbol Diester Receptor Down modulation	96
EL-4 mouse thymoma	Protein kinase C substrates	63
FELC, mouse friend erythroleukemia	Membrane lipid fluidity	35
Balb/3T3 mouse	K+/Na+/Cl- transport	97
Mouse Swiss/3T3	Mitogenic response	12-14,48
JB6	Mitogenic response	26,28
Swiss/3T3	Gene amplification response	49
HL-60	Differentiation responses	71
FELC	Differentiation responses	108
LC-7 mouse keratin- ocyte cell lines	Terminal differentiation	47,109,110
EL-4 thymoma	Interleukin-2 induction	63
Ad-5 rat embryo fibroblasts	Transformation promotion response	34,36
JB6 mouse epidermal	Transformation promotion response	18,40

Receptor Variants.

Hormone resistant variants identified in the human population or by selection of heterogeneous cell cultures have frequently included a subset whose resistance can be attributed to hormone receptor deficiency. Receptorless variants have, for example, been found for epidermal growth factor (EGF) (88) and for insulin (87). In the case of phorbol ester receptors, however, no variants have been found for either reduced number or reduced binding affinity (20,19,35). This implied that the consequences of receptor loss would be lack of viability, but did not provide information on specific functions that were receptor dependent. Nevertheless, since virtually all biochemical and biological responses to tumor promoting phorbol esters occur at the low concentrations characteristic of receptor mediated events, this suggests the essential nature of receptor binding for all the biologic responses to phorbol esters. Variants for receptor down modulation have been described in the case of HL-60 cells resistant to TPA-induced differentiation (96). The mechanism and significance of this phorbol ester receptor down modulation are otherwise unknown.

Receptor-associated protein kinase variants.
The preponderance of available data establishes the identity of the phorbol ester receptor as the calcium-dependent phospholipid dependent protein kinase, or C kinase (4,59,80). As in the case of binding activity, C kinase variants have to date not emerged.

Kinase substrate variants.
A number of C kinase substrates for serine or threonine phosphorylation have been elucidated including tyrosine hydroxylase (1) EGF receptors (17,53) and ribosomal components such as EIF2B (81), and ribosomal protein S6 (67) as well as several unidentified proteins using in vitro assays. Recently, Kramer and Sando (63) have described a variant of EL-4 mouse thymoma cells that is resistant to 12-0-tetradecanoyl-phorbol-13-acetate TPA-induction of interleukin-2 (IL-2). The resistant variant differs from sensitive EL-4 cells in two C kinase substrates unique to the sensitive cells and two C kinase substrates unique to the resistant variant. These four substrates may be critical to the positive or negative regulation of the IL-2 induction response.

Other signal transduction variants.
Other signal transduction or second messenger events that have been postulated to be on phorbol ester response pathways include reactive oxygen generation (79), calcium mobilization (82), phospholipid turnover (82), and monovalent cation transport (97). Sussman and O'Brien (97) have described a Balb/c 3T3 preadispose cell mutant with decreased activity of a Na+/Cl- cotransport system. The mutant cells were also resistant to a TPA-induced volume decrease, presumably involving a cytoskeletal response. Variants for such a "shrinking" response have also been described in the case of Caenorhabditis elegans (70).

Mitogentic Response Variants.
TPA, like EGF, FGF, fibroblast growth factor and vasopressin, induces a mitogenic response in quiescent Swiss 3T3 fibroblasts in the presence of limited serum concentrations (12). Butler-Gralla and Herschman have described variants lacking a mitogenic

response to TPA (12) and teleocidin (48), another tumor promoter with high affinity binding to the phorbol ester receptor. The resistant variants were unaffected in their arachidonic acid and prostaglandin release (14) and glucose uptake responses (13), but showed resistance to TPA enhanced gene amplification (49). Although the basis for the resistance to TPA-induced mitogenesis is still being sought, these results do suggest that mitogenic stimulation is required for gene amplification by TPA.

Colburn et al. (26) have described variants of JB6 mouse epidermal cells that are resistant to induction of mitogenic stimulation by TPA. These variants showed diminished glucose uptake response (28) and lack of EGF receptors (20). That the latter may be required for mitogenic response to TPA in JB6 cells was suggested by the finding that reconstitution of the resistant variants with EGF receptors in the form of unpurified membranes, yielded a restoration of mitogenic response not only to EGF but also to TPA (23).

Differentiation response variants.
TPA and congeners like teleocidin induce differentiation in human HL-60 promyelocytic leukemia cells (71) and inhibit induced differentiation in mouse Friend erythroleukemia cells (108). Resistant variants of both cell lines have been reported (71,108), but the basis for resistance to the TPA induced differentiation response is not known. Another class of differentiation resistant cells has been described by Hennings et al. (47) and Yuspa et al. (110,109). These are putatively initiated mouse keratinocyte cell lines which are resistant to induction of terminal differentiation by high calcium or by TPA. Such variants may be valuable in elucidating a tumor promotion-relevant response to TPA.

Transformation (or promotion of transformation) variants.
A case of what may be sensitive variants for transformation promotion has been described for fibroblasts from humans showing a genetic predisposition to cancer, namely familial polyposis coli (60). In this case sensitivity to TPA induced progression to anchorage independence but not to tumorigenicity was demonstrated.

Rodent cell variants for induction of neoplastic transfor-mation by tumor promoters have been described. These include adenovirus-5 transformed (AD5) rat embryo fibroblasts described by Fisher et al. (36,34) and spontaneously initiated mouse epidermal JB6 cells described by Colburn et al. (18,40,42). The sensitive cells in each case are induced to undergo neoplastic transformation measured by anchorage independence and other parameters in response to tumor promoting (but not non-promoting) phorbol esters, teleocidin, and EGF. In each case the response is irreversible. The sensitive JB6 cell lines undergo an anchorage independent transformation response to TPA that is 100-fold greater than that in the resistant variants. The induced anchorage independent transformants are tumorigenic. Dominance of the sensitive phenotype (as occurs in vivo [29]) was demonstrated by cell fusion experiments (24). That genes specifying promotion sensitivity could be expected, was demonstrated by transfection of DNA from sensitive (P^+) donors into insensitive (P^-) recipient cells (25).

Transformation Promoting (pro) Genes: Cloning and Characterization

As indicated above, several lines of experimentation suggested that specific gene(s) might be responsible for and govern specific steps (events) in tumor promotion. Recently our group suceeded in molecular cloning of two new genes that appear to determine promotion of neoplastic transformation of the P^+ clonal lines of the JB6 lineage of mouse preneoplastic epidermal cells (22). Below we shall summarize the data now available on the pro genes and discuss their functions and involvement in the progression of preneoplastic cells to tumorigenicity.

A. Molecular cloning and structure of pro genes. Various techniques have been employed in the last few years to clone previously unknown genes. They involve either "search" or "rescue" strategies. Both require establishment of genomic or sub-genomic libraries in suitable vectors and subsequent isolation of the recombinant gene by (1) "tracking" it, using a biological assay (the sib selection technique [16]), or (2) screening the library with available probes. The only promising option we had to clone the pro genes was to use sib selction (16,43), because no data that would lead to a molecular probe was available at the time. The cloning steps are presented in Figure 1 and Table 2. First, a subgenomic size-selected (3–12 kb) library of BglII (shown not to destroy the pro activity) fragments of Cl 22 was constructed by ligation into the BamHI site of the pCD-X vector of Okayma and Berg (50). This vector was chosen on the following grounds: (i) it can accommodate inserts up to 15–17 kb; (ii) the inserts are placed between the SV40 early promoter and SV40 polyadenylation site; (iii) most of the pBR322 has been removed from the vector to increase copy number and to delete poison sequences interfering with trans-formation of eukaryotic cells (51). Second, five cycles of sib selection were carried out and finally the recombinant plasmids that contained the activated pro gene(s) were selected from a pool containing 7 different plasmids. At each cycle to insure a 99% probability of retaining the active plasmids in the pool, 10 times more colonies then the expected number of different recombinants were grown and used to prepare DNA for transfection into the P^- cells. It should be emphasized here that only the sib-selection protocol permits isolation of all the active genes

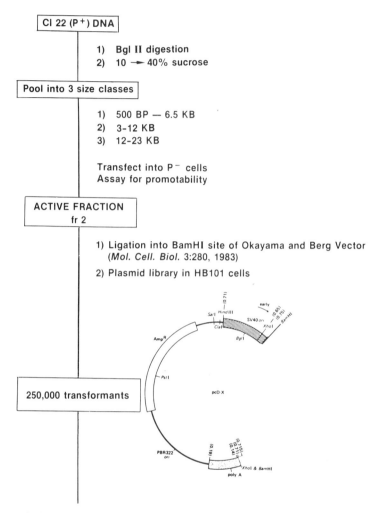

Active promoting sequences isolated by 6 cycles of sib selection

Fig. 1. A schematic outline of the cloning procedure for the pro genes.

TABLE 2.   Isolation of the pro genes by sib selection (16)

Cycle	No. Pools	Plates/ Pool	Trans- formants/ Pool	Colonies/ Pool	No. Active Pools	Pool No.(s) Selected
1	9	6	−25,000	−25,000	5	3,4,9
2	24	3	−3,125	−15,000	6	9−7
3	18	1	−175	2,000	4	18
4	10	2	−18	−200	2	8
5	10	1	−7	−200	3	3
6	1	1	−7	200	2 plasmids	−

of a similar kind present in a library, whereas screening with molecular probes could yield only homologues to probe sequences. We established (see below) that the two active plasmids (designated p26 and p40 respectively) contained different sequences. The p26 and p40 plasmids contained active genes that were designated pro-1 and pro-2, respectively (68). To date we have isolated an additional two active plasmids, but it remains to be seen whether they contained genes different from pro-1 and pro-2.

That pro genes are different at the DNA level is evident from lack of hybridization (68) and lack of heteroduplex formation between the p26 and p40 inserts (Fig. 2) difference in restriction maps (Fig. 3) and finally from absence of homology between the pro-1 and the pro-2 sequences (46). The absence of homology at the DNA level, however, does not preclude homology at the protein level. Protein homology seems possible because both pro genes appear to provide the P^+ cells and transfected P^-cells with an apparently similar function, namely, the ability to become transformed after TPA treatment. Limited homology on the protein level is an established feature for certain immortalizing genes including adenovirus Ela, c−myc, and c−myb (89) that do not show homology at the DNA level.

The structural features of the pro-1 gene recently sequenced (Fig. 4), are highly unusual in many respects. The gene is relatively small (1 kb in size) (Fig. 3 and Fig. 4) and resides in a highly repeated (and possibly unstable) genomic segment (Fig. 3), containing almost all known mouse repeated sequences. The pro-1 sequence itself appears as a fusion sequence assembled from two different types of middle repetitive elements, the BAM 5 and the Alu-type B1 repeat joined together by an apparently unique sequence of 64bp. The process that created such a structure is unknown. One possibility would be that the gene was created by exon shuffling (38), involving an ancestral gene and Alu DNA. The gene later gave rise to the BAM 5 repetitive

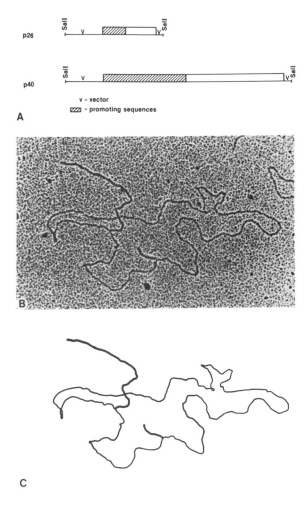

Fig. 2. Lack of heteroduplex formation between pro-1 and pro-2 gene sequences. Plasmids were linearized with Sal I and hybridization was carried out in 50% formamide, 100 mM Tris, pH 8.0, 6.4 mM EDTA, 56 mM Na+, and a final DNA concentration of 2.5 ug/ml at 37° for 45 minutes. The hybrid molecules were processed and examined as described (32).

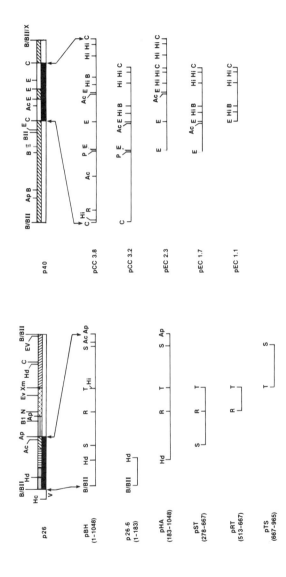

Fig. 3. Restriction and functional mapping of pro genes. The restriction sites mapped by standard procedures (55) and sequencing (56) are indicated. Mouse repeated sequences were mapped by Southern analyses using total DNA and cloned repeated sequences (B1, B2, BAM5, and R) as probes. To locate the pro genes fragments were assayed by transfection into JB6 C130 cells, then subcloned into pBR322 by normal DNA recombinant procedures (55).

AGATCTTCAGGTACTTCAGGTCCCTGGATGGTCATTCCTTCGGTCTCTGCTCCACATTTTGTCTCTGTAACTCTTTCATTGGGTATTTTGTTCTGC CTT A
CAAGAAG GACCAAAAT GTCCACACTTTGGTCTTCCTTCTTCCTGAGTTTCA TGTGGTTTG TGAACTGGATCTTGGGTATTCCAAGCTTCTGGGC TAATAA
CCATGTATTACTGAGGGCATGTCATGTATGTT CTTTTG AGACTAGGTTACCTCAATCAGGATGATATTTTCTAATCTGATCCATTTGCCTAAGGATTTCA
TAAATTCATTGTTTTAAATAGCTGAGTAGTACTCCATTGTGTAAATGTACCACATTTTCTGTACCCATACGCTGTTCAGAGACATCTGGGTT CTTCCAG

                        met tyr ile val glu his val ser leu leu asn val gly ala ser pro leu tyr ile pro gly ser gly ile
CTTCTAGCTACTATAAATAAGTCTTCTATGTACATAGTGGAACATGTGTCCTTATTAAATGTTGGAGCATCTCCTCTGTATATTCCCGGAAGTGGTATA

ala gly ser ser gly thr thr met ser asn phe leu ser ser his gln thr asp phe gln ser gly cys ala thr leu phe phe phe phe phe phe gly
GCTGGGTCCTCAGGTACTACTATGTCCAATTTTCTGAGTAGCCATCAAACTGATTTCCAGAGTGGTTGTGCCACTC TTTTTTTTTTTTTTTTTTTTT GGT

phe leu arg lys gly phe tyr val ***
TTTTTGAGAAAGGGTTTCTATGTATAACCCTAGCTGACCTAGCACTCCCTTTGTAGTCCAAGCTGGCCTCGAACTTAGGAATCTGCCTGCCTCTGCCTC
CCAAGTGCTGGG ATTAAA GTCATGAGCCAC CACA AAAAAAAAAAAAAGACAGATAGATAGATAGATAGATAGATAGATAGATAGATAGATAGATAGATAGA
TAGATAGGAAGGAAGAAAGAAAGAAAGAAAGAAAGAAAGAAAGAAAGAAAGAAGAAAGAAAGAAAGAAAGAAAGAAAGAAAGAAAGAAAGAAAGAAAGAAAA
GGAGAAATGAAAATTATCCACTTCATCCAGATTTTCCAGTTTTGTTGAGTATACACTTTTGTCTTTGGATCTGATAATTTTTTAAATTTTTTCCAT ATCT
                                                 1049
GTCGTTATGTCTCCCTTTCATTTCTCATTTTCTTAATTTACATACTGGGCCC

Fig. 4. Nucleotide sequence of the pro-1 gene. Sequencing was performed by the chemical degradation procedures of Maxam and Gilbert (74). The nucleotide sequence of 1049 bp between the BglII and ApaI sites (Fig. 3) is shown in bold letters with the predicted amino acid sequence above it. The termination codon is marked by asterisks. Consensus sequences common to RNA polymerase II transcribed genes: the "CCAAT" box positions 108–116), the "TATA" box (positions 195–200), the sequence "CTTTTG" associated with capping (positions 393–400); the polyadenylation signal "ATTAAA" (positions 727–730); and the cor enhancer SV40 type sequence "TGTGGTTTG" (positions 152–160) are boxed; the putative start of transcription is marked by an arrow. The dots at positions 1 and 510 demarcate the limits of homology to the mouse Bam 5 middle repetitive element, and at positions 574 and 732 to the Alu-type B1 element (homologies are to complemented and inverted sequences); tandemly repeated tetranucleotides "GATA" and "GAAA" are underlined.

element in a way similar to the creation of Alu family from the unique 7SL RNA gene (102).

The pro-1 sequence has all the landmark consensus sequences involved in accurate and abundant transcription employed by eukaryotic RNA polymerase II genes. The promoter elements ("TATA", "CAAT" boxes, a typical enhancer cor sequence, and a strong ribosomal binding site) are in an ordered spatial arrangement characteristic for pol II promoters; and a poly-adenylation hexanucleotide ("ATTAAA") along with a typical cleavage site are present in the sequence downstream to the translation terminator codon. The open reading frame (195bp) has a high probability of being a coding sequence according to the parameters given by Shepherd (93). This putative coding sequence is contiguous with no introns in the 5' and 3' regions of the gene. The lack of introns, and the presence of an uninterrupted oligo A stretch 3' to the polyadenylation signal are reminiscent of a processed gene. An alternative explanation for the lack of introns is that the gene may represent a highly conserved ancestral gene that did not acquire introns during evolution, or may have lost introns during a gene conversion event that did not affect the transcriptional control elements of the gene (6,85).

The predicted product of the pro-1 gene is a 65 amino acid protein (MW 7, 100 daltons) with a highly unusual composition. It contains 35% hydrophobic amino acids (Phe, Leu, Val, Ile), 24% of uncharged polar amino acids (Ser, Tyr, Thr) and is neutral. No significant homology between pro-1 protein and all vertebrate protein sequences in the Georgetown Protein Data Bank was detected.

It is noteworthy that most of the hydrophobic amino acids of the pro-1 protein are concentrated at the –COOH end, while the polar amino acids are scattered throughout the sequence (Fig. 4). This suggests that pro-1 may be a membrane protein, and its 3-D structure may be altered by secondary modification such as phosphorylation.

The genomic segment representing the pro-2 gene is 3.8 kb in size (Fig. 3) and is mostly a unique sequence except for a small highly repeated element present in the middle of the active gene (Fig. 3). This repeated element is unrelated to known mouse repeats. Sequencing of the entire 3.8 kb active genomic fragment representing the pro-2 gene is now almost complete and will be published elsewhere (46).

The obvious involvement of the pro genes in promotion of transformation prompted us to consider their relationship to known oncogenes. We searched for possibile homology to cloned viral and cellular oncogenes. Hybridization at conditions of higher or lower stringency showed that neither gene is homologous to 12 known viral oncogenes: abl, fes, fms, erbA, erbB, myb, myc, Ha ras, Ki ras, sis, src, and mouse c-mos (7). Sequence comparisons of the pro-1 sequence and the pro-2 sequence failed to reveal any homology to all oncogene sequences deposited into the Los Alamos Data Bank as of September, 1984. Analysis of the restriction maps of both pro genes showed that they are different from those of Nras (99), Blym (43), Tlym (66), Nmyc (61), raf/mil/mht (90), met (27), and mcf (33). Therefore, it appears likely that the pro genes are unrelated to known oncogenes. Nevertheless, based on their transformation promoting activity and the methodology used to isolate the pro genes, we are prompted to suggest that the pro genes may represent a novel class of oncogenes.

It is well established now that cellular oncogenes are highly conserved during metazoan evolution, implying that their products play a central role in cellular regulation and that their activation by either overproduction or mutational alterations may be critical for malignant transformation (78,104).

Southern analyses of human and mouse DNA's have shown that both pro genes are present and, therefore, conserved during human evolution. Human placenta and baboon lymphocyte DNA's produced a light smear of hybridization and a single band homologous to pro-1, suggesting that a small family or a single highly homologous copy is present. Consistent with this, screening $7x10^5$ phage of a human sperm library under highly stringent conditions revealed only two identical phage positive with probes from the pro-1 sequence (68). The size of the Cla I fragment containing the entire pro-2 gene in human DNA is only 3.2 kb as compared to 3.8 kb in the mouse. This size difference could arise from Cla I site polymorphysm or a loss of the 0.5 kb EcoRI fragment from the middle of pro-2 gene (Fig. 3) that contained a highly repeated mouse element. It is also possible that this repeated element was inserted after mouse and human diverged some 70 million years ago. We also observed that DNA from human nasopharyngeal carcinoma cell lines (CNE_1 and CNE_2) contained somewhat amplified pro-1 and pro-2 genes (20–30 phages in CNE_2 library homologous to pro-1 and 5 to pro-2 [69]). Together with the observation that DNA from CNE cells showed transformation promoting activity when transfected into mouse JB6 P- cells, this suggests that pro genes may be involved in human cancer induction.

The transformation promoting activity of the pro genes has so far been detected only by transfection into JB6 P- cell lines (Table 3). Transfection into NIH3T3 cells or secondary mouse keratinocytes did not transfer a P^+ response (25). On the other hand, transfection into human cancer prone fibroblast (BCNS cells) resulted in their lifespan extension (94).

2   Both cloned pro genes independently induced the P+ phenotype with specific activities similar to those of intact P+ DNA's (Table 3).

B. Pro genes: mode of activation, transcription, role in tumor promotion and carcinogenesis. The discovery of pro genes involved in promotion of transformation, and their highly conserved nature raise further questions: (a) how are the pro genes activated? (b) what are the products of pro genes? (c) what is the molecular basis of their activity? and (d) what is the relationship of pro genes and oncogenes?

TABLE 3. P+ activity of pro-1 and pro-2 cloned genes and genomic DNA's.

DNA	P+ Specific Activity (TPA-induced colonies per 10^5 cells per 10^{-17} moles pro gene equivalent transfected)
Genomic DNAs	
JB6 Cl 22	120
JB6 Cl 30	<1
Balb/c secondary mouse keratinocytes	<1
Balb/c mouse liver	<1
Human placenta	<1
Plasmids	
p26	101
pBH	152
p40	80
pCC3.8	117

P+ specific activity was determined from a concentration-response curve in which TPA-induced agar colony formation was assayed after transfection of 10^{-12} to 10^{-19} moles pro gene equivalents (10 ug to 1 pg plasmid DNA) per dish of JB6 Cl 30 P- recipient cells. Genomic DNA's were assayed at 15 ug (2×10^{-17} moles) per dish (2×10^5 cells) of Cl 30 recipient cells.

At the present time we have only partial answers to these basic questions.

Currently, two basic mechanisms for the activation of oncogenes have been proposed and in some cases proven. According to one mechanism, overproduction of an apparently normal oncogene product would, in some way, perturb normal cellular regulation and drive abnormal growth (78,104). This overproduction was shown to result from oncogene amplification, promoter activation through gene rearrangements or viral insertions, or both. Another mechanism involves structural alteration, such as point mutations, in the gene and its

product presumably resulting in different activity or regu-
latability of the product. Clearly, the lack of transformation
promoting activity in all normal mouse and human DNA's tested
and also in the JB6 P- cell (Table 3) suggests that the pro
genes found in JB6 P+ cells are somehow activated. Our current
hypothesis is that both basic mechanisms may be in use to
activate the transformation promoting potential of the pro genes
(68,69). First, normal alleles of both pro genes proved to be
inactive as revealed by transfection of DNA from mouse secondary
keratinocytes, mouse liver or human placenta (Table 3). Second,
of the mouse DNA's assayed, only DNA from mouse P+ cell lines,
or transformed tumorigenic lines derived from P+ cells by TPA
treatment, transferred promoting activity in the transfection
assay. DNA from human nasopharyngeal carcinoma cell lines
showed P+ activity, but it remains to be seen whether this
activity can be attributed to pro genes. Third, no rearrangements or significant amplification of pro-2 sequence was
observed in the P+ cell lines or tumor cell lines, or in mice
sensitive or resistant to tumor promotion (Fig. 5). The
homology to repeated sequences of the pro-1 gene precluded such
analysis in mouse P+ and tumor cells. An additional band,
however, hybridizing to pro-1 was found in human CNE tumor cell
lines when compared to normal human DNA. Whether this
additional band reflects some kind of rearrangement, or
restriction site polymorphism remains to be established.
Screening of a CNE$_2$ cell genomic library yielded 20–30 phage
containing pro-1 sequence, which may reflect an amplification of
the pro-1 gene whereas the germ line library yielded only one
phage. Fourth, both P$^+$ and P- cells treated with the TPA
respond with a transient increase in cytoplasmic RNA hybridizing
to pro-1 (52, and Table 4); this response is higher in P+ cells,
suggesting that overproduction of the gene product is possible.
Also, probing the chromosomal structure of pro genes has established that the pro genes reside in a transcriptionally active
chromatin (Table 5). Considered together these results suggest
that a small structural change, altering the gene product, may
account for the transformation promoting potential of the pro-2
gene; both alteration and overproduction of the pro-1 gene product may activate it. Direct comparison of normal and activated
alleles at the DNA sequence level will reveal the nature of any
change responsible for the activation of pro genes.

The products of oncogenes have been grouped into several
biochemical classes including tyrosine specific protein kinases,
growth factors and receptors, DNA binding proteins, and plasma
membrane proteins. On the other hand, two cooperating
functions, provided by different oncogenes, are sufficient to
transform primary rodent cells in culture (65). One function is
provided by immortalizing or establishing genes (locates to
nucleus) and the other by transforming genes (locates to
cytoplasm). This basic observation suggested that oncogene

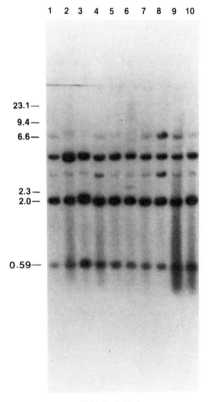

1. CI41 (cell line)
2. CI30 (cell line)
3. Sencar (liver)
4. C57/BL (liver)
5. DBA (liver)
6. BALB/c (liver)
7. JB8 (cell line)
8. D11a (cell line)
9. RT101 (cell line)
10. T-cell lymphoma (cell line)

Fig. 5. Lack of amplification or rearrangement of the pro-2 gene sequence in mouse cells. Total DNA was digested with EcoRI to completion, electrophorezed on 1% agarose gels and transferred to nitrocellulose filters by the method of Southern (73). The filters were hybridized under stringent conditions as described (68). The probe was the 3.2 kb insert of pCC3.2 (see Fig. 3, B).

TABLE 4.   TPA treatment of both P$^+$ and P$^-$ cells produces
           elevation of pro-1 RNA levels

| | Pro-1 Copies Per Cell | |
Cell Line	In Untreated Controls	In TPA Treated Cells (2 hrs)
JB6 Cl 22 (P$^+$)	36 $\pm$ 9	162 $\pm$ 18
JB6 Cl 30 (P$^-$)	17 $\pm$ 6	59 $\pm$ 13

Levels of cytoplasmic RNA that hybridized to a pro-1 probe
containing nucleotides 1-677 of pro-1 were determined by dot
blot analysis. Results are given   as the mean number of pro-1
copies $\pm$ half the range for 2 independent experiments in which
cells were exposed to TPA as indicated.

TABLE 5.   DNAse I sensitivity of the promoting (P$^+$) sequences
           in promotion sensitive (P$^+$) and transformed (Tx) cells

| | Promotion of Transformation after DNA Transfection into P- Cells* (TPA-Induced Soft Agar Colonies/1x10^5 Cells)**,*** | |
Units DNAse/ DNA Transfected	JB6 C141 (P+)	T^{3}6274 (Tx)
0	430	384
8	366	128
17	0	73
25	146	0
35	128	0

 *Recipient P- cells were JB6 C130
 **Solvent controls = 0
***TPA-treated P- cell background subtracted from each value.
Nuclei were isolated and assayed for DNAse I sensitivity
according to Wu (107). After treatment DNA was isolated and
assayed for pro gene activity by transfection into JB6 C130 P-
cells as described (25).

products act in a limited number of biochemical pathways. Pro
gene products may fall into one of the above classes. They
may be proteins involved in transcriptional or translational
regulation or certain growth factors which may or may not be
protein kinase C substrates. It is likely that the products of

<u>pro</u> genes are present in cells in small amounts and may function as transactivating factors inducing inappropriate transient expression of certain oncogenes or constitutive expression of certain others (Fig. 6), that function independently of TPA. In fact, we have recently described a novel transforming activity that appeared subsequent to <u>pro</u> gene activition (21).

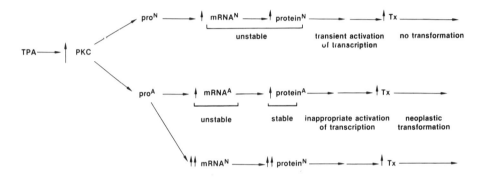

Fig. 6. A schematic presentation of the model showing the involvement of <u>pro</u> genes in carcinogenesis.

The discovery of two tumor promoter responsive <u>pro</u> genes supports the concept put forth by Boutwell (9) that a small set of genes whose expression is induced by tumor promoters are involved in tumor promotion. Tumor promoters may induce not only the expression of <u>pro</u> genes but also the expression of certain oncogenes (78,58). Preexisting heritable changes in their structure resulting in altered expression or altered products is postulated to be responsible for their tumor producing potential. The <u>pro</u> genes are clearly different from known oncogenes; together with other genes, like <u>myc</u> and <u>fos</u>, whose expression is also controlled by tumor promoters, they may provide the molecular basis of tumor promotion.

Genes Whose Expression is Modulated by Phorbol Esters and Other Tumor Promoters: Their Roles in Neoplastic Transformation

Many hormones and growth factors appear to exert their effects through transcriptional (or in some cases post-transcriptional) regulation of the expression of specific genes.

Since phorbol esters are apparently hormone–like in the sense that they work through specific receptors and trigger certain signals or second messengers, it seems reasonable to look for specific genes whose expression is modulated by them. A subset of these tumor promoter inducible (or repressible) genes can be expected to be promotion relevant. It is noteworthy that hypotheses for tumor promoters acting as gene regulators during preneoplastic progression have been set forth for many years (9, 52,105). What follows is a selective consideration of several classes of genes that might be candidates for transformation-relevant tumor promoter-regulated gene expression (see Table 6).

TABLE 6. Genes whose expression is modulated by phorbol esters
and other tumor promoters

Gene	Inducers	References
Cell Cycle Related		
c–myc	Con A, PDGF, TPA, EGF in quiescent cells	44,58,77
c–fos	Serum, PDGF, FGF, TPA	44,64,77
ODC	TPA, testosterone, serum	10,57,62
Secreted		
Collagen	TPA, EGF	30,95
MEP	TPA, PDGF, KSV	42
Plasminogen activator	TPA, EGF, RSV	76,106
Non–phorbolester Induced		
P1–450	TCDD	55,86
DNA Viral		
EBV	TPA, saccharin, DDT	54,56,98,111
BPV	TPA	2
Adenovirus 5	TPA	37,15
Genes for Some Unidentified proteins		
JD 15 (for p32)	TPA, PHA	51
p32	TPA	3
pp80 (hsp 80)	TPA	2,3,15,37,39, 41,54,56,92,98
pro–1	TPA	68

Genes involved in cell cycle traverse.
Considerable attention has been paid to finding rate-limiting events that control the G_0-to-G_1-to S phase progression (50). From studies of gene expression during mitogenic stimulation of lymphocytes or quiescent fibroblasts the finding has emerged that certain cellular oncogenes, in particular c-fos and c-myc, are transiently stimulated to produce elevated levels of mRNA and protein. In the case of mouse fibroblasts, whether the mitogenic stimulus is increased serum or added platelet derived growth factor (PDGF) or fibroblast growth factor (FGF), one finds a characteristic elevation of c-fos mRNA at 5 to 30 minutes after mitogen addition (44,64,77) and an elevation of c-myc mRNA at 1 to 4 hours post mitogen (78,79,84). Addition of TPA to quiescent fibroblasts under conditions that produced mitogenic stimulation also produced an identical time course of c-fos and c-myc mRNA elevation (44,64). The stimulation of tritiated thymidine incorporation into DNA occurred with an onset at 12-15 hours after mitogen exposure in each case (44,77). Greenberg and Ziff (44) showed by nuclear runoff transcription assays that the level of both fos and myc regulation was transcriptional. Whether stimulated fos and/or myc transcription were causally related to mitogenesis is not clear, but the possibility is suggested by the lack of fos transcriptional stimulation by the nonmitogen insulin and the low level of stimulation by the weak mitogen (for these cells) EGF (44,64). Stimulated fos transcription is not limited to conditions of mitogenic response, but has also been observed to occur preceding monocytic differentiation induced by TPA in HL-60 cells or in the monomyelocytic line U-937 (75). Granulocytic differentiation induced by DMSO was not preceded by fos mRNA elevation (75).

Another transiently induced cell cycle related gene is ornithine decarboxylase (ODC). ODC induction appears to be required in mouse skin tumor promotion by TPA (10). ODC is induced by a variety of inducers including TPA, transiently at the level of transcription with a subsequent elevation of the protein that is also transient. The time course of induction by testosterone shows a maximal ODC mRNA level at 24 hours (57,62) and by serum in quiescent cells shows a maximal ODC mRNA level at 2-10 hours (57).

Genes for secreted products.
Growth or differentiation regulatory genes can be considered likely targets for tumor promoter action. So too might certain genes for secreted products, considering that some of these products appear to be involved in invasion or metastasis (84), and others may be involved in autocrine regulation (100). In mouse JB6 cells, as in various other cells, TPA exposure produced a rapid decrease in translatable and hybridizable mRNA

for collagen (85). This decrease persisted in the continued
presence of TPA (30,85) in contrast to the transient effects
seen for fos, myc, and ODC.

Another protein whose mRNA levels are regulated by TPA is the
35 kilodalton major excreted protein (MEP) described by
Gottesman and Sobel (42). Maximal rates of MEP synthesis
occurred after incubating NIH/3T3 cells in TPA for 6 hours, with
a return to uninduced levels by 24 hours. Translatable MEP
mRNA levels were also elevated by PDGF exposure or infection
with Kirsten Sarcoma Virus. Finally, plasminogen activator (PA)
synthesis is stimulated in a variety of cells by tumor promoter
exposure, with a maximal effect at 6-24 hours (76,106). In
addition to TPA, EGF, retinoic acid, and Rous sarcoma virus
transformation have been found to be PA inducers (76).

Genes induced by nonphorbol tumor promoters.
Another class of tumor promoters found to regulate gene
expression are the halogenated aromatic hydrocarbons. The
pesticide 2,3,7,8 tetrachloro-dibenzo-p-dioxin (TCDD) induces a
set of drug metabolizing enzymes including aryl hydrocarbon
hydroxylase, and in some cases a set of genes involved in cell
division and differentiation (55,86).

DNA viral genes.
The observation that TPA induces Epstein-Barr virus (EBV) and
other oncogenic herpesviruses in genome-harboring cells, was
originally reported by Zur Hausen et al. (111). In virus
nonproducer cells, the tumor promoter induced EBV early antigen
(56). EBV early antigen was also induced by several nonphorbol
tumor promoters including some that do not interact with protein
kinase C (98). It is now clear that TPA treatment of certain
lymphoblast cell lines produces elevation of a 2.5 kb mRNA
containing an 11.3 tandem repeat of a 125 base pair G-C rich
unit (54). In addition, TPA has been shown to stimulate the
transcription of other DNA viral genes, including those of
bovine papilloma virus (2) and adenovirus 5 (Ad5)(37). TPA
specifically accelerates the appearance of early viral mRNA in
HeLa cells infected by Ad5 (15,37).

Other genes.
Thirty-two kilodalton proteins have been reported by two
laboratories to be induced by TPA (3,51). These are probably
different from MEP (42) and different from each other. Gindhart
et al. (39,41) reported induction by TPA of an 80 kd phospho-
protein likely to be a C kinase substrate. Rosengurt and
coworkers (5) also described a TPA inducible 80 kd phospho-
protein that may be the same protein.

Balmain et al. (5) have found elevated H-ras transcription in
papillomas and carcinomas induced in mouse skin by (7,12)

dimethyl benz[a]anthracene (DMBA)-TPA initiation-promotion, a finding not confirmed by others (101). In any case, TPA does not directly induce H-ras transcription in this system (75,101).

Finally, expression of the transformation promoting gene pro-1 described above, appears to be induced by TPA. A four-to-six-fold elevation of pro-1 RNA levels occurs 2 hours after JB6 promotion sensitive (P+) cells are exposed to TPA.

SUMMARY AND PERSPECTIVES

In summary, the use of genetic variants of established cell lines has been important in understanding certain genetic alterations; and has led us to the discovery and isolation of a novel class of genes, the pro genes, that are involved in cellular regulation and together with other genes provide the molecular basis of tumor promotion. Second, tumor promoters through a hormone-like receptor mechanism are regulating in a temporal fashion the activity of these tumor promotion related genes. We believe that deregulation of the temporal control of their activity results in perturbation of control mechanisms regulating growth and facilitates carcinogenic conversion. Third, it is clear that we have yet only unveiled the surface of a problem that is accessible to exploration.

ACKNOWLEDGEMENTS

We are grateful to Dr. M. Gonda for performing heteroduplex analyses, Mr. Eugene Lerman for the mathematical treatment of the sib-selection protocol, and Ms. Beverly Bales and Joyce Vincent for typing and organizing the manuscript.

REFERENCES

1. Albert, K.A., Helmer-Matyjek, E., Nairn, A.C., Muller, T.H., Haycock, J.W., Greene, L.A., Goldstein, M. and Greengard, P. (1984): Proc. Natl. Acad. Sci. USA,81:7713-7717.

2. Amtmann, E. and Sauer, G. (1982): Nature, 296:675-677.

3. Arya, S.K., Wong-Staal, F. and Gallo, R.C. (1984): Molec. Cell. Biol., 4:2540-2542.

4. Ashendel, C.L., Staller, J.M. and Boutwell, R.K. (1983): Cancer Res., 43:4333-4337.

5. Balmain, A., Ramsden, M., Bowden, G.T. and Smith, J. (1984): Nature, 307:658–660.

6. Baltimore, D. (1981): Cell, 24:592–594.

7. Blair, D.G., Wood, T.G., Woodworth, A.M., McGeady, M.L., Oskarrson, M.K., Propst, M.A., Tainsky, C.S., Cooper, R., Watson, B.M., Baroody, B.M. and Vande Woude, G.F. (1984): Cancer Cells, 2:281–292.

8. Boutwell, R.K. (1964): Prog. Exp. Tumor Res., 4:207–250.

9. Boutwell, R.K. (1974): CRC Crit. Rev. Toxicol., 2: 419–443.

10. Boutwell, R.K. (1982): Adv. Polyamine Res., 4:127–134.

11. Burns, F.J., Vanderlaan, M., Sivak, A. and Albert, R.E. (1978): In: Carcinogenesis, Vol. 2. Mechanisms of Tumor Promotion and Cocarcinogenesis, edited by T.J. Slaga, A. Sivak and R.K. Boutwell, pp. 91–96. Raven Press, New York.

12. Butler-Gralla, E. and Herschman, H.R. (1981): J. Cell Physiol., 107:59–67.

13. Butler-Gralla, E. and Herschman, H.R. (1983): J. Cell. Physiol., 114:317–320.

14. Butler-Gralla, E., Taplitz, S. and Herschman, H.R. (1983): Biochem. Biophys. Res. Commun., 111:1984–199.

15. Carter, T.H., Milovanovic, Z.Z., Babiss, L.E. and Fisher, P.B. (1984): Molec. Cell. Biol., 4:563–566.

16. Cavalli-Sforza, L.L. and Lederberg, J. (1956): Genetics, 41:280–289.

17. Cochet, C., Gill, G.N., Meisenhelder, J., Cooper, J.A. and Hunter, T. (1984): J. Biol. Chem., 259:2553–2558.

18. Colburn, N.H., Former, B.F., Nelson, K.A. and Yuspa, S.H. (1979): Nature, 281:589–591.

19. Colburn, N.H., Gindhart, T.D., Dalal, B. and Hegamyer, G.A. (1983): In: Organ and Species Specificity in Chemical Carcinogenesis, edited by R. Langenbach, S. Nesnow and J.M. Rice, pp. 189–200. Plenum Publishing Corp., New York.

20. Colburn, N.H., Gindhart, T.D., Hegamyer, G.A., Blumberg, P.M., Delclos, K.B., Magun, B.E., and Lockyer (1982): J. Cancer Res., 42:3093-3097.

21. Colburn, N.H., Lerman, M.I., Hegamyer, G.A., and Gindhart, T.D. (1985): Mol. Cell Biol., 5:890-893.

22. Colburn, N.H., Lerman, M.I., Hegamyer, G.A., Wendel, E., and Gindhart, T.D. (1984): In: Genes and Cancer, edited by M. Bishop, M. Graves and J. Rowley, pp. 137-155. A.R. Liss, Inc., No. 17, New York.

23. Colburn, N.H., Lerman, M.I., Srinivas, L., Nakamura, Y., and Gindhart, T.G. (1984): In: Cellular Interactions by Environmental Tumor Promoters, edited by H. Fujiki, pp. 155-166. Japan Sci. Soc. Press, Tokyo/VNU Science Press, Utrecht.

24. Colburn, N.H., Talmadge, C.B., and Gindhart, T.D. (1983): In: Progress in Nucleic Acid Research and Molecular Biology, edited by W.E. Cohn, pp. 107-118. Academic Press, New York.

25. Colburn, N.H., Talmadge, C.B., and Gindhart, T.D. (1983): Mol. Cell Biol., 3:1182-1186.

26. Colburn, N.H., Wendel, E.J., and Abruzzo, G. (1981): Proc. Natl. Acad. Sci. USA, 78:6912-6916.

27. Cooper, C.S., Park, M., Blair, D.G., Tainsky, M.A., Huebner, K., Croce, C.M., and Vande Woude, G.F. (1984): Nature, 311:29-33.

28. Copley, M., Gindhart, T., and Colburn, N.H. (1983): J. Cell Physiol., 114:173-178.

29. DiGiovanni, J., Prichett, W.P., Decina, P.C., and Diamond, L. (1984): Carcinogenesis, 5:1493-1498.

30. Dion, L.D., Bear, J., Bateman, J., DeLuca, L.M., and Colburn, N.H. (1982): J. Natl. Cancer Inst., 69:1147-1154.

31. Driedger, P.E. and Blumberg, P.M. (1980): Proc. Natl. Acad. Sci. USA, 77:567-571.

32. Elis, R.W., DeFeo, D., Shih, T.Y., Gonda, M.A., Young, M.A., Lowy, D.R., and Scolnick, E.M. (1981): Nature 292:506-508.

33. Fasano, O., Birnbaum, D., Edlund, L., Fogh, L., and Wigler, M. (1984): Mol. Cell Biol., 4:1695-1705.

34. Fisher, P.B., Bozzone, J.H., and Weinstein, I.B. (1979): Cell 18:695-705.

35. Fisher, P.B., Cogan, U., Horowitz, A.D., Schacter, D., and Weinstein, B. (1981): Biochem. Biophys. Res. Commun.,100:370-376.

36. Fisher, P.B., Dorsch-Hasler, K., Weinstein, I.B., and Ginsberg, H.S. (1979): Nature, 281:591-594.

37. Fisher, P.B., Young, C.S.H., Weinstein, I.B., and Carter, T.H. (1981): Molec. Cell. Biol. 1:370-380.

38. Gilbert, W. (1978): Nature, 271:501.

39. Gindhart, T.D., Nakamura, Y., Stevens, L.A., Hegamyer, G.A., West, M.W., Smith, B.M., and Colburn, N.H. (1985): In: Carcinogenesis - A Comprehensive Survey, Cancer of the Respiratory Tract: Predisposing Factors, edited by M.J. Mass, D.G. Kaufman, J.M. Siegfried, V.E. Steele and S. Nesnow, pp. 341-367. Raven Press, Vol. 8, New York.

40. Gindhart, T.D., Nakamura, Y., Stevens, L.A., Hegamyer, G.A., West, M.W., Smith, B.M., and Colburn, N.H. (1985): In: Tumor Promotion and Enhancement in the Etiology of Human and Experimental Respiratory Tract Carcinogenesis, edited by M. Mass, pp. 341-368. Raven Press, New York.

41. Gindhart, T.D., Stevens, L., and Copley, M.P. (1984): Carcinogenesis, 5:1115-1121.

42. Gottesman, M.M. and Sobel, M.E. (1980): Cell, 19:449-455.

43. Goubin, G., Goldman, D.S., Luce, J., Neiman, P.E., and Cooper, G.M. (1983): Nature, 302:114-119.

44. Greenberg, M.E. and Ziff, E.B. (1984): Nature, 311:433-437.

45. Hecker, E. (1968): Cancer Res., 28:2338-2349.

46. Hegamyer, G.A., Lerman, M.I., and Colburn N.H. (1987), submitted.

47. Hennings, H., Michael, D., Cheng, C., Steinert, P., Holbrook, K., and Yuspa, S.H. (1980): Cell, 19: 245–254.

48. Herschman, H.R. (1983): Carcinogenesis, 4:489–490.

49. Herschman, H.R. (1985): Mol. Cell. Biol., 5:1130–1135.

50. Hirschhorn, R.R., Aller, P., Yuan, Z–A., Gibson, C.W., and Baserga, R. (1984): Proc. Natl. Acad. Sci. USA, 81:6004–6008.

51. Hiwasa, C., Fujimura, S. and Sakiyama, S. (1982): Proc. Natl. Acad. Sci. USA, 79:1800–1804.

52. Hoffman–Liebermann, B., Liebermann, D., and Sachs, L. (1981): Int. J. Cancer 28:615–620.

53. Iwashita, S. and Fox, C.F. (1984): J. Biol. Chem., 259: 2559–2567.

54. Jeang, K. and Hayward, S.D. (1983): J. Virol., 48:135–148.

55. Jones, P.B.C., Miller, A.G., Israel, D.I., Galeazzi, D.R., and Whitlock, J.P., Jr. (1984): J. Biol. Chem., 259:12357–12363.

56. Jung–Chung, L., Shaw, J.E., Smith, M.C., and Pagano, J.S. (1979): Virology, 99:183–187.

57. Kahana, C. and Nathans, D. (1984): Proc. Natl. Acad. Sci. USA, 81:3645–3649.

58. Kelly, K., Cochran, B.H., Stiles, C.D., and Leder, P. (1983): Cell, 35:603–610.

59. Kikkawa, U., Takai, Y., Tanaka, Y., Miyake, R., and Nishizuka, Y. (1983): J. Biol. Chem., 258:11442–11445.

60. Kinsella, A.R. and Gainer, H.St.C. (1984): In: Cellular Interactions by Environmental Tumor Promoters, edited by H. Fujiki, pp. 261–272. Japan Sci. Soc. Press, Tokoyo/VNU Science Press, Utrecht.

61. Kohl, N.E., Kanda, N., Schreck, R.R., Bruns, G., Latt, S.A., Gilbert, F., and Alt, F.W. (1983): Cell, 35: 359–367.

62. Kontula, K.K., Torkkeli,T.K., Bardin, C.W., and Janne, O.A. (1984): Proc. Natl. Acad. Sci. USA, 81:731–735.

63. Kramer, C.M. and Sando, J.J. (1986): Cancer Res., 46: 3040–3045.

64. Kruijer, W., Cooper, J.A., Hunter, T., and Verma, I.M. (1984): Nature, 312:711–715.

65. Land, H., Parada, L.F., and Weinberg, R.A. (1983):Science, 2227–2231.

66. Lane, M.A., Sainten, A., Goherty, K.M., and Cooper, G.M. (1984): Proc. Natl. Acad. Sci. USA, 81:2227–2231.

67. Le Peuch, C.J., Ballester, R., and Rosen, O.M. (1983): Proc. Natl.Acad. Sci. USA, 80: 6858–6862.

68. Lerman, M.I., Hegamyer, G.A., and Colburn, N.H. (1986): Int. J. Cancer, 37:293–302.

69. Lerman, M.I., Sakai, A., Yao, K.T., and Colburn, N.H. (1987): Carcinogenesis, in press.

70. Lew, K.K., Chritton, S., and Blumberg, P.M. (1982): Teratogenesis. Carcinog. Mutagen., 2:19–30.

71. Lotem, J. and Sachs, L. (1970): Proc. Natl. Acad. Sci. USA, 76:5150–5162.

72. Lusky, M. and Botchan, M. (1985): Nature, 293:79–81.

73. Maniatis, T., Fritsch, E.F., and Sambrook, L. (1982): Molecular Cloning. Cold Spring Harbor, New York.

74. Maxam, A.M. and Gilbert, W. (1980): Methods Enzymol., 65:499–560.

75. Mitchell, R.L., Zokas, L., Schreiber, R.D., and Verma, I.M. (1985): Cell, 40:209–217.

76. Miskin, R., Easton, T.G., and Reich, E. (1978): Cell, 15: 1301–1312.

77. Muller, R., Bravo, R., Burckhardt, J., and Curran, T. (1984): Nature, 312:716–720.

78. Muller, R. and Verma, I.M. (1984): Curr. Top. Microbiol. Immunol., 112: 74–115.

79. Nakamura, Y., Colburn, N.H., and Gindhart, T.D. (1985):Carcinogenesis, 6:229–235.

80. Niedel, J.E., Kuhn, L.J., and Vandenbark, G.R. (1983):
    Proc. Natl. Acad. Sci. USA, 80:36-40.

81. Nishizuka, Y. (1984): Nature, 308:693-698.

82. Nishizuka, Y. (1983): Philos. Trans. R. Soc. Lond.
    Biol), 302:101-112.

83. Okayma, H. and Berg, D. (1983): Mol. Cell Biol., 3:
    280-289.

84. Ossowski, L. and Reich, E. (1983): Cell, 35:611-619.

85. Petes, T. and Fink, G.R. (1982): Nature, 300:216-217.

86. Poland, A., Knutson, J., and Glover, E. (1983): In:
    Human and Environmental Risks of Chlorinated Dioxins
    and Related Compounds, edited by R.E. Tucker, A.L.
    Young and A.P. Grey, pp. 539-559. Plenum Publishing
    Corp., New York.

87. Pollet, R.J. and Levey, G.S. (1980): Ann. Intern. Med.,
    92:663-680.

88. Pruss, R.M. and Herschman, H.R. (1977): Proc. Natl.
    Acad. Sci. USA, 74:3918-3921.

89. Ralston, R. and Bishop, J.M. (1984): Cancer Cells, 2:
    165-172.

90. Rapp, U.R., Bonner, T.I., and Cleveland, J.L. (1984):
    In: Retroviruses and Human Pathology, edited by R.C.
    Gallo, D. Stehelin and O.E. Varnier, pp. 449-472,
    The Humana Press, Inc., New Jersey.

91. Reiners, J., Davidson, K., Nelson, K., and Mamrack, M.
    (1983): In: Organ and Species Specificity in Chemical
    Carcinogenesis, edited by R. Langenbach, S. Nesnow and
    J.M. Rice, pp. 173-188. Plenum Press, New York.

92. Rosengurt, E., Rodriguez Pena, M., and Smith, K.A.
    (1983): Proc. Natl. Acad. Sci. USA, 80:7244-7248.

93. Shepherd, J.C.W. (1981): Proc. Natl. Acad. Sci. USA, 78:
    1596-1600.

94. Shimada, T., Dowjat, W.K., Lerman, M. I., Gindhart, T.D.,
    and Colburn, N.H. (1987): Int. J. Cancer, in press.

95. Sobel, M.E., Dion, L.D., Vuust, J., and Colburn, N.H.
    (1983): Molec. Cell. Biol., 3:1527-1532.

80. Niedel, J.E., Kuhn, L.J., and Vandenbark, G.R. (1983): Proc. Natl. Acad. Sci. USA, 80:36–40.

81. Nishizuka, Y. (1984): Nature, 308:693–698.

82. Nishizuka, Y. (1983): Philos. Trans. R. Soc. Lond. Biol), 302:101–112.

83. Okayma, H. and Berg, D. (1983): Mol. Cell Biol., 3: 280–289.

84. Ossowski, L. and Reich, E. (1983): Cell, 35:611–619.

85. Petes, T. and Fink, G.R. (1982): Nature, 300:216–217.

86. Poland, A., Knutson, J., and Glover, E. (1983): In: Human and Environmental Risks of Chlorinated Dioxins and Related Compounds, edited by R.E. Tucker, A.L. Young and A.P. Grey, pp. 539–559. Plenum Publishing Corp., New York.

87. Pollet, R.J. and Levey, G.S. (1980): Ann. Intern. Med., 92:663–680.

88. Pruss, R.M. and Herschman, H.R. (1977): Proc. Natl. Acad. Sci. USA, 74:3918–3921.

89. Ralston, R. and Bishop, J.M. (1984): Cancer Cells, 2: 165–172.

90. Rapp, U.R., Bonner, T.I., and Cleveland, J.L. (1984): In: Retroviruses and Human Pathology, edited by R.C. Gallo, D. Stehelin and O.E. Varnier, pp. 449–472, The Humana Press, Inc., New Jersey.

91. Reiners, J., Davidson, K., Nelson, K., and Mamrack, M. (1983): In: Organ and Species Specificity in Chemical Carcinogenesis, edited by R. Langenbach, S. Nesnow and J.M. Rice, pp. 173–188. Plenum Press, New York.

92. Rosengurt, E., Rodriguez Pena, M., and Smith, K.A. (1983): Proc. Natl. Acad. Sci. USA, 80:7244–7248.

93. Shepherd, J.C.W. (1981): Proc. Natl. Acad. Sci. USA, 78: 1596–1600.

94. Shimada, T., Dowjat, W.K., Lerman, M. I., Gindhart, T.D., and Colburn, N.H. (1987): Int. J. Cancer, in press.

95. Sobel, M.E., Dion, L.D., Vuust, J., and Colburn, N.H. (1983): Molec. Cell. Biol., 3:1527–1532.

96. Solanki, T.J., Slaga, M., Callahan, R., and Huberman, E. (1981): Proc. Natl. Acad. Sci. USA, 78:1722-1725.

97. Sussman, I. and O'Brien, T.G. (1985): J. Cell Physiol., 124:153-159.

98. Takada, K. and Zur Hausen, H. (1984): Int. J. Cancer, 33:491-496.

99. Taparovsky, E.K., Shimizu, K., Goldfarb, M., and Wigler, M. (1983): Cell, 34:581-586.

100. Todaro, G.J. (1982): Natl. Cancer Inst. Monogr., 60:139.

101. Toftgard, R., Roop, D.R., and Yuspa, S.H. (1985): Carcinogenesis, 6:655-657.

102. Ullu, E. and Tschudi, C. (1984): Nature, 312:171-172.

103. van Duuren, B.L. (1969): Prog. Exp. Tumor Res., 11:31-68.

104. Varmus, M.E. (1984): Ann. Rev. Genet., 18:553-612.

105. Weinstein, I.B., Gattoni-Celli, S., Kirschmeier, P., Lambert, M., Hsiao, W., Backer, J., and Jeffrey, A. (1984): In: Cancer Cells 1/The Transformed Phenotype, pp. 229-237. Cold Spring Harbor Laboratory, New York.

106. Wigler, M. and Weinstein, I.B. (1976): Nature, 256: 232-233.

107. Wu, K. (1982): Nature, 286:854-860.

108. Yamasaki, H., Enomoto, T., Hamel, E., and Kanno, Y. (1984): In: Cellular Interactions by Environmental Tumor Promoters, edited by H. Fujiki, pp. 221-233, Japan Sci. Soc. Press, Tokyo/VNU Science Press, Utrecht.

109. Yuspa, S.H., Ben, T., Hennings, H., and Lichti, U. (1982): Cancer Res., 42:2344-2349.

110. Yuspa, S.H. and Morgan, D.L. (1981): Nature (London), 293:72-84.

111. Zur Hausen, H., O'Neill, F.J., and Freeze, J. K. (1978): 373-375.

Tumor Promoters: Biological Approaches for
Mechanistic Studies and Assay Systems,
edited by Robert Langenbach et al.
Raven Press, New York © 1988.

RECEPTOR AND DNA PLOIDY CHANGES DURING PROMOTION
OF RAT LIVER CARCINOGENESIS

Karen Nelson*, Alison Vickers+, Geoffrey I. Sunahara*
and George W. Lucier*

*Laboratory of Biochemical Risk Analysis
National Institute of Environmental Health Sciences
Research Triangle Park, NC 27709, USA

and

+Sandoz LTD, 881
CH-4002
Basel Switzerland

ABSTRACT

In this study, the effects of two structurally different
liver tumor promoters, 17-α-ethinylestradiol (EE$_2$) and 2,3,7,8-
tetrachlorodibenzo-p-dioxin (TCDD), on rat hepatic glucocorticoid and epidermal growth factor (EGF) receptors and on DNA
ploidy distribution of liver cells have been investigated. The
two-stage tumor models were set up by initiating female rats
with a necrogenic dose of diethylnitrosamino (DEN) followed 90
days later by promotion with TCDD (1.4 µg/kg/day) or EE$_2$ (90
µg/kg/day). During TCDD promotion, a decrease in hepatic glucocorticoid receptor binding was produced in both DEN-initiated
and noninitiated rats. TCDD treatment had a differential effect
on the hepatic EGF receptor which resulted in a significant
reduction in EGF-receptor binding and autophosphorylation in
noninitiated rats but had little or no effect on the
EGF-receptor of DEN-initiated rats. Preliminary studies
suggested that modification of hepatic cAMP-dependent kinases
and protein kinase C may represent one mechanism by which TCDD
could be modulating the EGF- and glucocorticoid-receptor pathways. DNA ploidy analysis demonstrated that TCDD treatment of
DEN-initiated rats increased the proportion of diploid nuclei in
the liver; whereas, treatment of noninitiated rats did not
increase the diploid nuclei, but instead slightly increased the
number of tetraploid nuclei. During EE$_2$ promotion, hepatic
EGF-receptor binding and autophosphorylation were elevated; glucocorticoid receptor binding was not affected, and the proportion
of diploid hepatocytes was significantly increased in both
DEN-initiated and noninitiated rats. EE$_2$ and TCDD had

distinctly different effects on the EGF- and glucocorticoid-
receptor pathways that were not directly related to the changes
in the DNA ploidy of liver cells. However, the ability of these
structurally different liver tumor promoters to increase the
proportion of hepatic diploid nuclei in initiated rats may be an
important element in the mechanism of promotion for both TCDD
and EE_2.

INTRODUCTION

Promotion has been defined as the process by which initiated
cells are stimulated to develop into cancer and the agents that
accelerate this process are called promoters (11). The specific
characteristics that initiated cells have acquired which enable
them to clonally expand in response to a promoting environment
are not known. Properties of initiated hepatocytes that have
been proposed to influence their growth in response to tumor
promoters are the resistance to cytotoxic agents probably due to
induction of various metabolic enzymes, and/or the loss or
alteration of normal growth control (11,33,39). Alteration of
growth regulation may be an essential component of the
carcinogenic process as supported by recent evidence
demonstrating the interaction of oncogene encoded proteins as
well as some tumor promoters with elements along the mitogenic
pathway.
    The two-stage model of rat liver carcinogenesis is an
excellent system to study characteristics of both initiation and
promotion. One advantage of this system is that a number of
structurally diverse environmental contaminants and drugs are
promoters in the rat two-stage model; including some persistent
halogenated aromatic hydrocarbons, dichlorodiphenyltrichloroethane (DDT), some polychlorinated biphenyls (PCBs), phenobarbital, butylated hydroxytoluene, hexachlorocyclohexane and
steroid hormones such as synthetic estrogens (11,12,32,33,34,39,
41,43). Our laboratory is interested in determining whether
modification of receptor pathways associated with hepatocyte
growth control is important in the mechanism of action of a
number of structurally diverse liver tumor promoters. In our
present investigation, we are evaluating the promoting effects
of one of the most toxic halogenated aromatic hydrocarbons,
2,3,7,8-tetrachlorodibenzo-p-dioxin (TCDD), and a synthetic
estrogen, 17-α-ethinylestradiol (EE_2), on liver carcinogenesis
in rats initiated with diethylnitrosamine (DEN)(32,43).
Specific cellular receptors for EE_2 (estrogen receptor) and TCDD
(Ah receptor) are present in mammalian liver and the mechanism
by which these agents induce a number of specific liver
responses is thought to be through these distinct receptor pathways (12,30,34,41,43). As an initial step in our studies, we
are comparing the effects of TCDD and EE_2 on hepatic epidermal
growth factor (EGF) and glucocorticoid-receptors because considerable evidence exists which indicates that modulation of the

glucocorticoid and EGF-receptor pathways in hepatocytes and other cell types may be associated not only with growth regulation but also with the actions of carcinogens and promoters (5, 8,16,17,18,19,20,24,26,35,38). Also, we are investigating the role of protein kinases in the regulation of the function of these receptor pathways. Modification of these receptor pathways and protein kinases may be contributing factors that provide an environment suitable for the proliferation of initiated hepatocytes. Therefore, we have analyzed promoter-induced changes in DNA ploidy distribution of liver cells using flow cytometry to determine if a relationship exists between hepatic receptor modifications and changes in hepatocyte populations.

MATERIALS AND METHODS

Animal Treatment

Our protocol for TCDD promotion was a modification of the procedure used by Pitot et al. (32). Ovariectomized female Sprague-Dawley rats (8 weeks) were initiated by administration of a necrogenic dose (200 mg/kg, i.p.) of DEN (Sigma Chemical Company, St. Louis, Mo.) dissolved in saline (0.9% NaCl) and promoted biweekly with TCDD (1.4 µg/kg; gavage) (gift from Dr. J. McKinney, NIEHS, R.T.P., N.C.) dissolved in corn oil (Sigma Chemical Company). The four treatment groups were Saline/Corn Oil (SC), Saline/TCDD (ST), DEN/Corn Oil (DC) and DEN/TCDD (DT). For estrogen promotion, ovariectomized Sprague-Dawley rats (8-10 weeks) were initiated by a single dose of DEN (200 mg/kg, i.p.) in saline and promoted by subcutaneous implants of silastic capsules containing EE_2 (Sigma Chemical Company) mixed with a cholesterol carrier at various concentrations to produce estimated doses of 19, 37 and 90 µg/kg/day of EE_2. The treatment groups were DEN•Low EE_2 (19 µg/kg/day EE_2), DEN•Medium EE_2 (37 µg/kg/day EE_2), DEN•High EE_2 (90 µg/kg/day), and Saline•Cholesterol (SC).

EGF Receptor Assays

Hepatic plasma membranes were prepared by the method described by Neville (28) in the presence of protease inhibitors (20 µg/ml phenylmethylsulfonylfluoride [PMSF], 10 µg/ml leupeptin and 100 KU/ml aprotinin) (Sigma Chemical Company). EGF binding was carried as described by Carpenter (4) using varying concentrations of (0.02 - 2 nM) $[^{125}I]$-EGF (Meloy Labs, Springfield, VA) in the presence (non-specific) or absence (total) of 3 µM excess unlabelled EGF (Collaborative Research, Lexington, MA). Specific binding was calculated as the difference between the total and non-specific binding. Data were analyzed using the LIGAND procedure for best-fit.

To assay EGF-stimulation of receptor autophosphorylation, the receptor was solubilized by incubation of liver plasma membranes for 30 minutes at 0°C in the presence of 1% Triton X-100, 10% glycerol, 20mM Pipes pH 7.4 and then centrifuged at 100,000 xg for 30 minutes. The phosphorylation reaction was performed using the supernatant which contained the solubilized EGF-receptor by the method described by Rubin et al. (38). Aliquots of phosphorylated proteins were electrophoresed on 8% SDS-polyacrylamide gels overnight at 50 volts. Gels were stained with Coomassie Brilliant Blue, destained, dried and autoradiographed on Kodak XAR-5 film.

Glucocorticoid Receptor Assays

Liver cytosol for the glucocorticoid receptor analysis was prepared by homogenizing 3 g of minced liver in 9 ml of buffer (10 mM Tris pH 7.4, 2.5 mM EDTA, 5 mM dithiothreitol, 10% v/v glycerol and 20 mM Na molybdate) by 10 strokes in a motor driven Potter-Elvejeheim Homogenizer. All procedures were carried out at 4°C. Homogenates were centrifuged for 20 minutes at 10,000 x g followed by centrifugation at 105,000 x g for 65 minutes. The resulting cytosol supernatants were frozen at -70°C until assayed. The binding assays were performed by established methods (2,37,42,43) using 0.2 to 20 nM [^{3}H]-dexamethasone (Amersham) in the presence and absence of cold dexamethasone (Sigma Chemical Company) and incubated for 18 hours. Specific binding was calculated as the difference between the total and non-specific binding and the data were analyzed by linear regression.

Protein Kinase Assays

Crude membrane and cytosol preparations used for assaying protein kinase C were prepared and partially purified by DEAE chromotography using the methods described by Kikkawa et al. (21) and Forsbeck et al. (13). Protein kinase C assays were then performed on the fractions eluted with 150 mM NaCl from DEAE-sepharose as described by Kikkawa (21). Cyclic AMP-dependent protein kinases were assayed under conditions similar to those for protein kinase except that 5µM cAMP and 5 µM $MgCl_2$ were added instead of calcium, phospholipid and diolein (21).

Flow-cytometric measurements of DNA Content

The method described by Clark and Peck (6) was used to isolate nuclei either from liver slices (TCDD promotion) or from purified hepatocytes (Estrogen promotion) prepared by the collagenase perfusion technique. The nuclei were fixed in cold 70% ethanol and stored at 4°C until assayed. The DNA of the nuclei were stained with propidium iodide (0.1 mg/ml) for 30 minutes at 0°C. DNA analysis was carried out on a Becton Dickinson FACS 4 flow cytometer.

RESULTS AND DISCUSSION

I. TCDD Promotion

A. EGF-Receptor Binding and Phosphorylation

The results of Scatchard analysis of hepatic EGF-receptor binding after 22 weeks of TCDD promotion are shown in Table 1. TCDD treatment of noninitiated animals (ST) consistently results in a decrease in hepatic plasma membrane $[^{125}I]$-EGF-receptor binding with little or no change in Kd when compared to control (SC) animals. TCDD-mediated reduction of hepatic EGF-receptor binding levels in female rats is similar to that reported by Madhukar and coworkers (26) on TCDD effects in the male rat; however, we find that female Sprague-Dawley rats not only contain significantly lower levels (50%) of hepatic EGF-receptor but also are much more sensitive to TCDD with respect to the reduction of EGF-receptor binding and phosphorylation than male rats (data not shown). DEN treatment alone (DC) only caused a slight reduction of hepatic EGF-receptor binding in this experiment; however DEN treatment appeared to modify the liver's response to TCDD with respect to the EGF-receptor. As shown in Table 1, the hepatic EGF-receptor binding in animals initiated with DEN and promoted for 22 weeks with TCDD (DT) is not reduced as found in the noninitiated animals treated with TCDD (ST).

TABLE 1. Binding Kinetics of $[^{125}I]$-EGF Binding to Hepatic Plasma Membranes Following 22 Weeks of TCDD Promotion[a]

Treatment Group	Bmax($fmol$/mg)	Kd (nM)
Saline/Corn oil (SC)	2321	1.47
Saline/TCDD (ST)	1284 ± 161	1.54 ± 0.19
DEN/Corn Oil (DC)	1729 ± 497	1.21 ± 0.34
DEN/TCDD (DT)	2515 ± 434	1.78 ± 0.04

[a]The binding capacity (Bmax) and dissociation equilibrium constant (Kd) for the EGF-receptor were determined from pooled livers of 4 animals for the SC treatment group and for the other treatment groups. The results represent the mean and standard error obtained from separate determinations of 3 animals.

Another approach to study the EGF-receptor is the examination of the EGF-stimulation of the receptor's intrinsic tyrosine kinase an effect which leads to receptor autophosphorylation (10,23,30,31,38). As shown in Figure 1, the effect of TCDD promotion on the EGF-stimulated autophosphorylation of the solubilized EGF-receptor obtained from the various treatment groups

agrees well with the modification of EGF-receptor binding. TCDD
treatment of noninitiated animals (ST) results in a significant
decrease in hepatic EGF-receptor autophosphorylation when compared to control rats (SC) but has little effect on receptor
autophosphorylation of initiated animals (DT). This EGF-
stimulated phosphorylation is stable to base treatment, which
suggests that the phosphorylation is occuring at tyrosine residues. Solubilized rather than intact hepatic plasma membranes
were used for our phosphorylation studies because the background
phosphorylation of membrane proteins was elevated in intact
membranes obtained from TCDD treated animals, which often made
it difficult to demonstrate EGF-stimulation of EGF receptor
autophosphorylation.

EGF Dependent Phosphorylation
of EGF Receptors
22 Week TCDD Promotion

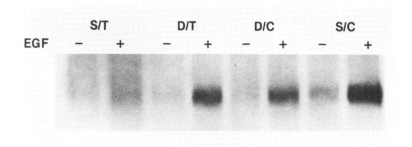

FIG. 1. EGF-dependent autophosphorylation of the EGF-receptor
of isolated hepatic plasma membranes after 22 weeks of TCDD
promotion. This figure shows an autoradiogram of a SDS-
polyacrylamide slab gel of EGF-receptor phosphorylation upon
incubation of solubilized plasma membrane preparations in the
presence (+) and absence (-) of EGF. EGF-stimulated phosphorylation of the hepatic EGF-receptor is 4 to 6 fold higher in
DEN/TCDD (DT) treated animals than found in the Saline/TCDD (ST)
treated rats. The differential effects of TCDD on the phosphorylation of the hepatic EGF-receptor of initiated and noninitiated
animals parallels its effect on the EGF-receptor binding.

The effect of TCDD on the [^{125}I]-EGF binding and phosphorylation of the hepatic EGF-receptor of noninitiated and initiated animals is similar to the differential response of initiated and noninitiated mouse keratinocytes to the phorbol ester tumor promoter, 12-0-tetradecanoylphorbol-13-acetate (TPA) (31,44). The differential effects of TPA on the EGF-receptor is just one of the biochemical parameters that are affected in initiated keratinocytes, which have a reduced response to differentiation signals. This defective differentiation is thought to be the basic mechanism for the selective clonal expansion of initiated keratinocytes that leads ultimately to the development of papillomas.

One explanation for the differential response of initiated keratinocytes to TPA is that the cellular receptor for TPA, now identified as protein kinase C, may be qualitatively different in the initiated cells than found in normal keratinocytes (44). Likewise, one possible explanation for our results is that DEN initiation of rat liver may also modulate the various receptor system(s) involved in TCDD action, and therefore, account for the differential effects of TCDD on the EGF-receptor as well as provide for the selective growth of initiated hepatocytes. DEN treatment may result in certain persistent biochemical changes which alter the liver response to tumor promoters. Chemical carcinogens and promoters have been reported to induce a number of biochemical changes in the liver (23,39). We have also found that DEN initiation induces very persistent changes in hepatic biochemistry lasting 30 weeks or longer; such as, increased concentrations of a cytochrome P-450 immunologically related to rabbit form 6 (Domin et al., in preparation), and the abnormal occupancy of the nuclear estrogen receptor (A. Vickers, in preparation).

B. Glucocorticoid Receptor Analysis

Our recent studies have indicated that a single treatment of TCDD can cause a significant reduction of up to 50% in hepatic glucocorticoid receptor levels in both adrenalectomized and normal female rats. The decrease in glucocorticoid receptor levels occurs between 6 and 24 hours after TCDD treatment, at doses as low as 0.001 μg/kg in adrenalectomized rats and persists over 42 days (manuscript in preparation). A representative Scatchard analysis showing a decrease in glucocorticoid receptor binding but no change in affinity 10 days following a single treatment with TCDD (10 μg/kg) is presented in Figure 2.

During TCDD promotion for 30 weeks at 100 ng/kg/day, the hepatic cytosolic glucocorticoid receptor levels are also decreased in both DEN-initiated and noninitiated rats (Figure 3). DEN treatment alone also induces a slight but not significant decrease in the glucocorticoid receptor binding in the liver. In addition to a reduction in binding, long term treatment with the low TCDD doses, used in our liver promotion studies, causes a decrease in the dissociation constant (Kd) of

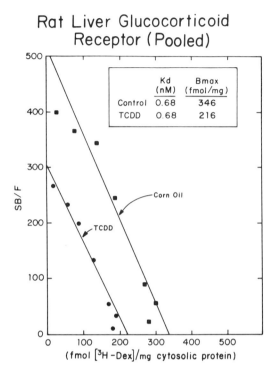

FIG. 2.   Scatchard plot of [3H] dexamethasone binding to receptors in liver cytosol pooled from control animals (Corn Oil) and
TCDD treated animals (10μg/kg; 1x) 10 days after treatment. The
concentration (Bmax) of the hepatic glucocorticoid receptor in
the TCDD treated animals is significantly lower than in the
control group, but the dissociation equilibrium constant (Kd) is
not altered.

the glucocorticoid receptor of the liver. In contrast, single
TCDD treatments at high doses do not consistently affect the Kd.

C. Protein Kinase Analysis
We are now focusing our research on the possible mechanism by
which TCDD is causing the glucocorticoid- and EGF-receptor
changes. Evidence suggests that phosphorylation and
dephosphorylation of hormone systems by specific protein kinases
may be a major mechanism by which cellular responsiveness to a
variety of signals is regulated. Furthermore, recent observations have demonstrated that both the glucocorticoid and

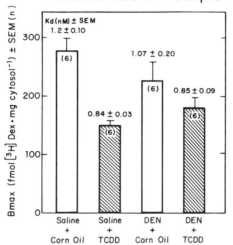

30 Weeks TCDD Promotion*
Adult Female Rat Liver Cytosolic
Glucocorticord Receptor

* Initiation — 200mg/kg DEN (i.p.)
Promotion — 100ng/kg day TCDD (gavage)

FIG. 3. A summary of the rat liver cytosolic glucocorticoid
receptor concentration (Bmax) and dissociation equilibrium
constant (Kd) of the various treatment groups following 30 weeks
of TCDD promotion. There were six animals per group and the
bars represent the mean ± the standard error. Long-term TCDD
treatment results in a reduction in the Bmax and Kd of the liver
glucocorticoid receptor in both the initiated and noninitiated
animals. DEN treatment alone (DEN + Corn Oil) also slightly
reduced the binding capacity of the hepatic glucocorticoid
receptor.

EGF-receptors are targets for protein kinases which regulate
their binding capacity and/or affinity (7,10,14,29,38,42).
   Interestingly, the effects of TCDD on the glucocorticoid and
EGF-receptors are similar to that produced by the potent phorbol
ester tumor promoter, TPA, suggesting a common mechanism of
action (7,8,15,26). The mechanism by which phorbol ester tumor
promoters elicit cellular responses is at least in part through
the activation of protein kinase C, a key enzyme of a major

signal transduction pathway that utilizes inositol phospholipids (7,10,29,31). Studies have shown that protein kinase C phosphorylation of threonine-654 of the EGF-receptor correlates with phorbol ester inhibition of EGF binding and tyrosine kinase activity (7,10). However, unlike TPA's effects on the EGF-receptor which occurs within minutes, through the activation of protein kinase C, it has been proposed that TCDD and certain polycyclic aromatic hydrocarbons inhibit EGF-receptor binding indirectly via the Ah receptor pathway. The latter mechanism requires cytoplasmic and nuclear events in order to produce membrane changes that mimic those induced by TPA, which may account for the longer latency period (24 hours or more) required for maximal effects on the EGF-receptor by these compounds (15,18).

Evidence suggesting that modification of protein kinases may be one mechanism of TCDD action was presented recently by Bombick and co-workers (3). They report significant increases in both cAMP dependent and independent protein kinases (10-20 fold) as well as in protein kinase C (2-fold) in isolated rat hepatic plasma membranes 10 to 20 days after TCDD treatment. In light of these observations, we wanted to determine whether TCDD could modify both cytosolic and membrane protein kinase early after treatment when alterations in the glucocorticoid and EGF-receptors are first observed. It is important to investigate both cytosolic and membrane protein kinases because evidence suggests that modification of the subcellular localization of protein kinases may be an important component of their regulation (22,25,29). For example, translocation of protein kinase C from cytosol to membranes has been reported to occur upon phorbol ester activation (1). Also, during liver regeneration, there is an intracellular redistribution and marked nuclear accumulation of cAMP-dependent protein kinase catalytic and regulatory subunits of both the type I and II isozymes (22). Therefore, we have measured both cAMP dependent kinase and protein kinase C in partially purified cytosolic and membrane fractions, 24 hours after TCDD treatment.

As shown in Table 2, TCDD treatment results in a ten-fold increase in hepatic protein kinase C associated with membranes but only a slight increase in its cytosolic activity. In addition, there is over an 8-fold increase in membrane associated cAMP-dependent protein kinase activity and a corresponding decrease in its cytosolic activity. Further study will be required to determine whether this dramatic modification of cAMP-dependent kinase activity is due to changes in the actual levels of catalytic and regulatory subunits in the membrane and cytosolic compartments, or due to changes in various activators or inhibitors of cAMP-dependent protein kinases (25). Regardless of the mechanism, it is obvious that TCDD has dramatic effects on the regulation of cAMP-dependent protein kinases inducing changes that may be similar to those found to occur in regenerating liver (22).

TABLE 2. Protein kinase C and cAMP-dependent kinase activity associated with hepatic membrane and cytosolic fractions 24 hours after TCDD (25µg/kg) treatment[a]

	Cytosolic		Membrane	
	Control	TCDD	Control	TCDD
Protein kinase C	218	519	298	3141
cAMP-dependent kinase	113	13	73	650

[a]Protein kinase C and cAMP-dependent kinase were assayed in cytosolic and membrane fractions obtained from pooled livers of 4 rats using the protocol described in the Materials and Methods. The results are presented as specific activities which represent the amount of enzyme that incorporates 1 µmol of phosphate from ATP into histone per minute per milligram of protein at 30°C.

Our data suggest that TCDD can influence the regulation of cAMP-dependent protein kinase and protein kinase C within 24 hours after treatment; both are key enzymes of two different major signal transduction pathways that play a crucial role in mediating a number of cellular responses to extracellular signals (29). We have not yet assayed the protein kinases after long term TCDD treatment following an initiating dose of diethylnitrosamine. It is possible that modification of these regulatory protein kinases by DEN may account for the differential effects of TCDD on the EGF-receptor.

D. DNA Ploidy Analysis

Recent observations have suggested that an early step and possibly an essential prerequisite stage in the development of liver cancer induced by hepatocarcinogens in the rat may be the selective outgrowth of diploid hepatocytes which are thought to be enriched with preneoplastic cells (40). The ability of most tumor promoters to increase the tumor incidence and to decrease the latency period may also in part be due to the selection of preneoplastic diploid populations. Therefore, we have investigated TCDD effects on the cellular ploidy of liver after 60 weeks of promotion of initiated and noninitiated rats. Flow cytometric analysis of the DNA content measured in nuclei isolated from liver cells obtained from animals of the various treatments is shown in Figure 4. The DNA histogram of isolated nuclei obtained from noninitiated (SC) and initiated (DC), are similar with approximately 33% and 36% of the nuclei as diploid, respectively, and 45% and 41% as tetraploid, respectively. The high proportion of diploid nuclei in normal rat liver has been shown to reflect the presence of a large number of tetraploid cells that are binucleated (40). Prolonged treatment of noninitiated animals with TCDD (ST) caused only a slight increase (19%) in the number of hepatic tetraploid nuclei. Whereas,

HEPATOCYTE DNA PLOIDY FOLLOWING
60 WEEKS OF TCDD PROMOTION

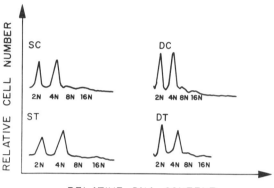

FIG. 4. DNA histograms of nuclei isolated from pooled livers of
4 rats obtained from the various treatment groups after 60 weeks
of TCDD Promotion. The DNA histograms were analyzed for the
percentage of nuclei in different classes relative to the total
number of nuclei measured and the results are as follows: SC -
33% 2N, 4% S, 45% 4N, 9% 8N and 9% 16N; ST - 30% 2N, 6% S, 49%
4N, 6% 8N and 9% 16N; DC-36% 2N, 7% S, 41% 4N, 9% 8N and 7% 16N;
and DT - 40% 2N, 8% S, 36% 4N, 11% 8N and 5% 16N. The class of
nuclei between 2N and 4N represents the percentage of nuclei in
DNA synthesis or "S" phase. A 16% decrease in the number of
diploid nuclei is found in the livers of the noninitiated animals treated with TCDD (ST); whereas, a 34% increase in the
diploid hepatic nuclei occurs in the initiated animals upon TCDD
treatment (DT).

treatment of initiated animals with TCDD (DT) results in a
significant increase in hepatic diploid nuclei by 34% over
control values. In addition, the percentage of nuclei undergoing DNA synthesis as measured by flow cytometry is higher in
livers obtained from the initiated (DC) and initiated-promoted
animals (DT) than the controls, but is not significantly
affected in the animals treated only with TCDD (ST). The ability of TCDD to increase the number of diploid nuclei present in
initiated livers may be an important component of TCDD's promotion of liver tumors. The biochemical mechanisms by which TCDD

brings about these changes in the liver populations are not clear. Modification of receptor pathways associated with hepa-tocyte growth control, especially the differential effects of TCDD on the hepatic EGF and glucocorticoid receptors (initiated versus noninitiated animals), may be one mechanism of action of TCDD by which a cellular milieu is produced that is conducive for the expansion of the diploid hepatocytes, leading to the possible selection of preneoplastic initiated cells. Further studies are needed to determine if changes in EGF-receptor, glucocorticoid receptor and cellular ploidy are occurring in preneoplastic cells and/or in normal surrounding tissue.

II. 17-α-Ethinylestradiol (EE$_2$) Promotion

A. Receptor Analysis
Modification of hepatic EGF- and glucocorticoid-receptors during EE$_2$ promotion of hepatocarcinogenesis differs from those receptor changes occurring during promotion with TCDD. After 30 weeks of estrogen promotion using low (19 µg/kg/day), medium (37 µg/kg/day) and high (90 µg/kg/day) doses of EE$_2$ there is a significant increase in hepatic [^{125}I]-EGF-receptor binding capacity at the medium and high doses of EE$_2$ when compared to the saline-cholesterol treated controls, but no consistent change in the dissociation constant (Kd) (Table 3). EE$_2$ treatment also increases the EGF-stimulated autophosphorylation of solubilized EGF-receptor (Figure 5).

In support of our observation, Madhukar et al. (26) report that multiple treatment of a single animal with DDT, a compound that has estrogenic activity (36), increased hepatic EGF-receptor binding by approximately 20%. Studies of Mukku and Stancel (27) have demonstrated that 17-β-estradiol administration to immature female rats increased uterine EGF-receptor binding and EGF-stimulated receptor autophosphorylation. Their data suggest that a distinct relationship may exist between increased EGF-receptor binding and estrogen stimulation of uterine growth. Other studies using human breast cancer cells have demonstrated that estrogen may regulate growth by the induction of polypep-tides related to epidermal growth factor which act as autocrine or paracrine growth factors (9). Similar to breast and uterus, liver growth is also significantly stimulated by estrogens (30). The mechanism of estrogen-dependent growth in the liver is not known but may be similar to that found in the uterus and breast, a process which involves the regulation of EGF-receptor levels and production of EGF-like growth factors. One explanation for our data is that the increase in hepatic EGF-receptor levels during EE$_2$ promotion may be associated with the greater proli-ferative capacity of estrogen-treated hepatocytes.

From our preliminary studies, we have found no consistent effects on the binding capacity or affinity constant of the hepatic glucocorticoid receptor during EE$_2$ tumor promotion (data not shown). In addition, the effects of EE$_2$ promotion on hepatic

TABLE 3.   The Effects of 30 Weeks of EE$_2$ Promotion on EGF
           Binding to Hepatic Plasma Membranes[a]

Treatment Group	Bmax (^{fmol}/mg)	Kd (nM)
Saline/Cholesterol	1165	1.06
DEN/Low EE$_2$	1015 ± 174	0.86 ± 0.06
DEN/Medium EE$_2$	1630 ± 103	1.19 ± 0.18
DEN/High EE$_2$	1449 ± 118	1.06 ± 0.18

[a]The binding capacity (Bmax) and dissociation equilibrium
constant (Kd) for the hepatic EGF-receptor of the saline/
cholesterol treatment group were determined in plasma membranes
isolated from pooled livers of 4 animals, and for the EE$_2$
treatment groups the results represent the mean and standard
error obtained from separated determinations of 3 animals.

EGF-Stimulated Phosphorylation
of the EGF-R

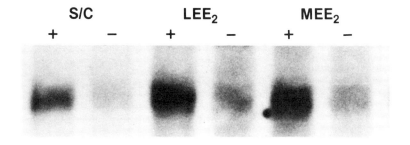

FIG. 5. An autoradiogram of an SDS-polyacrylamide gel showing
the effects of EE$_2$ promotion on EGF-receptor phosphorylation
upon incubation of solubilized plasma membrane preparations in
the presence (+) or absence (-) of EGF. EE$_2$ treatment of initiated animals at low (LEE$_2$; 19 µg/kg/day) and medium (MEE$_2$; 37
µg/kg/day) doses significantly enhances EGF-stimulation of
receptor phosphorylation when compared to controls (S/C).

cytosolic and membrane protein kinases has yet to be determined.

B. Hepatocyte DNA Ploidy Analysis

Flow cytometric analysis of the DNA content of isolated hepatocyte nuclei taken from animals of each treatment group demonstrates that treatment of initiated (DE) and noninitiated (SE) animals for 30 weeks with EE_2 induces a dramatic shift in the ploidy distribution of hepatocytes towards diploidy and away from higher ploidies (Figure 6). In addition, the number of nuclei in DNA synthesis is increased in the estrogen treated animals. This is consistent with a recent report which demonstrated that EE_2 induced liver growth mainly by hyperplasia, which is brought about by the stimulation of hepatocyte DNA synthesis and mitosis (30). The ability of EE_2 to increase both the diploid nuclei and the proliferative capacity of the liver probably plays an essential role in the mechanism by which EE_2 promotes liver carcinogenesis. Modification of EGF-receptor levels by EE_2 may reflect the changes in the ploidy distribution of the hepatocytes as well as represent one mechanism by which EE_2 may enhance the growth potential of the hepatocytes possibly by increasing their sensitivity to growth factors.

SUMMARY

The cellular alterations occurring during liver tumor promotion are complex. It is not clear whether the mechanism of promotion is similar or different for various classes of liver tumor promoters. There may be multiple pathways of promotion and each class of promoter may act through a different mechanistic battery with some common and different components. Treatment of liver with different promoters induces a variety of biochemical responses, many of which are associated with the ability of most tumor promoters to induce liver growth and to modify hepatic function by initiating specific gene programs such as drug metabolism (30,39). An example which suggests that the mechanism of action for the various tumor promoters may be different is the recent observation that estrogens differ from other tumor promoters such as TCDD and phenobarbital in that the estrogens do not induce hepatic mono-oxygenases but instead produce very specific changes in hepatic function through the induction of estrogen-responsive genes (12,30,43). However, one property that is probably essential for promoting activity and is shared by most liver promoters is the ability to induce liver growth (39). Therefore, the aim of our present study was to determine if two structurally different liver tumor promoters (TCDD and EE_2) could modify receptor pathways (EGF and glucocorticoid) associated with hepatocyte growth regulation and to relate these receptor changes to promoter-induced effects on the DNA ploidy distribution of liver cell populations. Our results demonstrate that TCDD and EE_2 have distinctly different effects on the EGF-and glucocorticoid-receptors of the liver.

ESTROGEN EFFECTS ON
HEPATOCYTE DNA PLOIDY

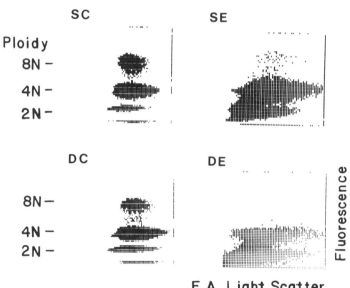

FIG. 6. Flow cytometric analysis of the DNA content of nuclei isolated from purified hepatocytes after 30 weeks of EE_2 promotion. Treatment of noninitiated and initiated animals with EE_2 (SE and DE) results in a significant increase in the number of diploid nuclei in the hepatocytes which is accompanied by a decrease in the proportion of nuclei at higher ploidies. In addition, the number of hepatocyte nuclei undergoing DNA synthesis is enhanced significantly in the EE_2 treatment groups when compared to controls (SC) or DEN-initiated animals (DC).

During TCDD promotion, there was a marked reduction in receptor binding for glucocorticoids in both initiated and noninitiated animals. TCDD treatment decreased hepatic EGF-receptor binding and receptor autophosphorylation in noniniti-ated rats but had little or no effect on the EGF-receptor in DEN-initiated rats at early stages of production. Modification of hepatic cAMP-dependent kinases and protein kinase C with significant increases associated with crude membranes was also found following a single TCDD treatment of noninitiated rats. These kinases have been shown to regulate peptide and steroid receptor function and, therefore, may represent one mechanism by which TCDD modulates the EGF- and glucocorticoid receptor systems. Although dramatic receptor changes were induced by TCDD in the livers of noninitiated animals, ploidy analysis revealed only a slight increase in the number of tetraploid nuclei. In contrast, TCDD increased the proportion of diploid nuclei in the livers of DEN-initiated animals; where DEN-initiation alone did not affect the DNA ploidy. The emergence of diploid hepatocytes has been proposed to be an important step in liver carcinogenesis. The mechanism by which TCDD increases the diploid liver nuclei only in initiated animals is not known but may involve in part modulation of receptor pathways.

In contrast to TCDD, EE_2 treatment induces similar effects on the livers of both noninitiated and initiated rats. During EE_2 promotion, EGF-receptor binding and autophosphorylation levels are elevated, glucocorticoid receptor binding is not affected, the proportion of diploid hepatocytes is significantly increased and the number of nuclei undergoing DNA synthesis is enhanced. The pronounced ability of EE_2 to enhance the diploid population and growth of the liver may be an essential component of its promoting activity, and may be reflected by the increase in the hepatic EGF-binding.

To conclude, our data indicate that EE_2 and TCDD have distinctly different effects on the EGF and glucocorticoid receptor pathways. There is not a clear relationship between promoter-induced modification of these receptor pathways and the changes in the DNA ploidy of liver cells. Our data also suggest that the mechanism of promotion and stimulation of growth by these tumor promoters may involve different receptor pathways than those involved in the regulation of liver regeneration. For example, the reduction in hepatic glucocorticoid- and EGF-receptors, and the effects on cAMP dependent kinases following TCDD treatment is similar to the changes reported to occur in regenerating liver; however, our preliminary results indicate that long-term treatment with TCDD does not significantly increase the number of cells in DNA synthesis. Although EE_2 treatment and partial hepatectomy increase the diploid popula-tion of the liver, EE_2 promotion elevates EGF-receptor binding and has no consistent effect on the glucocorticoid receptor which is in direct contrast to the effect of partial hepatectomy on these receptor systems. Our data support other observations which indicate that the growth response occurring during liver regeneration is different from that produced in response to tumor promoters; possibly because tumor promoters have the capacity to induce not only liver growth but also to induce dramatic changes in specific hepatic function (40).

ACKNOWLEDGEMENTS

We express our thanks to Tracy Sloop and Diane Campen for treating the animals, and to Gorgon Wiegand for the DNA analysis.

REFERENCES

1. Baribault, H., Leroux-Nicollet, L., and Marceau, N. (1985): J. Cell. Physiol., 122:105-112.
2. Beato, M. and Feigelson, P. (1972): J. Biol. Chem., 247:7890-7896.
3. Bombick, D.W., Madhukar, B.V., Brewster, D.W., and Matsumura, F. (1985): Biochem. Biophys. Res. Commun., 127:296-302.
4. Carpenter, G. (1985): Meth. Enzymol., 109:101-110.
5. Chester, J.F., Gaissert, H.A., Ross, J.S., and Malt, R.A. (1986): Cancer Res., 46:2954-2957.
6. Clark, J.H., and Peck, Jr. E.J. (1981): In: Laboratory Methods for Hormone Action and Molecular Endocrinology, edited by W.T. Schrader and B.W. O'Malley, pp.1-68. Houston Biological Association, Texas.
7. Davis, R.J. and Czech, M. (1986): Biochem. J., 233:435-441.
8. Davidson, K.A. and Slaga, T.J. (1983): Cancer Res., 43:3487-3851.
9. Dickson, R.B., Huff, K.K., Spencer, E.M., and Lippman, M.E. (1986): Endocrinology, 118:138-142.
10. Downward, J., Waterfield, M.D., and Parker, P.J. (1985): J. Biol. Chem., 260:14538-14546.
11. Farber, E. (1982): Am. J. Pathol., 106:271-296.
12. Forman, D., Doll, R., and Peto, R. (1983): Br. J. Cancer, 48:349-354.
13. Forsbeck, K., Nilsson, K., Hansson, A., Skoglund, G., and Ingelman-Sundberg, M. (1985): Cancer Res., 45:6194-6199.
14. Gruol, D.J., Campbell, N.F., and Bourgeois, S. (1986): J. Biol. Chem., 261:4909-4914.
15. Hudson, L.G., Toscano, Jr. W.A., and Greenlee, W.F. (1985): Toxicol. Appl. Pharmacol., 77:251-259.
16. Isohashi, F., Tsukanaka, K., Terada, M., Nakanishi, Y., Fukushima, H., and Sakamoto, Y. (1979): Cancer Res., 39:5132-5135.
17. Ivanovic, V. and Weinstein, I.B. (1981): Nature, 293:404-406.
18. Ivanovic, V. and Weinstein, B. (1982): Carcinogenesis, 3:505-510.

19. Josefsberg, Z., Carr, B.I., Hwang, D., Barseghian, G., Tomkinson, C., and Lev-Ran, A. (1984): Cancer Res., 44:2754-2757.
20. Kensler, T.W., Busby, Jr. W.F., Davidson, N.E., and Wogan, G.N. (1976): Cancer Res., 36:4647-4651.
21. Kikkawa, U., Minakuchi, R., Takai, Y., and Nishizuka, Y. (1983): Meth. Enzymol., 99:288-298.
22. Laks, M.S., Harrison, J.J., Schwoch, G., and Jungmann, R.A. (1981): J. Biol. Chem., 256:8775-8785.
23. Lev-Ran, A., Carr, B.I., Hwang, D.L., and Roitman, A. (1986): Cancer Res., 46:4656-4659.
24. Loeb, J.N. and Rosner, W. (1979): Endocrinology, 104:1003-1006.
25. Lohman, S.M. and Walter, U. (1984): Adv. Cyclic Nucleotide and Protein Phosphorylation Res., 18:63-111.
26. Madhukar, B.V., Brewster, D.W., and Matsumura, F. (1984): Proc. Natl. Acad. Sci. USA, 81:7407-7411.
27. Mukku, V.R. and Stancel, G.M. (1985): J. Biol. Chem., 260:9820-9824.
28. Neville, D.M. (1968): Biochem. Biosphys. Acta., 154:540-552.
29. Nishizuka, Y. (1986): Science, 233:305-312.
30. Ochs, H., Düsterberg, B., Günzel, P., and Schulte-Hermann, R. (1986): Cancer Res., 46:1224-1232.
31. Parkinson, E.K. (1985): Br. J. Cancer, 52:479-493.
32. Pitot, H.C., Goldsworthy, T., Campbell, H.A., and Poland, A. (1980): Cancer Res., 40:3616-3620.
33. Pitot, H.C. and Sirica, A.E. (1980): Biochem. Biophys. Acta, 605:191-215.
34. Poland, A. and Knutson, J.C. (1982): Ann. Rev. Pharmacol. Toxicol., 22:517-554.
35. Raab, K.H. and Webb, T.E. (1969): Experientia, 25:1240-1242.
36. Robison, A.K., Mukku, V.R., Spalding, D.M., and Stancel, G.M. (1984): Toxicol. Appl. Pharmacol., 76:537-543.
37. Rosner, W. and Polimeni, S.T. (1978): Steroids, 31:427-438.
38. Rubin, R.A., O'Keefe, E.J., and Earp, H.S. (1982): Proc. Natl. Acad. Sci. USA, 79:776-780.
39. Schulte-Hermann, R. (1985): Arch. Toxicol., 57:147-158.
40. Schwarze, P.E., Pettersen, E.O., Shoaib, M.C., and Seglen, P.O. (1984): Carcinogenesis, 5:1267-1275.
41. Vickers, A.E.M., Sloop, T.C., and Lucier, G.W. (1985): Environ. Health Perspect., 59:121-128.
42. Weinberg, R.A. (1985): Science, 230:770-776.
43. Yager, Jr. J.D. and Yager, R. (1980): Cancer Res., 40:3680-3685.
44. Yuspa, S.H. (1984): In: Cellular Interactions By Environmental Tumor Promoters, edited by H. Fujiki, E. Hecker, R.E. Moore, T. Sugimura, and I.B. Weinstein, pp.315-326. Japan Scientific Societies Press, Tokyo, Japan.

Tumor Promoters: Biological Approaches for
Mechanistic Studies and Assay Systems,
edited by Robert Langenbach et al.
Raven Press, New York © 1988.

TCDD RECEPTOR: MECHANISMS OF ALTERED GROWTH REGULATION IN NORMAL AND TRANSFORMED HUMAN KERATINOCYTES

R. Osborne, J.C. Cook, K.M. Dold, L. Ross,
K. Gaido, and W.F. Greenlee

Department of Cell Biology
Chemical Industry Institute of Toxicology
Research Triangle Park, NC 27709

BACKGROUND

2,3,7,8-Tetrachlorodibenzo-p-dioxin (TCDD) is the extensively studied prototype for a large group of halogenated aromatic compounds (HACs) which include the dibenzofurans, biphenyls and biphenylenes, azo- and azoxybenzenes, and naphthalenes (1-3). Studies in various animal models and in human and animal cells in culture indicate that TCDD and isosteric analogs can act directly on the epithelia from several target organs to produce a diverse spectrum of pathologic lesions ranging from epidermal hyperplasia and hyperkeratinization to thymic atrophy (1,3,4). The skin is a particularly sensitive target for TCDD and related HACs in humans. Histologic examination of sequential skin biopsies from individuals exposed to TCDD-contaminated 2,4,5-trichlorophenol revealed that the acinar base cells of the sebaceous glands are reprogrammed to differentiate into keratinocytes (4). Plugging of the follicular orifice occurs simultaneously with the sebaceous gland duct hyperkeratinization, ultimately resulting in the formation of persistent keratinous cysts (4).

Many of the actions of TCDD on target cells are mediated by a specific intracellular binding protein, the TCDD receptor (also called the $\underline{Ah}$ or dioxin receptor) (3,5). This protein was first detected in hepatic cytosol from inbred mice (6) and subsequently has been found in almost all tissues examined (3,7). In most cells the TCDD receptor mediates the TCDD-dependent expression of a battery of genes coding for cytochrome P_1-450 and other enzymes primarily involved in xenobiotic metabolism (3). In certain target cells, including murine and human epidermal keratinocytes, the TCDD receptor is postulated to regulate a second gene battery encoding proteins involved in the control of cell proliferation and differentiation (3,5).

RESPONSES OF HUMAN EPIDERMAL KERATINOCYTES AND SQUAMOUS CELL CARCINOMA LINES TO TCDD

Cultures of normal human epidermal cells and human squamous cell carcinoma (SCC) lines have been used in this laboratory as $\underline{in}$ $\underline{vitro}$

models to study the mechanisms of TCDD-induced alterations in epithelial cell growth and differentiation (see ref. 5 for review). Treat-

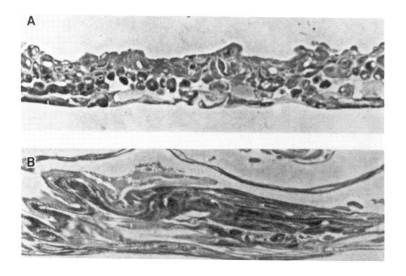

FIG. 1. Enhanced stratification in cultures of normal human epidermal cells treated with 10 nM TCDD for 4 days. Cross-sections of solvent control (A) or TCDD-treated (B) cultures are shown; the cell layer that was adjacent to the culture dish is toward the bottom of each panel. X250. Taken from Osborne and Greenlee (9).

TABLE 1. Actions of TCDD on Selected Parameters of Cell Growth and Differentiation[a]

	Control	TCDD
Total Cell Number $(X10^{-6})$	1.9 ± 0.2	2.0 ± 0.1
Small (basal) Cell Number $(X10^{-6})$	0.80 ± 0.06	$0.37 \pm 0.02^*$
Spontaneous Envelopes $(X10^{-4})$	1.5 ± 0.02	$3.5 \pm 0.2^*$
Envelope Competent Cells $(X10^{-6})$	0.92 ± 0.06	$1.9 \pm 0.05^*$

[a]Newly confluent cultures of normal human epidermal cells were treated for 4 days with 0.01% DMSO (control) or 10 nM TCDD. At the end of the treatment period the parameters indicated were measured. The mean $\pm$ SEM of values from triplicate dishes are given. Asterisks indicate values significantly different from control (p < 0.05). Taken from Osborne and Greenlee (9).

ment of human epidermal cell cultures in log-phase growth (8) or at confluency (9) with TCDD results in enhanced stratification and a decrease in numbers of basal cells (FIG. 1). The observed morphologic changes are accompanied by increases in several markers of terminal differentiation, including envelope competency, cross-linked envelopes and staining with keratin-specific dyes (9) (TABLE 1). Increased terminal differentiation is the predominant response to TCDD in at least one human SCC line, SCC-12F (5). In glucocorticoid-supplemented medium TCDD increases proliferation in another SCC line, SCC-9 (8,10). Supplementation of medium with glucocorticoids diminishes, but does not eliminate, TCDD-dependent differentiation in SCC-12F cultures (8,11). These observations suggest that the response of a given human epithelial target cell in culture to TCDD is dependent both on the programming of that cell and exogenous factors in the growth medium.

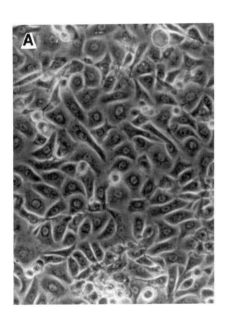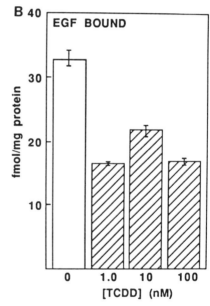

FIG. 2. (A) Phase-contrast photomicrograph of basal cells selected from a confluent culture of normal human epidermal cells in calcium-depleted medium (X200). (B) EGF specific binding in epidermal basal cells treated with the indicated concentrations of TCDD for 72 hr. EGF binding was measured as described previously (12). The mean ± SEM of values from triplicate dishes are shown. Levels of EGF binding in TCDD-treated cells were significantly lower than in control cells ($p < 0.05$).

Evidence for Involvement of the EGF Receptor

Epidermal growth factor (EGF) stimulates the proliferation of both mesenchymal and epithelial cells, including epidermal keratinocytes, through interaction with a specific receptor protein (13). TCDD decreases the level of binding of EGF to high-affinity receptors in both normal human epidermal (9) and SCC-12F cells (12). Several lines of evidence indicate that TCDD-dependent down modulation of EGF receptor binding in these cells is responsible at least in part for TCDD-stimulated differentiation: (i) TCDD decreases high affinity EGF binding in basal cells in growth medium containing a reduced concentration of Ca^{2+} (FIG. 2) (11); (ii) the decrease in EGF receptor binding activity precedes the morphologic transition of proliferating basal cells to intermediate and advanced stages of terminal differentiation (9); (iii) TCDD treatment inhibits keratinocyte responsiveness to EGF-dependent cell proliferation (8,11,12); and (iv) modulation of EGF binding by TCDD is biologically specific; i.e., among the human SCC lines examined, decreased EGF binding correlates with TCDD-induced differentiation (11).

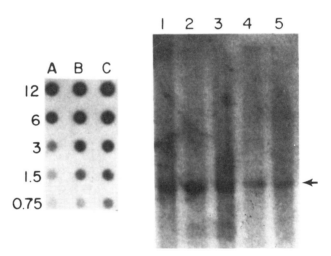

FIG. 3. Analysis of EGF receptor gene expression in SCC-12F cells. (Left) Total RNA prepared from control and TCDD-treated (10 nM, 48 hr) cells was applied to nitrocellulose filters, hybridized to a ^{32}P-labelled cDNA probe encoding the 3' end of the human EGF receptor gene (17), and analyzed by autoradiography. Lane A, no treatment; Lane B, 0.01% DMSO (control); Lane C, 10 nM TCDD. The numbers in the first column indicate the amount of RNA (µg) applied to each well in the corresponding row. (Right) Northern analysis of total RNA. Lane 1, no treatment; Lane 2, 0.01% DMSO (48 hr); Lane 3, 10 nM TCDD (48 hr); Lane 4 0.01% DMSO (72 hr); Lane 5, 10 nM TCDD (72 hr). The arrow indicates EGF receptor mRNA (6 kb). The EGF receptor probe (phEGFR-1) was kindly provided by Dr. Frank Simmen (see ref. 14).

The available data indicate that the observed TCDD-dependent regulation of keratinocyte terminal differentiation and EGF receptor binding activity are mediated by the TCDD receptor protein (8,11,12). The mechanism for the regulation of EGF binding activity by the TCDD receptor is not known. Based largely on the similarity between the values for the calculated half-life (20 hrs) for the reduction in high affinity EGF binding in TCDD-treated SCC-12F cells (12) with the reported half-life for the EGF receptor in human A431 cells (15), it has been postulated that TCDD may repress the EGF receptor gene (5). However, this hypothesis is not supported by the analysis of EGF receptor gene expression in SCC-12F cells which indicates that TCDD treatment does not alter EGF receptor gene transcription or processing of the RNA transcript (FIG. 3). Potential post-transcriptional actions of TCDD on EGF receptor turnover have not been examined.

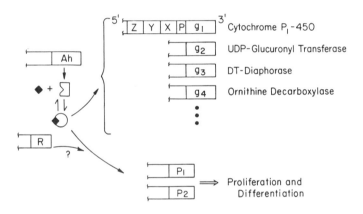

FIG. 4. Model for the regulation of multiple structural genes by the TCDD receptor. Upstream (5'-ward) promoter and regulatory regions are designated for the cytochrome P_1-450 gene: P, promoter; X, inhibitory domain; Y and Z, TCDD receptor responsive elements (see refs. 21 and 22). P_1 and P_2 designate putative genes involved in altered growth responses.

Several laboratories have reported on the role of site specific phosphorylation in the regulation of EGF receptor binding activity and function (see refs. 16 and 17 for reviews). The binding of EGF to its receptor results in the activation of a tyrosine kinase present within the cytoplasmic domain of this protein. This activated tyrosine kinase catalyzes autophosphorylation of the EGF receptor as well as the phosphorylation of other cellular protein substrates (17). The phosphorylation of threonine 654 on the EGF receptor by activated protein kinase C has been implicated in the regulation of high affinity EGF binding and the activity of the receptor tyrosine kinase domain (16,18,19). Protein kinase C can be directly activated by tumor promoting phorbol esters or indirectly by agents (e.g., platelet derived growth factor) which stimulate the phosphoinositol pathway (17).

Regulation of EGF receptor phosphorylation may represent an important mechanism for the observed actions of TCDD. However, in contrast to the tumor promoting phorbol esters, the actions of TCDD on the EGF receptor are characterized by a delayed onset (11,12), suggesting a mechanism other than direct activation of an EGF receptor-specific kinase. In mouse skin TCDD toxicity is regulated by two genes, Ah (the putative structural gene for the TCDD receptor) and hr (20). The hr locus appears to be required for TCDD receptor-dependent regulation of a gene battery encoding proteins involved in the control of cell growth and differentiation (3,20). A similar mechanism has been postulated for the actions of TCDD on human keratinocytes (5) (see Fig. 4).

Differences in Sensitivity to TCDD in Human Epidermal Cell Strains

Preliminary studies in strains of normal human epidermal cells derived from different individuals have shown differences in sensitivity for responses mediated by the TCDD receptor (23). Comparison of the induction of the cytochrome P_1-450-mediated monooxygenase activity, 7-ethoxycoumarin O-deethylase (ECOD), by TCDD in 4 strains of normal human epidermal cells indicated that 3 of the 4 strains were approximately equally sensitive (EC_{50} values = 2 nM), whereas one strain (designated strain G) was 10-fold more sensitive (EC_{50} = 0.2 nM) (FIG. 5A). The differences in sensitivity for the induction of ECOD activity were paralleled by differences in sensitivity for TCDD-dependent decreases in EGF binding (FIG. 5B), a specific biochemical response believed to be involved in TCDD-induced differentiation (5) (see above). Strain G cells also showed the largest magnitude response for regulation of both ECOD activity and EGF receptor binding (FIG. 5).

These data indicate that epidermal cells derived from different individuals can differ in their sensitivity to TCDD for receptor-mediated responses. One potential mechanism of interindividual differences in human sensitivity to TCDD is the presence of TCDD receptor isotypes that differ in affinity for HACs, as appear to occur in inbred mouse strains (6). The proposal that sensitivity to TCDD in human cells is determined at the level of the TCDD receptor is supported by the apparent correlation between sensitivity for TCDD induction of ECOD activity and levels of TCDD receptor binding activity in human SCC lines (24).

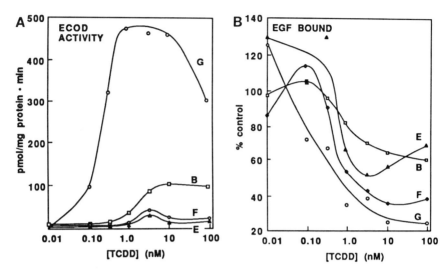

FIG. 5. Concentration dependence for the modulation of ECOD activity (A) and EGF specific binding (B) by TCDD. Confluent cultures of 4 strains of normal human epidermal cells were treated with the indicated concentrations of TCDD for 3 days prior to the measurement of ECOD activity (24) and EGF specific binding (12). Control levels of binding in strains B, E, F, and G were 9563 ± 460, 829 ± 33, 1593 ± 47, and 1082 ± 42 cpm/mg protein, respectively.

TUMOR PROMOTING ACTIVITY OF TCDD IN ANIMAL MODELS: POTENTIAL RELEVANCE TO CARCINOGENICITY IN HUMANS

TCDD has been shown to be a potent carcinogen in several animal species (3). Although the genotoxic potential of TCDD has been the subject of controversy, the bulk of the experimental evidence indicates that TCDD acts as a tumor promoter with little or no detectable initiating activity. TCDD promotes tumor formation in a two-stage model of liver carcinogenesis in the rat (25) and induces papilloma formation when painted on the skin of HRS/J hairless mice initiated with N-methyl-N'-nitro-N-nitrosoguanidine (MNNG) (26). In vitro TCDD promotes formation of transformed foci in MNNG-initiated C3H10T1/2 cells (27). Comparison of promotion by TCDD and 12-O-tetradecanoyl phorbol acetate (TPA) in mouse skin and C3H10T1/2 cells indicates that TCDD is 100- and 10,000-fold more potent than TPA, respectively (26,27). Characterization of the promoting actions of TCDD in these models suggest involvement of the TCDD receptor; however, specific events mediated by the interaction of TCDD with its cognate receptor relevant to the promotional response have not been elucidated.

In contrast to the findings in animal models, epidemiologic investigations of human populations inadvertantly exposed to TCDD have not shown a definitive link between human tumors and TCDD exposure. In most cases interpretation of the data is complicated by the relatively small size of the cohorts studied, and the complexity of the mixtures of chemicals to which the individuals were exposed. A mortality study of workers thirty years after exposure to TCDD contaminated trichlorophenol at an American plant found no significant increase in the overall incidence of deaths due to cancer (28). A U.S. Air Force study of personnel potentially exposed to TCDD in Agent Orange in Vietnam showed a significant increase in the incidence of basal cell carcinomas of the skin, but this study may not have been controlled adequately for exposure to sunlight in the test population (29). Swedish lumber workers exposed to chlorophenols and a phenoxyherbicide were reported to display an increased incidence of soft tissue sarcomas (30), but analysis of data from herbicide sprayers in New Zealand did not support that the phenoxy herbicide as used caused soft tissue sarcomas (31). Controversies have arisen over the diagnosis of soft tissue sarcomas (32), and in the case of American workers exposed to TCDD, the methods used for epidemiologic analysis (33).

The analysis of TCDD receptor-dependent responses in the human epithelial models presented in this report indicate that TCDD has the capacity to alter physiologic regulation of cell proliferation and differentiation. This is of potential relevance to the evaluation of the human carcinogenic potential of TCDD and related HACs. Yuspa and co-workers (34) have presented a model in which the dual actions of the phorbol ester tumor promoters on the differentiation of normal cells and the clonal outgrowth of initiated cells play a role in tumor promotion by phorbol esters in mouse skin. If the TCDD-induced alterations in cell proliferation and differentiation are relevant to tumor promotion in human cells, TCDD must be considered as having the potential to act as a tumor promoter in humans. It is likely, however, that this putative promotional activity of TCDD is under the same constraints, such as expression of tumor supressor genes, that renders human cells relatively insensitive to transformation by viruses or chemical carcinogens (35).

REFERENCES

1. Poland, A., Greenlee, W.F., and Kende,; A.S. (1979): Ann. N.Y. Acad. Sci., 320:214-230.
2. Goldstein, J.A. (1980): In: Halogenated Biphenyls, Terphenyls, Naphthalenes, Dibenzodioxins, and Related Products, edited by R. Kimbrough, pp.151-190. Elsevier/North-Holland, New York.
3. Poland, A. and Knutson, J.C. (1982): Ann. Rev. Pharmacol. Toxicol., 22:517-554.
4. Suskind, R.R. (1985): Scand. J. Work Environ. Health, 11:165-172.
5. Greenlee, W.F., Osborne, R., Dold, K.M., Hudson, L.G., Young, M.J., and Toscano, W.A., Jr. (1986): In: Reviews in Biochem.

Toxicol., edited by E. Hodgson, J. Bend, and R.M. Philpot, (in press). Elsevier/North-Holland, New York.

6. Poland, A., Glover, E., and Kende, A.S. (1976): J. Biol. Chem. 251:4936- 4946.

7. Gasiewicz, T.A. (1983): Proc. Annu. Conf. Environ. Toxicol. 13th, Dayton, Ohio, pp. 259-269.

8. Greenlee, W.F., Osborne, R., Dold, K.M., Hudson, L.G., and Toscano, W.A., Jr. (1985): Environ. Health Perspect., 60:69-76.

9. Osborne, R. and Greenlee, W.F. (1985): Toxicol. Appl. Pharmacol., 77:434-443.

10. Rice, R.H. and Greenlee, W.F. (1982): The Toxicologist, 2:463.

11. Hudson, L.G., Toscano, W.A., Jr., and Greenlee, W.F. (1986): Toxicol. Appl. Pharmacol., 82:481-492.

12. Hudson, L.G., Toscano, W.A., Jr., and Greenlee, W.F. (1985): Toxicol. Appl. Pharmacol., 77:251-259.

13. Carpenter, G. and Cohen, S. (1979): Annu. Rev. Biochem., 48:193-216.

14. Simmen, F.A., Gope, M.L., Schulz, T.Z., Wright, D.A., Carpenter, G., and O'Malley, B.A. (1984): Biochem. Biophys. Res. Commun., 124:125-132.

15. Krupp, M.N., Connolly, D.T., and Lane, M.D. (1982): J. Biol. Chem., 257:11489-11496.

16. Gill, G.N., Bertics, P.J., Thompson, D.M., Weber, W., and Cochet, C. (1985): In: Cancer Cells/3, edited by J. Feramisco, B. Ozanne, and C. Stiles, pp. 11-18. Cold Spring Harbor, New York.

17. Schlessinger, J. (1986): J. Cell Biol., 103:2067-2072.

18. Davis, R.J. and Czech, M.P. (1985): Proc. Natl. Acad. Sci. USA, 82:1974-1978.

19. Hunter, T., Ling, N., and Cooper, N.A. (1984): Nature(Lond.), 314:480-483.

20. Knutson, J.C. and Poland, A. (1982): Cell, 30:225-234.

21. Jones, P.B.C., Galeazzi, D.R., Fisher, J.M., and Whitlock, J.P., Jr. (1985): Science (Washington, D.C.), 227:1499-1502.

22. Jones, P.B.C., Durrin, L.K., Fisher, J.M., and Whitlock, J.P., Jr. (1986): J. Biol. Chem., 261:6647-6650.

23. Osborne, R., Dold, K.M., and Greenlee, W.F. (1985): Fed. Proc., 44:8385.

24. Hudson, L.G., Shaikh, R., Toscano, W.A., Jr., and Greenlee, W.F. (1983): Biochem. Biophys. Res. Commun. 115:611-617.

25. Pitot, H.C., Goldsworthy, T., Campbell, H.A., and Poland, A. (1980): Cancer Res., 40:3616-3620.

26. Poland, A., Palen, D., and Glover, E. (1982): Nature (London), 300:271-273.

27. Abernethy, D.J., Greenlee, W.F., Huband, J.C., and Boreiko, C.J. (1985): Carcinogenesis, 6:651-653.

28. Zack, J.A. and Suskind, R.R. (1980): J. Occup. Med., 22:11-14.

29. An Epidemiologic Investigation of Health Effects in Air Force Personnel following Exposure to Herbicides--Baseline Morbidity

Study Results, 24 February 1984. Epidemiology Div., Data Sciences Div., USAF School of Aerospace Medicine, Brooks Air Force Base, TX.

30. Hardell, L. and Sandstrom, A. (1979): Brit. J. Cancer, 39: 711-717.

31. Smith, A.H., Pearce, N.E., Fisher, D.OP., Giles, H.J., Teague, C.A., and Howard, J.K. (1984): JNCI, 73:1111-1117.

32. Hajdu, S.I. (1983): In: Public Health Risks of the Dioxins, edited by W.J. Lowrance, pp. 173-186. The Rockefeller University, New York.

33. Hay, A. and Silbergeld, E. (1985): Nature (London), 315:102 (Correspondence).

34. Yuspa, S.H., Hennings, H., Kulesz-Martin, M., and Lichti, U. (1982): In: Carcinogenesis and Biological Effects of Tumor Promoters. Carcinogenesis--A Comprehensive Survey, Vol. 7, edited by E. Hecker, N.E. Fusenig, W. Kunz, F. Marks, and H.W. Thielmann, pp. 217-230. Raven Press, New York.

35. Sager, R. (1986): Cancer Res., 46:1573-1580.

Tumor Promoters: Biological Approaches for Mechanistic Studies and Assay Systems,
edited by Robert Langenbach et al.
Raven Press, New York © 1988.

REFLECTIONS ON THE DECLINING ABILITY OF THE SALMONELLA ASSAY TO
DETECT RODENT CARCINOGENS AS POSITIVE

John Ashby

Imperial Chemical Industries PLC
Central Toxicology Laboratory
Macclesfield
Cheshire

SUMMARY

It is suggested that urgent attempts should be made to define and
gain general agreement for the existence of two classes of animal
carcinogen, those which are genotoxic and those which are not.
In the absence of such a step, attempts to validate in vivo
genotoxicity assays, and to derive a meaningful structure
activity database for chemical carcinogenesis, will be
frustrated. These suggestions are supported by the preliminary
findings of a detailed analysis of the carcinogen database
accrued by the United States National Toxicology Program.

The possibility that many non-genotoxic carcinogens should be
regarded as tumour-promoting agents is considered.

DISCUSSION

Genotoxic Carcinogens

A decade ago there seemed to be ample confirmation of the fact
that the Salmonella mutation assay was capable of detecting as
positive about 90% of the animal carcinogens known at the time,
while maintaining an equally high specificity for non-
carcinogens. The low (~10%) incidence of 'false' positive
responses was deemed acceptable given that the available cancer
bioassays on such mutagenic non-carcinogens were often less than
definitive. The low (~10%) incidence of carcinogens that
remained undetected was perceived as a cause for concern, and
that led to several collaborative studies whose aim was to
discern a generally acceptable in vitro assay with which to
complement the Salmonella test. At that time (~1976) it was
appreciated that a small minority of carcinogens may have
elicited tumours in animals via their protracted disturbance of
normal body homeostasis, as opposed to via their direct

interaction with DNA; however, there seemed to be few such agents and they were consequently deemed to present a neglible problem. Examples of these presumed non-genotoxic (epigenetic) carcinogens were provided at that time by thioruea (rat thyroid) and DDT (mouse liver).

A decade later it fell to Zeiger and Tennant (1986) of the United States National Toxicology Program (NTP) to confirm with data a growing perception that the Salmonella assay was not as efficient at detecting carcinogens as had once been thought. In particular, they demonstrated a reduced sensitivity (53%) for this assay to 130 carcinogens and equivocal carcinogens defined by the NTP, together with a reduced specificity of 71% to 80 non-carcinogens. More recently, Tennant et al (1987) have concluded that the employment of additional mammalian cell genotoxicity assays as complements to the Salmonella assay does little to increase the overall detection rate for NTP carcinogens. The situation appears bleak - the standard in vitro genotoxicity assays appear to offer little more than a random sensitivity to the NTP rodent carcinogens, or put another way, the earlier and seemingly minor problem of non-genotoxic carcinogens seems to have reappeared in force in the developing NTP carcinogen bioassay program. The failing fortunes of in vitro genotoxicity assays appear in stark contrast to the progress which has been made in molecular biology over the past few years, the data from most of which studies appear to enhance the credibility of the somatic mutation theory of carcinogenesis.

It is suggested here that the declining sensitivity of the Salmonella assay to carcinogens is the direct result of a change in the design and sensitivity of the rodent cancer bioassay protocols, rather than of a change in the intrinsic sensitivity of the assay itself. In fact, rather than decreasing, the sensitivity to mutagens of the Salmonella assay protocol has increased over the past few years. The cancer bioassay protocols employed by the NTP involve the lifetime administration of chemicals to mice and rats at the maximum tolerated dose-level (MTD). Further, these studies are accompanied by extensive pathological assessment of the treated animals and are assessed using statistical models in cases where a clear carcinogenic effect is not observed. It is suggested that such exhaustive protocols, while enabling the detection of weak genotoxic carcinogenic effects, also offer an optimised environment in which to observe chemical-induced modulations (promotion) of spontaneous tumour incidences. Agents in the latter category, when classified as carcinogens, are essentially indistinguishable from genotoxic carcinogens in the absence of ancilliary information. Therefore, if an amplification of the earlier class of non-genotoxic carcinogen has taken place in the NTP program over the past decade, the only way to appreciate this change will be to employ classical structure activity relationships (SA), coupled to knowledge of the activity of the test agent as a genotoxin. This, of course represents one of the purest cases of cyclic logic, but it is felt to be worthy of consideration given the magnitude of the current problems faced by in vitro genotoxicity assays. In fact, it is initially difficult to understand why the detractors of in vitro genotoxicity assays have not made more capital out of the present poor performance of the Salmonella assay, for it would require little literary skill to use the carcinogen predictivity figures published by Zeiger and Tennant (1986) to destroy the fundamental premise that carcinogens are mutagens (McCann et al 1975). The fact that this has not happened probably indicates a shared perception that something other than the Salmonella assay has changed.

The need to understand the present situation is made the more important by the fact that efforts to study and predict new tumour-promoting agents may currently be being hampered by unqualified use of the word carcinogen. Thus, it is suggested later in this article that many of the non-genotoxic NTP 'carcinogens' may in fact be tumour-promoting agents, and that as such their classification as 'carcinogens' presents the dual problem of forcing genetic toxicologists to doubt the validity of their assays, and of depriving workers in tumour-promotion of chemicals which could perhaps act as their primary reference agents for study. A further danger resides in our current failure to distinguish genotoxic from non-genotoxic carcinogens, that is, that many investigators are currently attempting to evaluate the value of short-term in vivo genotoxicity assays - mainly as a means to discern which new in vitro genotoxins are likely to also be mutagenic/carcinogenic in vivo. As a part of such evaluations it is legitimate to ask questions about the general sensitivity of these in vivo assays to carcinogens before they are employed to qualify predictions of potential activity for a chemical based on observations made in vitro. Yet, if one were to attempt a validation of any of these in vivo genotoxicity assays against the NTP carcinogen database, one would as surely devalue them as has recently occurred with the in vitro assays.

One therefore either has to accept that genotoxicity assays are of little value for the prediction of animal carcinogencity, or one has to look in detail at the NTP carcinogen database, and to speculate regarding its true nature and status.

A detailed reanalysis of the NTP carcinogen database (~300 chemicals) was recently undertaken in cooperation with Dr Raymond Tennant of the NTP. The results of that study will be published in a special issue of Mutation Research, but in the meantime, some of its main conclusions are discussed here as they enable some of the rather diffuse concepts discussed above to be formalized. Our analysis was based on the bringing together of three separate studies. The first was to collect together chemicals which had been evaluated for carcinogencity

in Fischer 344 rats and B6C3F1 mice in studies deemed acceptable
by the NTP peer review group (223 chemicals). Conclusions of
carcinogenicity were accepted and the supporting tumour database
tabulated. The carcinogens thus identified were segregated into
six groups according to their level of carcinogenicity. The
highest level was accorded to agents found carcinogenic to both
species and producing tumours at two or more sites. The lowest
categories were agents only found to be active at a single site
in a single sex of a single species, and agents deemed to give
only equivocal evidence of carcinogencity. Eighty eight non-
carcinogens were also identified. The second study involved
classifying the resultant 223 agents according to structure-
activity (SA) relationships established for carcinogens prior to
1976, ie, according to whether their chemical structure
indicated genotoxicity or not. This was a relatively
uncomplicated exercise based upon recently published criteria
(Ashby 1985). Finally, Dr Errol Zeiger of the NTP made
available to us the Salmonella mutation assay data which he had
for most of these agents.

It is not intended to present the results of that tridentine
study here, rather, the following points are selected as
relevant to the present debate:

1)   The overall sensitivity of the Salmonella assay to the 109
     unequivocal carcinogens was 56%, and its specificity for
     the non-carcinogens was 69%. These figures reflect those
     published earlier by Zeiger and Tennant (1986) and confirm
     the need for the present discussion.

2)   The level of concordance between the Salmonella assay and
     SA was consistently high (85-98% agreement across the
     several levels of carcinogenic response). This suggests
     that the electrophilic theory of carcinogenesis advanced by
     the Miller's, and the ability of the Salmonella assay to
     discern electrophiles as positive, remain unchanged for the
     NTP database.

3)   Trans-species/multi-site carcinogens (eg TRIS, Fig 1) were
     detected by the Salmonella assay in 37 of 51 cases (73%),
     and there was 92% concordance with SA for these compounds.
     The figure of 73% sensitivity for the Salmonella assay for
     these agents would probably have been higher had all of the
     experiments been conducted according to the more sensitive
     pre-incubation test protocol. Whatever, the data indicate
     a much more encouraging performance for this assay than is
     seen across the whole database.

4)   The overall specificity of the Salmonella assay (69%)
     reflects the fact that 26 of 84 (31%) non-carcinogens were
     mutagenic <u>in vitro</u>, 21 of which were also classed as
     positive based upon structural considerations. This would
     seem to confirm that <u>in vitro</u> genotoxicity assays are

intrinsically over-sensitive, as befits their role as screening tests. But of much greater significance is the fact that a similar proportion of Salmonella mutagens were of carcinogen with low levels of carcinogencity, yet in those cases it is regarded as the 'sensitivity' figure for the Salmonella assay to these 'carcinogens', as opposed to the incidence (%) of false positive predictions for the non-carcinogens. For example, for the 20 chemicals recorded as selectively carcinogenic to a single tissue of potentially electrophilic structure, and 7 of these 8 comprised the only agents from among the 20 (35%) which were mutagenic to Salmonella. One construction to place on these figures is that the Salmonella assay only predicted 35% of the carcinogens of this class. An alternative construction is that as a class, these agents had the same proportion of in vitro mutagens as possessed by the class of non-carcinogens, and that these were 20 selective 'carcinogens' all of which had modified the tumour incidence in the test animals by a non-genotoxic mechanism. Two examples are provided to illustrate these concepts. In Fig 2 the data for the non-mutagenic rat thyroid carcinogen DETU are shown. The critical question presented is 'should one penalise the Salmonella assay for failing to detect as positive this carcinogen -rather, should not its non-mutagenicity, taken together with its non-electrophilicity, alert to an alternative mechanism of carcinogenic action? Similar questions could be asked regarding the profile seen for Dicofol, one of the chemicals present in the species/sex/site specific group of carcinogens (Fig 3).

If one collects together the 20 equivocal carcinogens, the 20 which affected only a single site of a single species, and the further 20 which only affected a single site of a single sex of a single species of animal, then a group of 60 compounds is formed. The performance of the Salmonella assay for these 60 agents does not differ significantly from its performance with the 84 non-carcinogens for which Salmonella data were available (Fig 4). The fact that structural considerations support the low overall assay sensitivity observed (37%) indicates that these 60 agents are not just weak examples of the trans-species/multi-site carcinogens discussed in 3) above.

Of course, the present analysis leads to the definition of provocative examples which lie across the borders of the two proposed classes of carcinogen. One such is shown in Fig 5, 4-acetamido-2-ethoxyaniline (AEA). This agent has a structure which is consistent with its mutagenicity to Salmonella, yet it is uniquely and weakly carcinogenic to the thyroid of the female B6C3F1 mouse. At present there are no data to indicate if this represents a highly selective genotoxic carcinogenic response, or an example of a non-genotoxic endocrine carcinogen which happens to be,

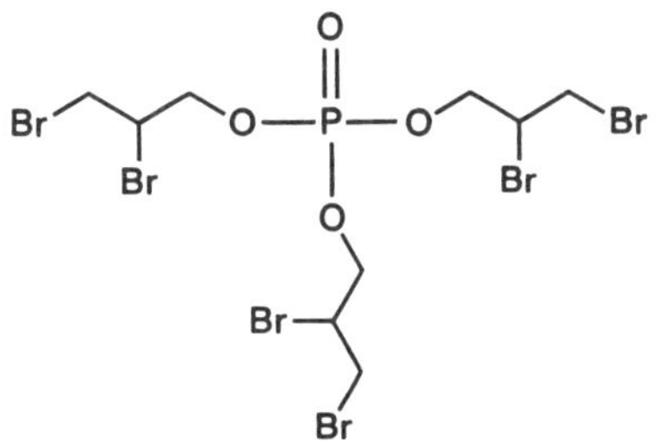

TRIS

Salmonella	+ve	
♀/♂ rat	+ve	} NTP
♀/♂ mouse	+ve	

Kidney, forestomach, liver, lung
mouse ≫ rat

Fig 1. NTP mutagenicity and carcinogenicity data for
tris(2,3-dibromopropyl)phosphate (TRIS).

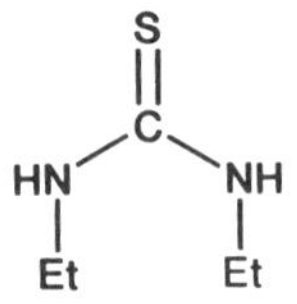

DETU

Salmonella	−ve	
♀/♂ mouse	−ve	} NTP
♀/♂ rat	+ve	

	C	Low	High
Thyroid, foll. cell. carc.	0	2	23% TBA ♂
foll. cell. aden.	0	9	37% TBA ♀

Fig 2. NTP mutagenicity and carcinogenicity data for
N,N'-diethylthiourea (DETU). TBA = tumour bearing animals in
control (c), low (L) and high (H) dose levels.

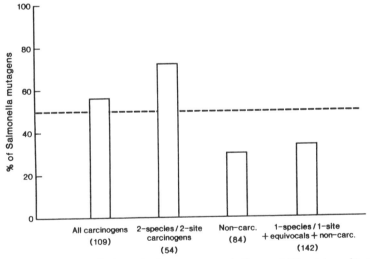

DICOFOL

Salmonella	−ve
♀/♂ rat	−ve
♀ mouse	−ve
♂ mouse	+ve

	C	Low	High
Hepatocellular carc.	17	44	74% TBA

Fig 3. NTP mutagencity and carcinogencity data for Dicofol. See legend to Fig 2.

Fig 4. Abstract of data being prepared for publication (Ashby and Tennant, 1987). For 109 NTP carcinogens and 84 non-carcinogens, the carcinogenicity data for which is adequate in both F344 rats and B6C3F1 mice, the Salmonella assay appears to have a sensitivity of 56% and a specificity of 69%. However, for the 54 2-species multiple-site carcinogens, an enhanced sensitivity was evident, while the proportion of Salmonella mutagens among the selective carcinogens, equivocal carcinogens and non-carcinogens (142 compounds) was essentially the same as for the non-carcinogens, suggesting an alternative mechansim of carcinogenic action.

in common with 26 of 84 NTP non-carcinogens, mutagenic to Salmonella.

In summary, it is speculated that the NTP database of 109 chemicals adequately tested in 2 species and concluded as unequivocal carcinogens contains a significant sub-group (40; 37%) of non-genotoxic carcinogens. The performance of the Salmonella assay is acceptable when testing the trans-species/multi-site carcinogens, and is no more sensitive to the 40 selective and the 20 equivocal carcinogens than it is to the non-carcinogens.

Non-genotoxic carcinogens/tumour promoting agents

Evaluation of the 60 selective or equivocal NTP carcinogens for tumour promoting properties in those species/sexes/tissues in which tumours were observed may prove to be more rewarding than their repetitive testing in increasingly esoteric, and increasingly unreliable in vitro genotoxicity assays. Certainly, such agents should temporarily be excluded from consideration when extending the already impressive database supporting the validity of certain of the available in vivo genotoxicity assays.

Attempts to study the possible tumour promoting properties of these 60 chemicals should take account of two factors:

i)   That as with genotoxicity assays, in vitro assays for promotional activities may be over-sensitive, ie, they may involve the generation of a significant incidence of false positive responses. Thus, for a chemical to interrupt inter-cellular communication among cultured cells may not mean it will elicit a similar effect in vivo.

ii) The selective carcinogenic (promotional?) effects observed for the above 60 agents may be uniquely associated with enhancement of the 'spontaneous' tumour incidences in the appropriate tissues of the species/strains/sexes of the animals used in the NTP cancer bioassay program. The promotional influence may be sufficient to reveal 'spontaneous' tumours in tissues normally not observed to carry control tumours -initiated cells may nonetheless be present (c.f. Fig 2).

Rosenkranz et al (1986) have aknowledged the need for separate computer databases for carcinogens and Salmonella mutagens. That problem is probably due to two separate factors:

i)   the hypersensitivity of in vitro assays, as illustrated by the results of the above mentioned study, ie, a significant proportion of non-carcinogens will be genotoxic in vitro yet be non-genotoxic in vivo and non-carcinogenic (genotoxic carcinogenesis).

ii) the possibly incorrect classification of a range of tumour-producing agents as carcinogens.

AEA

Salmonella	+ve	
♀/♂ rat	−ve	NTP
♀ mouse	−ve	NTP
♂ mouse	+ve	NTP

	C_1	C_2	Low	High
Thyroid, foll. cell. carc.	0	0	0	16% TBA

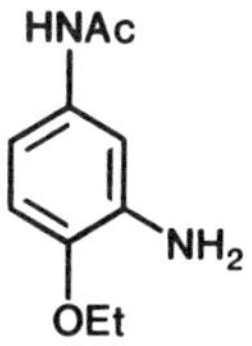

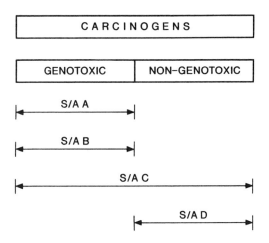

Fig 5. NTP mutagenicity and carcinogencity data for 4-acetamido-2-ethoxyaniline (AEA). See legend to Fig 2.

Fig 6. Stylized illustration of the effect upon structure-activity (S/A) relationships in chemical carcinogenesis of segregating genotoxic from non-genotoxic carcinogens. S/A A represents the relationships established by ~1976, and these are generally consistent with those observed in genotoxicity assays (S/A B). If a diverse set of new S/A relationships exist for non-genotoxic carcinogens (as seems likely, S/A D), then this will confuse S/A relationships for all 'carcinogens' (S/A C; cf, Rosenkranz et al 1985 and Ashby 1985).

The second of these two factors is potentially the most serious as it will eventually lead to a corruption of the carcinogenicity databases by benign structures such as thiourea and Dicofol (Fig 6). These concerns endorse further the need to define and agree two distinct classes of chemical carcinogen. Tennant has suggested the terms inductive and adaptive carcinogens to describe these two classes, the latter of which terms would replace the excess of terms currently in use eg, non-genotoxic/epigenetic/hormonal/ambivalent, etc carcinogen and tumour promoting agent.

It is suggested to be unlikely that any single assay, be it conducted in vitro or in vivo, will be sufficient to detect all non-genotoxic carcinogens. Attempts to anticipate such agents would seem to be best made in the whole mammal, and as such they could form part of the normal evaluation of a chemical for general toxicity. Thus, it may be, for example, that the most relevant alert to the rodent 'carcinogencity' of the following non-mutagens may be provided by the forms of toxicity they are known to elicit (shown in parenthesis):

Sodium saccharin	(rat bladder hyperplasia)
Thiourea, AEA, DETU, etc	(hyperplasia of both c-cells and follicular cells in the thyroid)
Nitrotriacetic acid	(heavy metal ion disturbances in the kidney and bladder)
Diethylhexylphthalate	(disturbances in lipid metabolism in the liver)
Butylated hydroxyanisole	(selective toxicity to the rodent stomach)
Dicofol, TCDD and analogs	(interruption of cell-cell communication in the liver)

Testing Strategies

The above considerations impinge upon the design of test batteries, in particular, on the proposals made on that subject a year ago (Ashby 1986). First, in relation to the need for in vitro assays to act as a complement to the Salmonella assay; second, in relation to false positive in vitro responses. The need for a reliable complementary assay remains as real yet as small as it has been for the past five years - a few genotoxic (electrophilic) carcinogens and in vivo mutagens remain undetected by the Salmonella assay, however advanced the test protocol employed. These include benzene, hexamethylphosphoramide, urethane and, perhaps the best example, as recently emphasized by Gatehouse and Tweats (1986), procarbazine. These agents require detection as genotoxins in vitro and no in vitro battery can be regarded as effective until its sensitivity to them is established. The imminent danger is that the performance of complementary assays will be judged against the 60 NTP non-genotoxic 'carcinogens' referred to above. As has been suggested earlier, no genotoxicity assay is likely to detect these agents, and if agents such as these are employed as standards, the important need for an efficient complementary assay for gentoxins may be devalued. If that happens, it will do a great disservice to the science. Second, the incidence of Salmonella mutagens which fail to prove carcinogenic (and non-mutagenic in vivo where evaluated) is too high (~30%) for sole reliance to be placed on in vitro assays in any screening strategy.

This emphasises a critical role for in vivo genotoxicity assays, but they, like in vitro complementary assays, could easily be wrongly discredited by their failure to detect as positive 'carcinogens' such as diethylthiourea (Fig 2) and Dicofol (Fig 3). The continuing validation of in vivo genotoxicity assays should be, at least initially, undertaken with significant genotoxic carcinogens such as Tris (Fig 1).

This article is built on the implicit assumption that trans-species/multi-tissue/genotoxic carcinogens are of maximum potential hazard to man, while selective and non-genotoxic carcinogens (tumour promoting agents?) present a neglible hazard in the particular. This is partially supported by the fact that agents in latter category already have limited evidence to suggest that their carcinogenicity in one species is not predictive of their activity in a second. It may be that repeated exposure of humans to a range of tumour promoting agents could increase the spontaneous cancer incidence, and generalisations should be considered carefully should they involve the assumption, for example, that the non-genotoxic carcinogen TCDD presents a negligible human hazard. Nonetheless, it remains true that an individual is unlikely to discern initially his exposure to a carcinogenic dose-level of benzidine, yet might become alerted by the consequences to health of exposure to sub-carcinogenic doses of thiourea or chloroform, etc. The Salmonella assay, used as part of a small battery of in vitro and in vivo genotoxicity assays, continues to alert to carcinogens such as benzidine - the failure of such a battery to alert to Dicofol and diethylthiourea may eventually be seen as an advantage.

CONCLUSIONS

After a decade of continuing attempts to force genotoxicity assays to detect all rodent carcinogens as positive, it has become clear that this is not to be. It is suggested that future validation studies of genotoxicity assays should take account of changes taking place in perceptions of the word carcinogen. When a unique role for rodent genotoxicity assays in the detection of possible human mutagens and carcinogens was initially proposed (Ashby, 1983), the relevant database appeared as shown in Fig 7. Were a corresponding in vivo genotoxicity database for the NTP carcinogens to be aquired (say by 1988) it would probably appear as shown in Fig 8. Hopefully, by that time we will have agreed a name for the non-genotoxic carcinogens which will prevent them from being used to

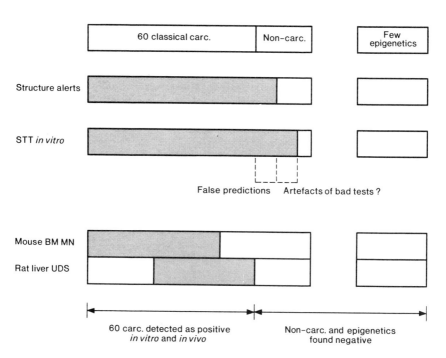

Fig 7. Summary (stylized) of the situation apparent in 1983 concerning the activity of 'classical' carcinogens in in vitro and in vivo genotoxicity assays. Most carcinogens (about 60 studied) were potentially electrophilic in structure and genotoxic in vitro. Some non-mutagenic (epigenetic?) carcinogens were known and some non-carcinogens were genotoxic in vitro. Some of the latter responses may have been due to artefacts of the test or its protocol (that remains true in 1987). In 1983 the data available suggested that the combination of two in vivo genotoxicity assays would isolate the carcinogens as positive, thus their role in testing. Shaded areas represent positive responses - the scale of these histograms is purely illustrative and is not precise.

1988

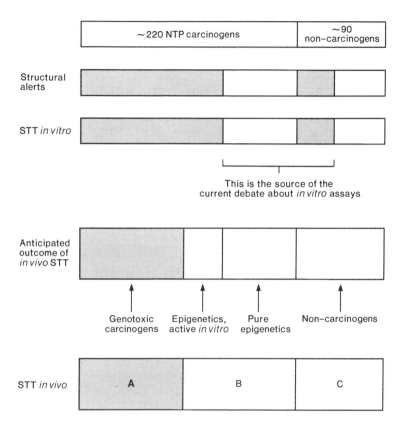

Fig 8. Summary (stylized) of the situation which may prevail in 1988 if the NTP carcinogens are fully evaluated for genotoxicity in vivo. The present debate concerning the value of short-term tests (STT) in vitro is evident and exagerated as compared to in 1983 (Fig 7). Aquisition of in vivo genotoxicity data will lead to a large number of carcinogens being found to be inactive. These may be the epigenetic carcinogens referred to herein. Whatever, selection of chemicals from group A or group B will enable in vivo genotoxicity assays to be 'validated' or devalued. Selection from groups A or B could be based on structural alerts and genotoxic activities observed in vitro. Nonetheless, the original aim (Ashby 1983) would have been fulfilled -the isolation of genotoxic carcinogens as a maximum hazard sub-group. Assays for tumour-promotion may be required to detect group B agents. Shaded areas represent positive activity and the scale is not precise.

'validate' (undermine?) genotoxicity assays. If we have not, then it will have to be accepted that genotoxicity assays have little to offer for the prediction of rodent carcinogenicity, irrespective of how well they may define potential and/or actual rodent mutagens.

REFERENCES

Ashby J (1985), Fundamental structural alerts to potential carcinogencity or non-carcinogenicity, Environ. Mutagen, 17, 919-921.

Ashby J (1986), The prospects for a simplified and internationally harmonized approach to the detection of possible human carcinogens and mutagens, Mutagenesis, 1, 3-16.

Ashby J (1983), The unique role of rodents in the detection of possible human carcinogens and mutagens, Mutation Research, 115, 117-213.

Ashby J and Tennant R W (1987), Categorization of 223 chemicals evaluated by carcinogenicity in rats and mice according to structural criteria, mutagenicity to Salmonella and level of carcinogenicity, Mutation Res., in preparation.

Gatehouse D G and Tweats D J (1986), Letter to the Editor, Mutagenesis, 1, 307-309.

McCann J, Choi E, Yamasaki E and Ames B N (1975), Detection of carcinogens as mutagens in the Salmonella/microsome test: Assay of 300 chemicals, Proc.Nat.Acad.Sci. USA, 72, 5135-5139, and 73, 950-954.

Rosenkranz H S, Mitchell C S and Klopman G (1985), Artificial intelligence and Bayesian decision theory in the prediction of chemical carcinogens, Mutation Research, 150, 1-11.

Tennant et al (1987). To be completed within 10 days.

Zeiger E and Tennant R W (1986), Mutagenesis, Carcinogenesis: Expectations, Correlations and Relations, Genetic Toxicology of Environmental Chemicals, B, 75-84, Alan P. Liss Inc.

Tumor Promoters: Biological Approaches for
Mechanistic Studies and Assay Systems,
edited by Robert Langenbach et al.
Raven Press, New York © 1988.

PROMOTION AND TUMOR PROGRESSION

Philippe Shubik

Green College, Oxford, OX2 6HG, UK

I will begin this talk with a brief review of the historical
background to studies that are now commonly called two stage
carcinogenesis experiments (even though there has been uncontrolled proliferation of the number of stages by some investigators
to as many as seven stages, I have heard tell).

I think that it is of some importance that we recall the reasons for which these studies were undertaken since, as time has
gone on, in-depth investigations of one area or another using
"model systems" has, at times, resulted in a loss of overall perspective.

There were originally three series of studies undertaken for
entirely different reasons that arrived at the conclusion that
skin carcinogenesis could be demonstrated to involve two separate
stages, hypothetically involving different mechanisms. The studies of Berenblum began with a desire to determine whether or not
"chronic irritation" played a secondary role in carcinogenesis.
The view that chronic irritation was not able to induce cancer by
itself appeared to have been laid to rest once and for all by the
discovery that coal tar was not just an irritant but contained
active principles - one of which was benzo(a)pyrene.

I am sure that some of you realize that the view that chronic
irritation in a generalized non-specific sense is still thought
of by some as a cause of cancer just as there are still members
of flat earth societies. Berenblum's logically constructed program of studies was, of course, preceded by both the studies and
pronouncements of others. I have always been totally fascinated
by the incredible prescience of the father of experimental pathology, Julius Cohnheim, the first man to describe the dynamics
and significance of inflammation. In discussing the role of injury and irritation in cancer in his lectures in the 1870's, Cohnheim remarks that although a few cases of injury and irritation
appear to be associated with cancer clinically, it is obvious
that the majority of instances of injury are not precursors of
cancer. Therefore, he postulated that it must be a matter of

injury having its effect on an abnormal tissue that gives rise
to such an effect. He then postulated that the abnormal tissue
arises as a result of incomplete embryological development and
that embryonic rests are the "initiated tissues".

When the first chemical carcinogen, coal tar, became available, the Belgian scientist Deelman combined applications of it
with wounding in the skin of the mouse and found an enhancing
effect. Berenblum then proceeded to study various irritant
chemicals in this system (and later with pure polycyclic hydrocarbons) and found a variety of different results. Mustard gas,
for example, inhibited the action of other carcinogens; croton
oil greatly increased the number of tumors when applied simultaneously; Berenblum then undertook a key experiment in which he
applied benzo(a)pyrene (B(a)P) and croton oil sequentially and
induced tumors this way. Mottram refined this by applying a
single application of B(a)P first followed by and preceded by
croton oil. This was the basis for the series of experiments
that I was privileged to undertake with Berenblum; in our first
study we found that we could not confirm the enhancing effect of
croton oil reported by Mottram but managed to induce tumors with
a single application of B(a)P or 7,12-dimethylbenz(a)anthracene
(DMBA), etc., followed by croton oil. Since then several others
- but notably Pound - have reported that the pretreatment with
croton oil does have an effect. This is one of numerous anomal-
ous reports in the literature for which the reasons for the anom-
alies in this regard concern the intervals between the different
treatments.

Another controversial issue that must be resolved for any of
these studies to be considered seriously concerns the carcinogenicity of croton oil or the phorbol esters. Had croton oil induced tumors alone in the original studies, I am quite sure that
these would never have been published. The key fact that was
reported was that tumors could be induced by the sequential application of a carcinogen at a dose that could not induce tumors
followed by repeated applications of an agent that alone could
not induce tumors at any dose. This is the basis of the conclusion that two different mechanisms - initiation and promotion -
could combine to give rise to tumors. If the promoter and the
initiator can both produce tumors alone, it would seem quite impossible to aver that they represent different mechanisms of
action. Over a period of several decades there have been a series of claims that croton oil alone or phorbol esters are carcinogenic alone. The first of these claims was made by the well
known group at the McArdle Laboratory at the University of Wisconsin. At the time of this finding I was deeply involved in
these skin studies in mice and was much concerned. Had I been
able to confirm these results, I would have stopped work in the
area forthwith and concluded that the original studies had no
merit.

I was graciously given a sample of croton oil used by Drs
Rusch and Boutwell in Wisconsin and tested this on the Swiss mice

that we were using in Chicago. The source of the croton oil they were using was different from ours and it seemed only reasonable to believe that the differences in results could be due to some impurity. No tumors were induced with this material alone. We therefore decided to investigate the only other variable that was amenable to study in those pre-GLP days - namely the animals used. The Wisconsin group then used a mouse not, as far as I have been able to ascertain, used by anyone else in this field. This was a hybrid albino mouse called the "Sutter strain" that was the product of a small commercial animal breeder in Missouri. With some difficulty we managed to obtain a small number of these mice and, since they were all infected with Salmonella, put them in isolation and decided to breed them and use the F1 generation for our tests. To our great astonishment the mice started to develop multiple skin tumors in the untreated state. We ascertained (again with considerable difficulty) that these mice had been bred in wooden boxes and had almost certainly been exposed to creosote. Peyton Rous had had occasion to unearth a similar episode some years before.

I only resurrect this study because it has some bearing on recent observations (those who ignore history are destined to relive it). Dr Iversen has recently made a great deal of fuss about his ability to induce skin tumors with phorbol esters alone and it is interesting to note that the presence of wood has once again reared its head; in this instance Iversen's mice are said to reside on wood chips. In view of the previous observations and of the association of nasal sinus cancers in wood workers, it would seem as well to exclude this possible source of initiating agents before deriving any drastic conclusions.

Secondly and by no means less important is the question of the specificity of both the strains and species in such studies. The vast majority of studies in two stage carcinogenesis in the skin undertaken during the past 15 years have used mice labelled as Sencar which originated from the Wisconsin group and are extremely difficult to define. These are not inbred or outbred mice but are animals with a special sensitivity to skin tumor induction for no known reason. It is rumoured that inbred Sencar mice are to become available but we have been unable to locate a source of these animals. The existence of these special mice has complicated this problem for the moment but perhaps in the long run it will be useful.

There are again a number of controversies surrounding the specificity of croton oil as a mouse "promoting agent". In my original studies I could not induce any tumors in the skin of the rabbit, rat, or hamster with croton oil as a promoting agent. I did eventually induce some tumors in the rat with TPA when this became available but these were in very small number and the results were in no way comparable to those seen in the mouse.

Goerttler has claimed that TPA can promote melanotic tumors in the skin of the hamster. Saffiotti and I originally wondered if croton oil could induce a slight increase in these tumors that are induced in profusion with a single dose of DMBA of only 50 micrograms. It would be extremely difficult to demonstrate a promoting effect of any magnitude in this system. In any event there is no promoting effect seen in this species concerned with epidermal tumors, although croton oil and TPA induce massive hyperplasia of this tissue.

One must conclude from the literature that croton oil and TPA can be classified as non-carcinogenic and active in the mouse in a manner that is not seen in other species. There is, apart from the hamster experience, extremely convincing data that in this system hyperplasia induction and promoting action cannot be equated.

To continue with the second reason that these studies were undertaken, we must turn to the fine series of studies that began to examine the life history of the tumors induced in the skin of the rabbit with coal tar. Rous made the surprising discovery that when tumors were induced in the skin of the rabbit with coal tar, cessation of treatment would result in the regression of many of the tumors. When treatment was resumed these regressed tumors could be made to reappear. This observation was then followed with the study that links these investigations to those with croton oil. It was found by Rous and his group that these regressed tumors could be made to reappear by wound healing or by applications of turpentine. From this study the terms "Initiation", "Promotion", and "Latent Tumor Cell" were introduced. It is unfortunate that these studies have not been extensively repeated and followed up. I repeated some of them some while ago and only published the results in a thesis; I managed to obtain some effects with wounding but not as marked as those reported by Rous et al., and had concluded that only benign lesions occurred. I could not confirm the turpentine results, even using the turpentine provided to me by Rous.

Efforts have been made to analyse the components of wound healing that might be responsible for promotion but I believe these need to be redone with more modern techniques for the in vivo studies so far undertaken as well as in vivo application of in vitro studies undertaken comparing epidermal growth factor and promoting agents such as TPA. There seems to be every reason for believing that wounding can play a role as a "promoting agent" and if this is the case it must be taken into account in all studies. Many of the agents reported to induce "promotion" are often quite damaging at the doses used and before concluding that some new chemically specific effect has been found this non-specific component needs to be excluded.

In my first studies with Berenblum I observed that a great majority of the lesions induced with a single application of carcinogen followed by croton oil regressed. This occurred because these papers formed a major part of a doctorate thesis and necessitated much more detailed descriptions than in the papers of those days. The charts of all those individual tumors were included in the thesis but not in the paper. Subsequently the behaviour of the tumors were recorded in a separate paper and a series of publications then described the comparative life histories of tumors induced in mouse skin using different dosages and regimes of carcinogens with and without croton oil.

I have pointed out on several occasions that three fundamentally distinct patterns of tumor behaviour can be caused at will in the skin of mice. A single, large dose of a carcinogen will induce many carcinomas and many regressing lesions; a single low dose followed by croton oil or TPA will give rise to many regressions, many benign tumors and a relatively low incidence of carcinomas; lastly, repeated applications of the carcinogen alone will give rise to many benign and malignant tumors and few regressions. I reiterate this only to emphasize that if one cannot escape from the conclusion that a variation in carcinogenic induction procedures influences not only the number of tumors induced but also the biological characteristics of the individual neoplasm (i.e., does it remain benign, become malignant or regress) then our simplistic views of transformation of the normal cell to a cancer cell must be entirely erroneous.

I think it is now time for me to apologize for not addressing the primary topic of this meeting, namely the use of _in vitro_ systems in these studies. I have been known to make uncomplimentary remarks about these systems in the past but am pleased to be able to report that I have finally mellowed a little in this regard. It is now difficult for even the most iconoclastic whole animal biologist to ignore the key role that certain _in vitro_ procedures are now playing in investigating the mechanisms involved at the molecular biological level.

Unfortunately, as far as I am aware, no _in vitro_ system has been devised that can allow the research worker to investigate varying stages of neoplasia (benign, malignant, regressing) effectively. It certainly seems not beyond the imagination to design systems _in vitro_ to mimic the various stages of neoplasia that are seen in the whole animal. Indeed, while preparing this talk, I wondered whether someone would tell me at this meeting that this had already been done. If it has not, I hope that someone will start on it right away.

The benign tumor, that is far and away the commonest endpoint in "two stage studies", is an orphan in the cancer research literature. There is little, if any speculation on the nature of benign tumors amongst current cancer research workers. This is largely a result of the prejudice amongst early carcinogenesis workers that one either induced a genuinely malignant, invasive, metastasizing transplantable tumor or the result was valueless.

Nowadays the only discussion of these lesions appears to be confined to the toxicologists. Here the argument ranges at what can only be described as a mindless level; the more extreme "concerned citizen" group maintains that benign tumors in rodents are exactly the same as malignant tumors for "regulatory purposes" whereas the group concerned with the sale of the products maintains that benign and malignant tumors are entirely different

entities. No one appears to believe that it might be worthwhile
wondering about their significance to an understanding of neoplasia.

I believe that of all the initial experiments undertaken, the
most impressive was one in which we initiated the animals with a
subeffective dose of DMBA and did not start applications of croton oil until 43 weeks later in one group. These animals developed precisely the same number of tumors as those in which the
promoting treatment was begun only one month later. This study
seems to indicate that the initiation process gave rise to an
irreversible change. Subsequent repetition of this study by Van
Duuren and by Roe cast doubt on this result. Although none of
these studies concluded that all the initiated cells disappeared
they did conclude that many of these changed cells did so. Most
recently Stenback, Richard Peto and myself published a large
study in which we repeated these experiments. Our studies were
designed to determine not only the effect of an interval between
initiation and promotion but also the effect of age of the mouse
on their sensitivity to the chemicals found that mice progressively became less sensitive as they aged and that after an interval between initiation and promotion of 60 weeks the mice that
were over 70 weeks of age were only half as sensitive to the effect of the promoter as young adult mice. When this factor was
taken into account the original conclusions that initiation results in an irreversible cellular change seemed to be substant-
iated. Thus, whatever the mechanism of promotion, at least these
studies have been able to delineate the nature of the initiation
step with some clarity.

In most two stage studies the phenomenon of regression of induced tumors plays a major role. I noted this occurrence in my
first studies with Berenblum when we were inducing tumors with a
polycyclic hydrocarbon initiation and recorded this fact in subsequent papers. I have continued to write about my views of the
meaning of these tumors and will bore you with some of these later. Rous and later Foulds were particularly concerned with this
occurrence and I must confess that I find it utterly astonishing
that this fact is of so little general interest. In more recent
years there have been a few investigators who have actually not-
iced that regression occurs and have bothered to record it. In
the instance of skin tumors induced with croton oil or the phorbol ester it seems quite remarkable that this should have been
overlooked since in many experiments as many as 80% of all the
lesions induced may regress. I regret having to say that this
unhappy fact was brushed under the carpet initially because the
experiments would have seemed much less convincing in a day when
pathologists rule the experimental field.

The third series of studies that concluded that carcinogenesis
involved at least two stages were those of Al Tannenbaum in his
original studies on the effects of diet on various kinds of carcinogenesis. When Tannenbaum presented his first findings to the
American Association for Cancer Research (AACR) in 1940 Rous had

not yet published his concept of Initiation and Promotion and when Tannenbaum announced that he had found that caloric restriction had different effects at different times in chemical tumor induction and that he had named these stages "genesis" and "development" he was vigorously attacked by Rous.

Remaining within the confines of skin carcinogenesis, certain key facts seem to me to merit continuous reiteration:

1. Croton oil and/or the phorbol esters derived from it are far and away more potent as "promoting agents" than any other compounds discovered.

2. Of the remaining agents that are classified as "promoting agents" very few, if any, approach croton oil activity levels and most are also carcinogenic.

3. Evidence for the carcinogenicity of croton oil/phorbol esters is tenuous at best.

4. The species specificity of croton oil/phorbol ester is very marked.

5. There is no correlation between ability to induce hyperplasia and promoting action.

6. Wound healing can act as a "promoter".

7. The vast majority of recent skin experiments on promoting action have made use of special strains of mice - notably "Sencar". These mice are exceptionally sensitive to skin carcinogenesis for entirely unknown reasons. Results obtained in these animals cannot be extrapolated to other strains of mouse, let alone other species.

8. In spite of all these reservations, there is good evidence leading to the hypothetical conclusion that neoplasms can be induced sequentially by agents acting in different ways. Of course the mechanism of neither step being known makes this hypothesis tenuous.

Up to this point I have dealt with this problem within the confines of the rigid structure of the original experiments. The area has advanced in quantum leaps since that time and a huge number of experiments have been performed that claim to be investigations of a two or more stage process in carcinogenesis. The majority of studies undertaken since the original skin studies were performed have used a variety of combinations, most of which have involved both initiators and promoters that induce tumors alone - usually if the dose is increased above that used in the two stage studies. A primary question to be answered is whether or not such studies can justifiably be said to permit for a conclusion that different mechanisms of carcinogenesis can be said to be involved in the two stages. From the original skin studies it was concluded that carcinogens were both initiators and promoters and were often more or less potent in one or the other of these categories. More recently efforts have been made to classify carcinogens as either primarily initiators or primarily promoters. I have even heard that somewhat confusing term a "promoting carcinogen" used recently.

There is not the slightest question that studies along these
lines are amongst some of the most promising in the field of
carcinogenesis. However, it is an unfortunate fact of life that
carcinogenesis has become a major part of toxicology in recent
years and, as a result, there has been a considerable added con-
fusion in the field engendered by regulatory problems. Efforts
to suggest that "promoting agents" are special forms of carcinogen that require regulation are, in my view, quite premature and
likely to make an already muddy area even more obscure.

I shall only say a few words about two or more stage studies
in carcinogenesis in the liver. These studies parallel those in
the skin in many ways. Unfortunately the primary "promoting agent" used in the liver studies, phenobarbital, is unequivocally
carcinogenic alone. Mere prolongation of treatment longer than
that used in the usual two stage study results in many tumors.
Again, the kind of rat or mouse used is a major determinant and
perhaps the suggestions of Watanabe et al. about an oncogene
determinant is important. However, as in mouse skin, wounding
with regeneration appears to have an effect although this is, as
in the mouse skin, an inconstant and low level effect. Once
again, in-depth study of mechanism is still needed. The hepat-
omas regress when treatment is stopped. The relationship of
regression to different modes of induction still requires further elucidation.

The use of the urinary bladder as a model system is of considerable interest but extremely confusing as a result of the use
of numerous systems whose variations illustrate many of the difficulties inherent in the entire field. Hicks must be given cre-
dit for designing an imaginative system that would, hopefully,
parallel the original mouse skin studies. She instilled NMU into
the urinary bladder of rats and followed this after an interval
with systemically administered saccharin or cyclamate. In her
first study the NMU was essentially non-carcinogenic alone as
were the two "promoters". Unfortunately, repetition of this
study revealed that her chosen dose of NMU was a potent carcinogenic level for the bladder and, of course, saccharin is carcinogenic to the bladder alone but not under her conditions. Cyclamate has not been found carcinogenic except in an old and complicated study. Subsequently Cohen and his colleagues found that
cancer in the bladder could be induced by first administering the
potent bladder carcinogen FANFT systemically followed by much
abused saccharin; these studies are confounded by many tumors
with the FANFT alone and major change in tumor incidence when the
interval between the FANFT and the saccharin is introduced. The
same and more complexities confuse the results obtained by Ito
and his group who used the bladder carcinogen BBN followed by
saccharin and other compounds. Most of Ito's interesting studies
are quite short term and rather than involving actual tumor induction use hyperplasia as an end point. In view of the fact that
Hicks' original studies engendered considerable discussion on
whether or not tumors were tumors or hyperplasias, this point is

of considerable importance. It is now said frequently that perhaps saccharin is a promoting agent. This would seem to me to be
a singularly meaningless statement that serves well to illustrate
the sort of useless employment of undefined terms that has become
commonplace. Saccharin mysteriously gives rise to bladder tumors
in certain strains of rat when administered at an early age at
high doses. How this non-metabolized compound does this is anyone's guess at the moment. The occurrence of these tumors is not
associated with the induction of hyperplasia. These simple well
established facts are glossed over by those who would wish to
place this perhaps non-genotoxic compound into a nice category
that must have some meaning to someone.

It is just possible that I have a vested interest in seeing
that the scientific basis for an approach to understanding the
intimate details of neoplasia is not lost.

Tumor Promoters: Biological Approaches for
Mechanistic Studies and Assay Systems,
edited by Robert Langenbach et al.
Raven Press, New York © 1988.

Tumor Promotion: A Discussion of Current Topics,
Available Assay Systems and Research Needs

Robert Langenbach[1], Raymond W. Tennant[1], and J. Carl Barrett[2]

[1]Cellular and Genetic Toxicology Branch and
[2]Laboratory of Molecular Carcinogenesis
National Institute of Environmental Health Sciences
Research Triangle Park, North Carolina 27709

Carcinogenesis is a complex process, which has operationally
been divided into stages termed initiation, promotion, and
progression. Environmental chemicals can contribute to the process at one, some, or all of these stages. The stage at which a
chemical exerts its effect is of mechanistic importance for
understanding the process and also of possible regulatory importance for limiting human exposure. Based on increased
understanding of the carcinogenesis process, there is a belief
that chemicals which act at the promotion stage (promoters) may
play a significant role in human carcinogenesis. However, to
date, no chemical has been unequivocally identified as a human
tumor promoter, although stages in human cancer development are
known to exist (5,6). Therefore, to elucidate the significance
of tumor promotion in human carcinogenesis and to identify chemicals which influence this stage there is a need to continue developing systems which will expand our understanding of the
promotion stage of cancer.

A major goal of this meeting was to determine the current
status of systems which can be used to identify tumor promoters
and to study their biological mechanisms. Most chemical carcinogens are identified by their ability to induce or increase
the incidence of tumors in rodents. However, the rodent
bioassays generally do not provide evidence as to the mode of
action by which a chemical influences the carcinogenesis process.
Short term, in vitro systems have proven useful for studying the
mechanism(s) of action of chemical carcinogens, and also for
identifying some classes of chemical carcinogens. For example,
genetic toxicology assays, such as the Ames bacterial mutation
assay (1), have performed fairly well in identifying carcinogens
which act by direct interaction with DNA. However, chemicals
which are carcinogenic but act by mechanisms other than covalent
interaction with DNA are not always detected in currently
available in vitro systems. In fact, absence of genetic toxicity
in these systems has sometimes been used to ascribe a mode of
action to a known carcinogen. Tennant et al. (15) reported that
about 50% of the carcinogens identified by the National

441

Toxicology Program (NTP) from 1979 to 1985 were not detected in a battery of standardized in vitro genetic toxicology assays. If short-term tests are to be of value in the identification of all classes of chemical carcinogens, then assays which can detect nongenotoxic carcinogens such as tumor promoters must be developed and used to supplement the genetic toxicology assays. In addition, the results from such systems should provide valuable information on the modes by which these chemicals manifest their carcinogenic activity.

The definition of "tumor promotion" was discussed at this meeting but no single definition was agreed upon. It should be noted that initiation, promotion and progression are operational terms and the lack of discrete boundaries between them contributes in part to the difficulty in defining any stage independently. Some chemicals (complete carcinogens) effectively complete all three stages, while other chemicals seem to influence predominantly only one stage. However, whether any chemical can act at only one stage is not clear with our current knowledge. Specifically for chemicals regarded as promoters, there is always the problem of distinguishing between a chemical without initiating activity but which promotes spontaneously initiated cells and a chemical with weak initiating activity and strong promoting activity. Thus, with current technologies, it is not possible to classify a chemical as a "pure" promoter. The inability to define promotion is probably in part also due to the fact that it is an observable phenomenon with no currently known single underlying mechanism. Different classes of chemicals presumably promote via different mechanisms and even the same chemical may promote by different mechanisms in different tissues. Furthermore, promotion in skin has been subdivided into at least two stages (4), which further illustrates the complexity of the process. Therefore, given the number of possible mechanisms involved and our current understanding of the process, a promoter can at this time best be described in terms of the chemical treatments involved and the observable outcomes.

While a concensus definition of a tumor promoter is difficult to achieve, certain biological characteristics have been ascribed to the promotion stage. Reversibility, which is the regression of premalignant lesions in the absence of continued chemical treatment, is one important characteristic . Many promoter-induced papillomas or preneoplastic foci are dependent on continued chemical treatment. By contrast, initiation and progression are believed to be irreversible events, and once the event has occurred the presence of the chemical is no longer needed. The mechanisms by which regression occurs have received little attention, but it appears that the papilloma or foci regresses to some non-detectable clonal size. Clonal expansion will recur if promoter treatment is resumed. Inherent in the concept of reversibility has been the theory that promoters have no permanent effect on cells. However, recent data has accumulated which indicated that cells do have a memory for promoter treatment (Kinzel, et al., Fusenig, et al., Lerman and Colburn, this volume). Additionally, in mouse skin, the papillomas reappear rapidly when promoter treatment is resumed which also indicates a lasting effect of the first promoter treatments. Reversibility may be more a characteristic of the premalignant state of the lesions than a property of the chemical used to induce them. For example, preneoplastic lesions in rat tracheas induced by the complete and potent carcinogen DMBA, also regress when treatment ceases (16). Further research on the mechanisms by which regression occurs and the nature of the latent lesion are clearly need.

Related to reversibility of tumor promotion is the concept of threshold. The manifestation of the threshold phenomenon can be subdivided into threshold for treatment dose and threshold for treatment frequency. The current view is that initiators are active at a single low dose, whereas promoters need to be administered at a certain dose and at a certain frequency. Below this dose and/or frequency of promoter treatment no tumors are observed. However, thresholds are experimentally determined and their observation is dependent on the biological system being studied. Furthermore, the threshold dose for the initiator and threshold dose for the promoter may be inter-related. Thus, an increase in the dose of one can reduce the dose of the other needed to manifest the biological response. In addition many chemicals have multiple effects (i.e. complete carcinogens) which further complicates the concept of threshold when considering hazard from environmental chemicals. The conceptual existence of thresholds for tumor promoters, but not for tumor initiators, does have possible implications for regulatory purposes. However, more studies are needed with model promotion systems to verify the concept of threshold as it relates to initiators and promoters and to determine how the existence of thresholds (or lack of) may be used when regulating human exposure.

Cell proliferation and toxicity are often associated with tumor promotion. In mouse skin the induction of regenerative hyperplasia is a common feature of tumor promoters (DiGiovani et al., this volume). In liver systems where toxicity does appear to be a factor, the reduced sensitivity of initiated hepatocytes to the toxic effects of the chemical is a means by which selective expansion of an altered cell population can occur (7). However, other liver promoters such as phenobarbital apparently operate via minimally toxic mechanisms (8). Thus toxicity and regenerative hyperplasia may be mechanisms to allow clonal expansion of the initiated cells; however, since other mechanisms also exist (i.e. dietary effects, responsiveness to hormones, etc.), toxicity is not always necessary or sufficient for tumor promotion.

Tumor promoters exhibit very dramatic organ, strain and species specificities (DiGiovani et al., this volume), but the basis for this specificity is virtually unknown. To illustrate the extent of the organ/species differences which can occur, TPA and phorbol will be used as examples. TPA is one of the most potent skin tumor promoters known for certain strains of mice, but TPA is not active in all mouse strains (DiGiovani et al., this volume). Furthermore, it is only weakly active on rat skin and inactive as a promoter on hamster skin. Biochemical responses can be elicited in sensitive and resistant strains/species so the varying sensitivities do not appear to be caused by simply dose or metabolism differences. Sustained hyperplasia in the skin, as opposed to transient hyperplasia, does correlate with species susceptibility (13) and resistance species may show some form of adaptive responsive to the promoter treatment. However, the mechanisms involved are unknown. The second example is phorbol, the deesterified product of TPA. Phorbol is inactive as a skin tumor promoter and is commonly used as a negative control for skin studies. However, in contrast to its inactivity in skin, phorbol has been demonstrated to be a promoter in the rat liver and mammary gland (2,3). With our current knowledge it appears that organ/species/strain specificities for tumor promoters may be even greater than for tumor initiators, and the basis for these differences needs to be further explored. Without some understanding of the causes of species differences, it will be extremely difficult, if not impossible, to extrapolate promotion activity observed in a test species to humans.

Of the in vivo systems which have been used to study tumor promotion, the mouse skin and the rodent liver models have been the most thoroughly studied (Pitot and Campbell, Fischer et al., this volume). However, other organ systems are also at various stages of development. These other systems include: mouse lung, rat mammary gland, bladder, kidney, colon, and thyroid (14). Further development of these systems is needed so that mechanisms of promotion and the basis of tumor promoter organ specificity can be elucidated. However, in relating these systems to promotion in animals or humans during environmental exposure, it must be considered that the model systems are designed to accentuate the promotion stage. Furthermore, the endpoints generally scored in these model systems are usually papillomas, foci or other pre-neoplastic lesions, and not malignant growths, although the conversion of preneoplastic lesions in these models is well documented. The relationship of results from these model systems to the overall carcinogenesis process needs to be further clarified, although their use for mechanistic studies is unquestionable.

All initiation-promotion systems are based on initial treatment of the target organ with an initiating carcinogen. However, it is doubtful that all "initiated cells" formed in the target organ are identical, and in fact it is likely that a spectrum of initiated cells is produced by a given carcinogen treatment (Hennings, this volume). Some initiated cells may progress to malignancies without further chemical treatment, although effects of dietary and other natural promoters cannot be ruled out. Other initiated cells may be promoted at varying rates to papillomas or altered foci by further treatment. These observations raise several interesting questions about promotion. For example, how do initiated cells differ so that they give varying responses to promoters? Promoter induced clonal expansion rates are known to vary within a given organ (Pitot and Campbell, this volume), but the causes for the different responses are unknown. Additionally, it is unknown why some papillomas or foci progress to carcinomas while others do not and may even regress.

Likewise, it would be interesting to determine if an individual initiated cell would respond to all promoters. Stated another way, can an initiated cell respond to one promoter but be refractory to a promoter of different chemical structure or with an alternative mode of action? These questions are of mechanistic as well as practical importance in understanding the process of promotion.

Recent studies have indicated several mechanisms which may be involved in tumor promotion. One mechanism which has received much attention is activation of protein kinase C (PKC) (O'Brien, et al., Ashendel, et al. this volume). PKC is a receptor for certain potent promoters (i.e. phorbol esters) and its enzymatic activity is also activated by the promoter binding. The activation of PKC results in increased phosphorylation of specific cellular proteins which may be an early event in the promotion process. However, not all promoters have an effect (at least directly) on PKC. TCDD, an extremely potent carcinogen, which is believed to act as a promoter, does not bind to PKC but rather binds to the Ah receptor and induces cytochrome P-450s and other drug metabolizing enzymes (Osborne et al., this Volume). The alteration of drug metabolizing enzymes could change the balance of endogenous chemicals (i.e. hormones) as well as the metabolism of exogenous environmental compounds. Peroxisomal proliferation may be another mechanism by which liver promotion can occur (12). These examples imply that alterations in metabolism of normal cellular constituents may contribute to promotion. While little is known about the mechanisms, altered caloric and dietary intake may also contribute to the promotion process. For example, high sucrose diets appear to promote mammary carcinogenesis and rat liver foci development (9,11). Additionally, it is known that certain promoters increase oxygen radical production in cells, a process that could contribute to the promotion and/or progression stages of carcinogenesis (17). Gene amplification, which may be induced by promoters, also provides a potential mechanism of action (18). Inhibition of intercellular communication via gap junctions, which possibly results in altered growth regulation, is another tumor promotion mechanism receiving considerable attention (Trosko and Chang, Welsch, Yamasaki and Fitzgerald, Elmore, et al., Tong and Williams, this volume). Closure of gap junctions can be caused by receptor mediated as well as nonreceptor mediated mechanisms. Indeed, activation of PKC is one mechanism believed to be involved in altered function of gap junctions. Blocked or altered differentiation of certain cell types is another event associated with tumor promoter treatment (Huberman, this volume). Additionally,

studies with oncogenes have indicated that under certain conditions they may alter a cell or tissue's response to promoters
(10). While it is conceivable that many events could lead to
tumor promotion, an underlying common mechanism is not readily
apparent.

In terms of relevance to human health, three fundamental
questions about tumor promoters exist: 1) how to identify them;
2) what are their potencies relative to each other and to tumor
initiators; and 3) what is their contribution to human carcinogenesis? The answers to these questions will require a better
understanding of promoters and the promotion stage of cancer than
we now possess. Thus, the development and refinement of systems
to answer these questions must continue. Two systems, the mouse
skin and the mouse or rat liver, have been used to identify most
of the known tumor promoters. The greatest number of chemicals
have been studied on mouse skin and this system can distinguish
between initiator and promoter activity. However, the quantitative separation of these activities has been accomplished in
the rat liver system (Pitot and Campbell, this volume) although
significantly fewer chemicals have been tested in this system. A
less rigorous method to identify tumor promoters has been to
assume that all chemicals which were carcinogenic in the rodent
bioassay, but negative in in vitro genetic toxicology assays, act
via promoting mechanisms. However, this assumption has not been
tested and probably will be incorrect for at least some chemicals. Limitations of the currently available genetic toxicology
assays may cause even some DNA reactive carcinogens to be missed
and thus cause their misclassification. Furthermore, even a DNA
reactive chemical could concieveably be a "pure" tumor promoter
since the DNA reactivity measured in vitro may not contribute to
initiation of carcinogenesis in vivo.

Two in vivo approaches which are not yet validated but may be
potentially useful for identifying tumor promoters are as
follows. One would be to treat the test animals with a
multiorgan initiator prior to testing the suspect (test) chemical
in a chronic study. The animals would receive a weak or non-
tumorigenic dose of initiator followed by continuous treatment
with the test chemical. An increased incidence and/or an organo-
tropic difference in tumors of initiated and promoted animals
compared to animals treated with the initiator alone or test
chemical alone would provide evidence of tumor promotion by the
test chemical. While this approach is not without limitations,
an advantage would be that multiorgan promotion effects could be
obtained from a single experiment. A second in vivo approach
would be to treat with the test chemical alone for a period of
time and then stop treatment in some groups. This construct
assumes that spontaneous lesions which were promoted by the test
chemical would regress when chemical treatment is terminated.
After proper validation of the approach, this method of testing
could provide valuable information about the mode of action of
the chemical with relevance for regulating human exposure.

There is little doubt that accurate in vitro short-term tests for tumor promoters would be very useful. The in vitro systems for detecting promoters which to date have received the most attention are described in this volume. However, because of the time required for promotion in vivo and the multiple and probably cascading events involved, it seems unlikely that a single in vitro system could mimic the phenomenon as it occurs in vivo. Therefore, most in vitro systems probably at best reflect only one of the possible mechanisms involved and it would be unrealistic to require any single in vitro system to detect all classes of tumor promoters. None of the in vitro systems described herein have been properly validated and therefore cannot be recommended for routine testing. However, many of these systems are useful for mechanistic studies and with proper validation may be useful for screening environmental chemicals.

The ultimate reason for studying tumor promotion is to determine its relative significance in human carcinogenesis and, if possible, to control human exposure to chemicals with promoting activity. As stated above, and throughout this volume, there is evidence to suggest that promoters act mechanistically differently than initators or progressors; but the differences may be more quantitative than qualitative. For example, initiation is considered irreversible, but some evidence suggests promotion also has long lasting effects. Possibly, the imprints left on the cell by initiators compared to promoters are different, with one (initiation) being of longer lasting biological significance. But with available data we simply cannot say with certainty. The same difficulties arise with most criteria which purport to separate the promotion stage from the other stages. Thus the question, can promoters as a subclass of carcinogens be regulated differently than carcinogens in general, must at present be answered 'No'. There is simply too little information presently available to give any other response. Possibly when adequate information is obtained to allow a better understanding of the mechanisms involved, we can reach a consensus definition of the term "promotion", and the answer will change.

Some areas of future research which may be helpful in elucidating the role of promotion in human cancer, and in carcinogenesis in general, are as follows. Mechanisms involved in promotion, such as PKC activation, P-450 enzyme induction, etc., require further study and possible underlying common mechanisms identified. The role and/or need for toxicity as a promotional stimulus should be examined. The significance of oncogenes in the promotion process requires further study. Systems which allow separation of the initiation, promotion and progression stages need to be further explored and, if possible, methods should be developed to determine the relative potencies of the test chemical at each stage. In vivo organ-specific and other whole animal approaches to identify tumor promoters, in addition to skin and liver, should be further developed. In vitro systems which can identify promoters are needed and could be used to supplement current short term tests. A better understanding of the basis for and the extent of species differences is needed. The identification of chemicals which act as promoters in humans requires more attention, and the importance of promoters as a contributing factor to human cancer should be elucidated.

In summary, the phenomenon of tumor promotion is observably real but it is mechanistically elusive. Further advances in the areas described in this text and related areas are needed to better understand the phenomenon and to determine its significance in human carcinogenesis.

REFERENCES

1. Ames, B.N., McCann, J., and Yamasaki, E. (1978) Mutation Res., 31: 347-364.
2. Armuth, V. and Berenblum, I. (1972): Cancer Res., 33: 2259-2262.
3. Armuth, V. and Berenblum, I. (1974): Cancer Res., 34: 2704-2707.
4. Boutwell, R.K. (1974): CRC Crit. Rev. Toxicol., 2: 419-443.
5. Day, N.E. (1982) In: Carcinogenesis: Cocarcinogenesis and Biological Effects of Tumor Promoters. Vol. 7, edited by E. Hecker, N.E. Fusenig, W. Kinz, F. Marks, and H.W. Thielmann, pp. 183-199. Raven Press, New York.
6. Doll, R. (1973): Cancer Res., 38: 3573-3583.
7. Farber, E. (1984): Cancer Res. 44: 4217-4223.
8. Goldsworthy, T., Campbell, H.A., and Pitot, H.C. (1984): Carcinogenesis, 5: 67-71.
9. Hei, T.K. and Sudilousky, O. (1985): Cancer Res. 45: 2700-2705.
10. Hsiao, W-L., Gattoni-Celli, S., and Weinstein, I.B. (1984): Science, 226: 552-555.
11. Klurfield, D.M., Weber, M.M., and Kritchevsky, D. (1984): Carcinogenesis, 5: 423-425.
12. Rao, M.S. and Reddy, J.K. (1987): Cancer Res., 8: 631-636.
13. Sisskin, E.E., Gray, T. and Barrett, J.C. (1982): Carcinogenesis, 3: 403-407.
14. Slaga, T., editor (1983): Mechanisms of Tumor Promotion: Tumor Promotion in Onternal Organs. Volume I. CRC Press, Inc., Boca Raton, Florida.
15. Tennant, R.W., Margolin, B.H., Shelby, M.D., Zeiger, E., Haseman, J.K., Spalding, J., Caspary, W., Resnick, M., Stasiewicz, S., Anderson, B. and Minor, R. (1987): Science, 236: 933-941.
16. Topping, D.C., Griesemer, R.A., and Nettesheim, P. (1979): Cancer Res., 39: 4829-4837.
17. Troll, W., and Wiesner, R. (1985): Ann. Rev. Pharmacol. Toxicology, 25: 509-528.
18. Varshawsky, A. (1981): Cell, 25: 561-568.

Subject Index

abl, 309,310
S-Adenosyl-L-methionine decarboxylase, 46
Adenovirus 5, 374,376
Adenovirus E1a, 363
    signal transduction and protein phosphory-
    lation, 332
Adhesion molecules, cell, 99
ADP ribosylation, 102
A431 cells, 411
Age and tumor progression, 436
Agent Orange, U.S. Air Force study, 414
AHH, 53,376
Ah locus, 412
    changes, hepatocarcinogenesis, 388
Alcian blue, 122
Allopurinol, 80
Alteration sequence, endometrial stromal
    cells, MNNG-treated, 293
Ames test. *See Salmonella* assay
Amobarbital, 153,154
Aneuploidy
    C_3H mouse keratinocytes, phorbol-ester-
        induced, 269
    mouse skin multistage carcinogenesis assay,
        24–26
Anthralin, 242
Antioxidants, 18,21,205–209
Antipain, chromosomal aberrations, C_3H
    mouse keratinocytes, 268,270
Antipromoters/antipromotion, 19,219
Arachidonic acid
    and calcium, protein kinase C in tumor pro-
        motion, 347–349
    cascade, 261,270
        cyclooxygenase pathway, 261
        lipooxygenase pathway, 20,261
        papilloma malignant conversion, mouse
        skin assay, 47
ARL cell system. *See* Metabolic cooperation
    assay, hepatocyte/liver epithelial (ARL)
    cell system
Aryl hydrocarbon hydrolase (AHH), 53,376
Asbestos-induced mesothelioma, 275
ATPase, 85
Autophosphorylation, EGF receptors, hepa-
    tocarcinogenesis, 389,391–393,400,403
5-Azacytidine, 82

BALB/C-3T3, *in vitro*, transformation–pro-
    motion assays compared, 238–242,244

Barbiturates, 80; *see also specific barbiturates*
Benign tumor progression, promotion and,
    435–436
Benzo(a)pyrene
    genetic factors and susceptibility to skin tu-
        mor promotion, mouse, 52–54,56
    in vitro transformation–promotion assays
        compared, 243
    oncogene activation, 306
    SHE cell transformation assay, 188–191,
        193,195,196,198
    tumor progression, promotion and, 432
Benzoyl peroxide, 26–27,102
    genetic factors and susceptibility to skin tu-
        mor promotion, mouse, 59–61
    metabolic cooperation assay, V79 cells,
        153,155
BHA, 91,426
    metabolic cooperation assay, 153,154,168,
        169
BHT, 80
    C_3H-$10T^1/2$ assay, 242
    metabolic cooperation assay, V79 cells,
        153,154
Bile acids, C_3H-$10T^1/2$ assay, 241
Bitumen road dust, SHE cell transformation
    assay, 197,198
Bovine pituitary extract (BPE), 276,277
BPL (β-propriolactone), oncogene activation,
    306
Butylated hydroxyanisole. *See* BHA
Butylated hydroxytoluene. *See* BHT

Cadmium, SHE cell transformation assay,
    196,242
Caenorhabditis elegans, 359
Caffeine, 190,191
Calcium
    and arachidonic acid, protein kinase C in tu-
        mor promotion, 347–349
    gap junction, effect on, 99–102,106,136
    keratinocytes
        TCDD receptor, 410
        TPA effects on oncogenes, 322–327
    lung cells, human, *in vitro*, carcinogenesis
        model, 279,280
    pro genes, 360
    retinoid inhibition of tumor promotion, 233
    signal transduction and protein phosphory-
        lation in tumor promotion, 332,335,337

Calcium/calmodulin-dependent protein kinase, 338,344–348
Calcium ionophore A23187, 337
Calorie restriction, 437
Carcinogen database, U.S. National Toxicology Program, 419,420
Carcinogen detection. *See Salmonella* assay
Carcinogenesis
   cell differentiation role, 247–255
   incomplete, 88
   cf. teratogenesis, 113
   see also Mouse skin multistage carcinogenesis assay
Carcinoma
   mouse skin multistage carcinogenesis assay, 11,12,24,25
   progression from papilloma, mouse skin assay, 25–27
   squamous cell, genetic factors and susceptibility to skin tumor promotion, mouse, 52
Catalase, 18–19
   $C_3H-10^2/2$ (clone 8) *in vitro* transformation assay, 205–206
Catechol, metabolic cooperation assay, V79 cells, 155,156
C57BL6 mouse, susceptibility to skin tumor promotion, 52,55–61,63–65
Cell adhesion molecules, 99
Cell–cell channel; cell–cell communication.
   See Gap junction *entries*; Intercellular communication disruption/inhibition
Cell differentiation in carcinogenesis, 247–255
   HL-60 leukemia cells, phorbol diesters, 252–255
   protooncogenes, 251,255
Cell memory, tumor promotion, summary, 442–443
Chinese hamster ovary (CHO) cells, 169
Chlordane, 165–167,172
Chondrogenic differentiation, human embryonal palate mesenchyme, 119–122
   inhibition, 120
Chromosomal aberrations, C_3H mouse keratinocytes, phorbol-ester-induced, 259–271
   aneuploidy, 269
   antipain, 268,270
   cytogenetics cf. primary culture, 262–264
   ETYA, 261,267,268,270
   HEL cell lines, 261–262,264
   markers, 264
   4-O-methyl TPA, 261,264,265
   oncogene, 267,269,270
   4-α-PDD, 261,264,265
   RPA, 260,261,264,265,270
   TPA, 259–262,264–270
   types of aberrations, 262,264,265,268

Chromosome changes, SHE cell transformation assay, 191,192
Chrysarobin, 59–61
$C_3H-10T^1/2$ (clone 8) *in vitro* transformation assay, 201–209,213–220,238–244,336–338,346
   antioxidants, 205–209
   assay endpoints, 215–219
      intercellular communication inhibition, 217–219
      Lucifer yellow transfer, 216,217
      uridine exchange, 215,216
   focus formation, enhanced, 219–220
      anti-promotion, 219
      3-methylcholanthrene (MCA), 218,219
      4-O-methyl-TPA, 214,216
      mezerein, 216
      protease inhibitors, 205–208
      schema, 209
      TCDD, 215–220
      TPA, 201–209,213–214,216–219
         regression of foci upon withdrawal, 214
      x-ray, 203–204,206–209
   see also Retinoids, inhibition of tumor promotion, $C_3H-10T^1/2$ (clone 8) assay
Cigarette smoke condensate
   BALB/C-3T3 assay, 242
   $C_3H-10T^1/2$ assay, 242
   lung cells, human, *in vitro* carcinogenesis model, 282–284
   SHE cell transformation assay, 195–198, 242
Cirrhosis and hepatocarcinogenesis, rat, 74
Clastogenicity, 23,24,88
Clomiphene, 346
Clone 8. *See* $C_3H-10T^1/2$ (clone 8) *in vitro* transformation assay
Clostridium perfringens, 20
Coal tar, 1
   SHE cell assay, 195–197,242
   tumor progression, promotion and, 432,434
Collagen, 374,376
Colony size effects, retinoid inhibition of tumor promotion, $C_3H-10T^1/2$ (clone 8) assay, 227–231
Communication. *See* Gap junction *entries*; Intercellular communication disruption/inhibition
Con A, 374
Connexons, 99
Conversion. *See* Papilloma malignant conversion, mouse skin assay
Cooperation. *See* Metabolic cooperation assay *entries*
Cortisone, $C_3H-10T^1/2$ assay, 241
Creosote, SHE cell assay, 195,196,242
Croton oil, 52,62,80,81
   gap junction effect, 133
   tumor progression, promotion and, 432–437

CSF-1 receptor, 314
Cyclamate, 438
  metabolic cooperation assay, V79 cells,
    153,155
Cyclic-AMP, 231–233
  gap junction effect, 99,100,106,136
    disruption, human embryonal palate
      mesenchyme, 119,122
    lung cells, human, *in vitro* carcinogenesis
      model, 276–278,281,285
    signal transduction and protein phosphory-
      lation in tumor promotion, 332
Cyclic-AMP-dependent protein kinase, 233,
    351,354
  hepatocarcinogenesis, rat, 396,397,403
  modulation of gap junction intercellular
    communication, 101,106
Cyclic-GMP and signal transduction/protein
    phosphorylation, 332
Cyclic-GMP-dependent protein kinase, 351
Cycloheximide effect, papilloma malignant
    conversion, 46–47
Cyclooxygenase, 47,261
Cytochrome P-450, 393,407,412,447

Dark basal keratinocytes and phorbol ester
    promotion, mouse skin, 3,57–59,65
DBA/2 mouse, genetic factors and susceptibil-
    ity to skin tumor promotion, 52,53–60,
    63,65
DB(c,h)ACR, oncogene activation, 306
DDT, 80,101,163–165,169,170,374
DETU, *Salmonella* assay, 421,422,426
Dexamethasone, 190,191,195,242,243
Diacylglycerol, 20,101,133,136,332–337
Diazepam, 171
Dibutyryl cAMP, 119,122
Dicofol, *Salmonella* assay, 421,423,426,427
Diethylhexylphthalate, 426
Diethylnitrosamine (DEN), 89,90
  hepatocarcinogenesis, receptor and DNA
    changes, 388,389,391,393,395,400,
    402,403
  immunologic modulation of initiated and
    promoted transformation, 184
  oncogene activation, 307
Diethylstilbestrol, C₃H-10T¹/2 assay, 241,
    242
Differentiation, cell. *See* Cell differentiation in
    carcinogenesis
Differentiation response variants, *pro* genes,
    360
α-Difluoromethyl ornithine, lung cells, *in vitro*
    carcinogenesis model, 277
1-α-25-Dihydroxy-vitamin D₃, 242,253,254
Dinitrofluorobenzene, metabolic cooperation
    assay, V79 cells, 155,156
Dioxin, 88,90,91; *see also* TCDD *entries*
DMBA, 260,269

hepatocarcinogenesis, rat, 82–83,88,90
mouse skin assay, 14–16,32–36,51,53,54–
    57,60
  papilloma malignant conversion, 40,41,
    44,46
oncogene activation, 306,308
tumor progression, promotion and, 432,434,
    436
DMCC, oncogene activation, 306,308
DMN-OME, oncogene activation, 306
DMSO, 326,375,410
  C₃H-10T¹/2 (clone 8) *in vitro* transforma-
    tion assay, 202,205–209
DNA
  adduct formation, genetic factors and sus-
    ceptibility to skin tumor promotion,
    mouse, 53,54
  ploidy, hepatocarcinogenesis, receptor and
    DNA changes, 390,397–399,401–403
  replication, papilloma malignant conver-
    sion, mouse skin assay, 47–48
  see also Hepatocarcinogenesis, rat, recep-
    tor and DNA changes
cDNA clone isolation, protein kinase C in tu-
    mor promotion, 348–354
  multigene family, 353–354
  probe, 349
  sequence analysis, 349,351,353
DNase I sensitivity, *pro* genes, 372
DNA viruses, 5
N-Dodecane, metabolic cooperation assay,
    V79 cells, 153,155,156
Double minute chromosome, phorbol-ester-
    induced, C₃H mouse keratinocytes, 262
Down regulation in tumor promotion, 337–
    339
Dye coupling, gap junction disruption, human
    embryonal palate mesenchyme, 120–
    125,127

EDTA, signal transduction and protein phos-
    phorylation in tumor promotion, 334,335
Eicosatetraynoic acid (ETYA), 47,261,267,
    268,270
Electrophilic theory, *Salmonella* assay, car-
    cinogen detection, 420
Embryo(s)
  fibroblasts, rat, TPA, 317–321
  Xenopus, 132
  see also Gap junction disruption, human em-
    bryonal palate mesenchyme, mouse;
    Syrian hamster embryo (SHE) cell
    transformation assay
Embryogenesis, gap junction role, 113–115,
    132,133
Endometrial stromal cells, human, MNNG-
    treated, 289–301
  alteration sequence, 293
  cf. endometrial epithelial cells, 290

Endometrial stromal cells *(contd.)*
γ-glutamyl transferase, 293,295,298–299
hormones, 290–291
  estrogen, 291
  progesterone, 291
initiation, 300
TPA, 289,290,294–300
dichotomous effect, 300,301
ENU, 25
oncogene activation, 306
Enzyme-altered foci, hepatocarcinogenesis,
  82–87,89–90
foci within foci, 87,91
Epidermal growth factor
BALB/C-3T3 assay, 242
binding, keratinocyte TCDD receptor, 409,
  410,413
$C_3H-10T^1/2$ assay, 242
lung cells, *in vitro* carcinogenesis model,
  276,277,282,283
pro genes, 358,359,374,375
Epidermal growth factor receptor, 337
hepatocarcinogenesis, receptor and DNA
  changes, 389–391,395,396,399–401,
  403
autophosphorylation, 389,391–393,400,
  403
oncogenes, 6
pro genes, 360
TCDD receptor, keratinocyte growth, 410–
  412
Epinephrine, lung cells, *in vitro* carcinogenesis model, 276–278,281,285,286
Epithelial cells. *See* Metabolic cooperation
  assay, hepatocyte/liver epithelial (ARL)
  cell system
Epstein-Barr virus, 374,376
erb-B, 309–310
17-β-Estradiol, 399
Estrogens, 80
MNNG-treated endometrial stromal cells,
  291
17-α-Ethinylestradiol, hepatocarcinogenesis,
  388–403
7-Ethoxycoumarin O-deethylene (ELOD),
  412,413
Ethyl phenylpropriolate, metabolic cooperation assay, V79 cells, 154,156
ETYA, 47,261,267,268,270
Experimental systems listed, 80–81

Familial polyposis coli, 360
FANFT, 438
Fat, unsaturated, 81
Feeder cell method, lung cells, *in vitro* car-
  cinogenesis model, 275–276
fes, 309,310
Fibroblast growth factor, 374,375
  pro genes, 359

Fibroblast-like cells, immunologic modulation
  of initiated and promoted transformation,
  179,180
Fibroblast, rat embryo, TPA effects, 317–321
  myc, 318–320
  ras, 318–321
Fibronectin, SHE cell transformation assay,
  194,195
Flow cytometry, hepatocarcinogenesis, receptor and DNA changes, 390,402
Fluocinolone acetonide, 35–36
fms, 310–314
Foci
enhanced formation, $C_3H-10T^1/2$ (clone 8)
  in vitro transformation assay, 219–220
anti-promotion, 219
enzyme-altered, hepatocarcinogenesis, 82–
  87,89–90
foci within foci, 87,91
regression upon TPA withdrawal, 214
Formaldehyde, $C_3H-10T^1/2$ assay, 241
Forskolin, 231
fos, 310,374–376
keratinocytes, TPA effects on oncogenes,
  322–327
Freeze-fracture, gap junction disruption, human embryonal palate mesenchyme, 126
Furan, oncogene activation, 307
Furfural, oncogene activation, 307

Gap junction(s), 97–106,131–133,140–142,
  445
calcium, 99–102,106
chemical inhibition, 102–104
cyclic-AMP, 99,100,106
diminished, correlation with transformation,
  136–140
distribution, 98
embryogenesis role, 113–115,132,133
functional operations, 98–99
incidence, human embryonal palate mesenchyme, 118
metabolic cooperation assay
  hepatocyte/liver epithelial (ARL) cell
    system, 162
  V79 cells, 157
modulation, 98–100
  oxygen radicals, 100–102
  protein kinases, 100–102
oncogenes, role in regulation of proliferation and differentiation, 99,104–105
pH, 99–101,106
promoter effect on, 133–136
retinoid inhibition of tumor promotion, 231–
  233
  permeability, control by phosphorylation,
    233
tetratogen disruption, 115–116
  cf. carcinogenesis, 113

TPA, 101,103
see also Intercellular communication disruption/inhibition
Gap junction disruption, human embryonal palate mesenchyme, 116–127
  chondrogenic differentiation, 119–122
  inhibition, 120
  cyclic-AMP, 119,122
  cyclic-AMP, dibutyryl, 119,122
  dye coupling, 120–125,127
  freeze-fracture, 126
  incidence, 118
  quantitative morphometry, 125–126
  retinoic acid, 117,119,120,122–127
  13-*cis*-retinoic acid, 120
  TPA, 116,118
Genes, structural, TCDD receptor, keratinocyte growth, 411
  Ah locus, 412
Genetic factors and susceptibility to skin tumor promotion, mouse, 51–66
  aryl hydrocarbon hydrolase (AHH), 53
  benzo(a)pyrene, 52–54,56
  carcinoma, squamous cell, 52
  conversion, 62
  DMBA, 51,53,54–57,60
  MNNG, 55,61
  mouse strains, 12,14–15,21–22,52
    C57BL6, 52,55–61,63–65
    DBA/2, 52,53–60,63,65
    SENCAR, 12,14,21,52,53,55–57,60–65
  non-phorbol esters, 59–62
  cf. other species, 51–52,54–55,63,64
  oxygen radicals, 64
  papilloma, 52,57,60
  phorbol esters, 54–59,61–65
  polycyclic aromatic hydrocarbons, 52–54
  promoters, first cf. second stage, 62, 64
  TPA, 51–66
  receptors, 65
  see also Oncogenes
Genetic variant studies of tumor promotion, *pro* genes, 358–361
Genotoxicity, 97–98
  assays, 149
  Salmonella assay, 417–425,428–430
Glucocorticoid receptor changes, hepatocarcinogenesis, 388,390,393–395,399,401, 403
Glucose-6-phosphatase, 85
γ-Glutamyl transferase, 72,85
  MNNG-treated endometrial stromal cells, 293,295,298–299
Glycerol, 80
Growth factor receptors, oncogenes, 6
GTPase, oncogenes, 6

HBT, metabolic cooperation assay, hepatocyte/liver epithelial (ARL) cell system, 168–170
HEL cell lines, chromosomal aberrations, phorbol-ester-induced, 261–262,264
Hepatitis B virus, hepatocarcinogenesis, 74
Hepatocarcinogenesis, rat
  chemical effects, quantitation, 87–91
  relative efficiencies, 89
  cirrhosis, 74
  enzyme-altered foci, 82–87,89–90
  foci within foci, 87,91
  hepatitis B, 74
  hepatocellular carcinoma, 72,86,87,88
  initiation, 79,82–83,88
    DMBA, 82–83,88,90
  index, 89–90
  nucleotide pools, 73–75
  phenobarbital, 71,73,82–86,90
  precancer, 72
  progression, 86–88
  promotion, 83–86,88,90
  orotic acid, 71–75
Hepatocarcinogenesis, rat, receptor and DNA changes, 387–404
  Ah receptor, 388
  diethylnitrosamine (DEN), 388,389,391, 393,395,400,402,403
  DNA ploidy, 390,397–399,401–403
  epidermal growth factor receptors, 389–391,395,396,399–401,403
    autophosphorylation, 389,391–393,400, 403
  17-α-ethinylestradiol, 388–403
  flow cytometry, 390,402
  glucocorticoid receptors, 388,390,393–395,399,401,403
  protein kinase C, 390,394–397,403
  signal transduction, 396
  TCDD, 388,389,391–399,401,403
Hepatocytes. *See* Metabolic cooperation assay, hepatocyte/liver epithelial (ARL) cell system
Hepatoma, 307
Heptachlor, metabolic cooperation assay, hepatocyte/liver epithlial (ARL) cell system, tumor promoter detection, 165–167, 172
HGPRT⁻ mutagenesis assay, 162–165,167, 169,170,172
Histopathologic grading, mouse skin multistage carcinogenesis assay, 24
History of study, tumor promotion, 1–7
HL-60 leukemia cells, 326
  phorbol diesters and cell differentiation in carcinogenesis, 252–255
  pro genes, 358–360,375
Hydrocortisone, 190,191
Hydrogen peroxide, 26–27

1-Hydroxy-2-3-dehydroestragole, 307
4-Hydroxyphenylretinamide, 226
Hyperplasia, 443,444
 and phorbol ester promotion, mouse skin,
  54,57–59,65

IAR-20 cells, rat liver, gap junctions, 141
Immunologic modulation of initiated and promoted transformation, 179–185
 diethylnitrosamine, 184
 fibroblast-like cells, 179,180
 guinea pig, 179–183
 leukoregulin, 182–185
 Syrian hamster, 179–185
Incomplete carcinogenesis, 88
Indomethacin, 46,47
Inflammation/irritation, chronic
 and phorbol ester promotion, mouse skin,
  57–59,65
 and tumor progression, 431
Initiated cells, 444–445
 INIT C_3H-10T^1/2 cells, retinoids, 226,227,
  229,230,232,234
Initiation
 endometrial stromal cells, MNNG-treated,
  300
 hepatocarcinogenesis, rat, 79,82–83,88
 immunologic modification, 179–185
 mouse skin multistage carcinogenesis assay,
  11,12
  cf. papilloma malignant conversion,
   mouse skin assay, 32–36,40–41
Initiators, listed, 80–81
Insulin, BALB/c-3T3 assay, 242
Intercellular communication disruption/inhi-
  bition
 C_3H-10T^1/2 (clone 8) *in vitro* transformation assay, 217–219
 metabolic cooperation assay, hepatocyte/li-
   ver epithelial (ARL) cell system, 161–
   162,165,169–170,172
 retinoids, inhibition of tumor promotion,
   C_3H-10T^1/2 (clone 8) assay, 231–234
 SHE cell transformation assay, 193,195
 see also Gap junction *entries*
Interlaboratory comparisons, metabolic co-
  operation assay, V79 cells, 152–157
 agents, listed, 154,155
Interleukin-1, 278,280
In vitro transformation–promotion assays
 compared, 237–244,441–444,447
 BALB/C-3T3, 238–242,244
 benzo(a)pyrene, 243
 chemicals, listed, 242
 C_3H-10T^1/2, 238–244
 MCA, 240,241
 MNNG, 240
 SHE cells, 238,239,242,243
 TPA, 240–243

 typical protocol, 239
In vivo systems
 cf. metabolic cooperation asay, V79 cells,
  156–158
 tumor promotion, 444,446–447

Keratinocytes
 dark basal, and phorbol ester promotion, 3,
  57–59,65
 rat primary, TPA effects on oncogenes,
  321–327
  calcium, 322–327
  fos, 322–327
  myc, 322–327
  protein kinase C, 326,327
  TCDD receptors, 407–414
Kirsten sarcoma virus, 374
kit, 309,310

Leukemia. *See* HL-60 leukemia cells
Leukoregulin, 182–185
Lime oil, 80,81
Lipoxygenase pathway, arachidonic acid cascade, 20,261
Lithocholic acid, 80
Liver
 IAR-20 cells (rat), gap junction effect, 141
 phenobarbital in, 438
 see also Hepatocarcinogenesis *entries*; Metabolic cooperation assay, hepatocyte/
  liver epithelial (ARL) cell system
Lucifer yellow, 120–124,216,217
Lung cells, human, *in vitro* carcinogenesis
  model, 275–286
 bovine pituitary extract (BPE), 276,277
 calcium, 279,280
 cigarette smoke condensate, 282–284
 cyclic-AMP, 276–278,281,285
 α-difluoromethyl ornithine, 277
 epidermal growth factor, 276,277,282,283
 epinephrine, 276–278,281,285,286
 feeder cell method, 275–276
 interleukin-1, 278,280
 nickel sulfate, 282,285
 oncogenes, 284–285
 ornithine decarboxylase, 276–278,282–283
 phorbol dibutyrate (PDBU), 283
 retinoic acid, 281
 squamous differentiation, 278–280,282,
  286
 TPA, 278,280,285
 transforming growth factor-β, 279–281
Lung, squamous metaplasia, smokers, 278

Malignant conversion. *See* Papilloma malignant conversion, mouse skin assay
Markers, chromosomal aberrations, C_3H
  mouse keratinocytes, phorbol-ester-induced, 264

Maximum tolerated dose, *Salmonella* assay, carcinogen detection, 418
MCA
  C_3H-$10T^1/2$ assay, 218,219
  retinoid inhibition, 225,226,232
  gap junction effect, 140
  in vitro transformation–promotion assays compared, 240,241
  oncogene activation, 306
MCF-7 cells, 347
"Memory," 442–443
  papilloma malignant conversion, mouse skin assay, 44
Menstrual cycle, 290,291
Mesenchyme, palate. *See* Gap junction disruption, human embryonal palate mesenchyme
Mesothelioma, asbestos-induced, 275
Metabolic cooperation assay, hepatocyte/liver epithelial (ARL) cell system, 161–172
  BHA, 168,169
  chlordane, 165–167,172
  DDT, 163–165,169,170
  HBT, 168–170
  heptachlor, 165–167,172
  intercellular communication disruption, 161–162,165,169–170,172
  gap junctions, 162
  polybrominated biphenyls (PBBs), 167–168
  retinoic acid, 171
  6-thioguanine resistant, 162–165,167,169–171
  TPA, 162,171,172
Metabolic cooperation assay, tumor promotion in V79 cells, 149–158
  amobarbital, 153,154
  benzoyl peroxide, 153,155
  BHA, 153,154
  BHT, 153,154
  catechol, 155,156
  cyclamate, 153,155
  dinitrofluorobenzene, 155,156
  N-dodecane, 153,155,156
  ethyl phenylpropriolate, 154,156
  flow chart, 151
  gap junction inhibition, 157
  interlaboratory comparisons, 152–157
    agents, listed, 154,155
  cf. *in vivo* data, 156–158
  pH, 157
  phenobarbital, 153,154
  phenol, 154,156
  saccharin, 153,154
  6-thioguanine, 150–152
  TPA, 152–154
  D(+)-tryptophan, 153,154
3-Methylcholanthrene. *See* MCA

4-O-Methyl-TPA, 188,189,214,216,261, 264,265
Mezerein, 15,23,34,39,242,318
  BALB/C-3T3 assay, 242
  C_3H-$10T^1/2$ (clone 8) *in vitro* transformation assay, 216
  SHE cell assay, 189,242
Mineral oil, SHE cell transformation assay, 197,198
Mitogens cf. mutagens, 100,101
MMS, oncogene activation, 306
MNNG, 25
  genetic factors and susceptibility to skin tumor promotion, mouse, 55,61
  in vitro transformation–promotion assays compared, 240
  trachael epithelial cells, rat, oncogene alteration during transformation, 305–307,314
  see also Endometrial stromal cells, human, MNNG-treated
Motor oil, SHE cell transformation assay, 197,198
Mouse skin multistage carcinogenesis assay, 3,11–28,71,188,191,213–214,238,260, 269,281,317,435–437
  aneuploidy, 24–26
  bioassay system, 11–15
  carcinoma, 306
  histopathologic grading, 24
  mechanisms, 15–27
  promoters, listed, 13
  see also Genetic factors and susceptibility to skin tumor promotion, mouse; Papilloma malignant conversion, mouse skin assay
Mutagenesis assay, HGPRT⁻, 162–165,167, 169,170,172
Mutagens cf. mitogens, 100,101
myb, 309,310,363
myc, 133,284,285,309,310,317,318,363, 374–376
  keratinocytes, rat primary, TPA effects, 322–327
  SHE cells, 191
  signal transduction and protein phosphorylation in tumor promotion, 332

neu, 306,308
N-HO-AFF, oncogene activation, 307
Nickel sulfate
  lung cells, *in vitro* carcinogenesis model, 282,285
  SHE cell assay, 196,197,242,243
Nicotinamide, 81
Nitrotriacetic acid, 426
NMRI mice, 39–49,62
NMU, 438
  oncogene activation, 306

NMU *(contd.)*
  tracheal epithelial cells, rat, oncogene alteration during transformation, 308
NTP, 441–442
Nuclear proteins and oncogenes, 6
Nucleotide(s)
  pools, hepatocarcinogenesis, rat, 73–75
  pyridine, 72
Nucleotide sequence, *pro* genes, 366

Oncogenes, 5,18,446
  activation by various carcinogens, listed, 306–307
  alteration during transformation, tracheal epithelial cells, 305–314
  and chromosomal aberrations, C_3H mouse keratinocytes, phorbol-ester-induced, 267,269,270
  and gap junctions, 133
  listed, 6
  lung cells, *in vitro* carcinogenesis model, 284–285
  in regulation of proliferation and differentiation, gap junction intercellular communication, 99,104–105
  signal transduction and protein phosphorylation in tumor promotion, 332–333
  TPA effects, rat primary keratinocytes, 321–327
  see also pro genes; *specific oncogenes*
Ornithine decarboxylase, 18,20,21,43,46,54, 65,72,374–376
  lung cells, human, *in vitro* carcinogenesis model, 276–278,282–283
Orotic acid, hepatocarcinogenesis, rat, 71–75
Ovary cells (CHO), Chinese hamster, 169
Oxygen radicals, 4,18–19,22–23,445
  gap junction intercellular communication, 100–102
  genetic factors and susceptibility to skin tumor promotion, mouse, 64
  protein kinase C in tumor promotion, 343

p27, 233
Palate mesenchyme. *See* Gap junction disruption, human embryonal palate mesenchyme
Papilloma, mouse skin, 11,12,24,25
  genetic factors and susceptibility to tumor promotion, 52,57,60
Papilloma malignant conversion, mouse skin assay, 25–27,31–36,39–49,62
  arachidonic acid metabolism, 47
  conversion distinct from TPA promotion, 35–36
  cycloheximide effect, 46–47
  DMBA, 40,41,44,46
  DNA replication, 47–48

heterogeneity of conversion protocol, 33–35,36
  cf. initiation, 32–36,40–41
  memory of skin, 44
  modulators, 44–46
  promotion, 32–34,40–41
   full, 42–45
   two-stage vs. full, 42
  RPA, 39–45,47,49,62
  schema, 48
  TPA, 39–49
PCBs, 80
PC12 cells, 324
PDD
  BALB/C-3T3 assay, 242
  SHE cell assay, 188–190,242
  signal transduction and protein phosphorylation in tumor promotion, 338,339
4-α-PDD
  chromosomal aberrations, C_3H mouse keratinocytes, 261,264,265
  SHE cell transformation assay, 188, 189
Peroxisome, 191,445
pH
  gap junction intercellular communication, 99–101,106
  metabolic cooperation assay, V79 cells, 157
Phenobarbital, 80,81,171,172
  and hepatocarcinogenesis, 71,73,82–86,90, 438
  metabolic cooperation assay, V79 cells, 153,154
  SHE cell transformation assay, 197, 198
Phenol, metabolic cooperation assay, tumor promotion in V79 cells, 154,156
Phenothiazines and protein kinase C in tumor promotion, 346,347
Phorbol dibutyrate (PDBU), lung cells, human, *in vitro* carcinogenesis model, 283
Phorbol esters, 3,5
  binding proteins, 339
  genetic factors and susceptibility to skin tumor promotion, mouse, 54–59,61–65
  see also specific phorbol esters
Phorbol-12-monomyristate (PMM), SHE cell transformation assay, 188,189
Phorbol 12-retinoate 13-acetate (PRA), gap junction effect and transformation, 138
Phosphodiesterase inhibitors, 190–191,195, 231
Phospholipase A_2, 20
Phospholipase C, 20,21
  signal transduction and protein phosphorylation in tumor promotion, 333
Phospholipid dependence, protein kinase C, 344–348

Phosphorylation, protein. *See* Signal transduction and protein phosphorylation in tumor promotion; *specific enzymes*
Platelet-derived growth factor, 374,375
  oncogenes, 6
  SHE cell transformation assay, 195
plt, 133
PMA, HL-60 cells, 252–255
Poly (ADP) ribosylation inhibitors, 82
Polybrominated biphenyls (PBBs), metabolic cooperation assay, hepatocyte/liver epithelial (ARL) cell system, 167–168
Polycyclic aromatic hydrocarbons, 15,396
  genetic factors and susceptibility to skin tumor promotion, mouse, 52–54
Polyposis coli, familial, 360
Potassium chromate, SHE cell assay, 242
pp60^{src}, 137–138,233
Precancer, hepatocarcinogenesis, 72
Procarbazine, 426
pro genes, 357–377
  activation, transcription, and role in tumor promotion, 368–373
    DNase I sensitivity, 372
  calcium, 360
  epidermal growth factor, 358,359,374,375
    receptors, 360
  fibroblast growth factor, 359
  genetic variant studies of tumor promotion, 358–361
    differentiation response variants, 360
    listed, 358
    protein kinase C, 359
    protein kinase C substrates, 359,372,376
    signal transduction, 359
  HL-60, 358–360,375
  molecular cloning and structure, 361–368
    novel oncogene family, 367–368
    nucleotide sequence, 366
    restriction and functional mapping, 365
  cf. other genes modulated by tumor promoters, 373–377
  teleocidin, 360
  TPA, 359,360,363,372–377
  vasopressin, 359
Progesterone and MNNG-treated endometrial stromal cells, 291
Progression, mouse skin multistage carcinogenesis assay, 11,12
Prolactin, 81
Promoters. *See* Tumor promoters
Promotion. *See* Tumor promotion
β-Propriolactone, 306
Prostaglandin F$_{2\alpha}$, 46,47
Protamine sulfate, 346
Protease inhibitors, 19,205–208
Protein kinase
  Ca/CaM-dependent, 338,344–348

cyclic AMP-dependent, 101,106,233,351, 354,396,397,403
cyclic GMP-dependent, 351
gap junction intercellular communication, 100–102
oncogenes, 6
Protein kinase C, 4,18,20,233,412,445,447, 343–354
  arachidonic acid, 347–349
  calcium dependence, 344–349
  cDNA clone isolation, 348–354
    multigene family, 353–354
    probe, 349
    sequence analysis, 349,351,353
  gap junction effect, 136
  hepatocarcinogenesis, rat, receptor and DNA changes, 390,394–397,403
    signal transduction, 396
  HL-60 cells, differentiation and carcinogenesis, 252,253,255
  inhibitors, 344–348
    phenothiazines, 346,347
    rhodamine 6G, 347–348
    tamoxifen and related thiphenylethylenes, 345–347
  keratinocytes, rat primary, TPA effects on oncogenes, 326,327
  modulation of gap junction intercellular communication, 101,102,106
  oxygen radicals, 343
  phospholipid dependence, 344–348
  pro genes, 359
  RPA, 344
  signal transduction in tumor promotion, 333–340
    abnormal regulation by TPA, 334–339
    down regulation, 337–339
  substrates, *pro* genes, 359,372,376
  TPA dependence, 345,346,348
Protein phosphorylation. *See* Signal transduction and protein phosphorylation in tumor promotion
Protooncogenes, cell differentiation in carcinogenesis, 251,255
Pyridine nucleotides, 72

raf, 284,310
ras, 133,140,183,191,269,284,306–307, 308–310,317,321,376–377
Receptors
  growth factor, 6
  promoter, 4,18
  see also Hepatocarcinogenesis, rat, receptor and DNA changes; *specific receptors*
Regression/reversibility, 214,434,436,443
Restriction and functional mapping, *pro* genes, 365
Retinoic acid, 35–36,326
  gap junction disruption, 115,116

Retinoic acid *(contd.)*
  gap junction disruption *(contd.)*
    human embryonal palate mesenchyme, 117,119,120,122–127
    lung cells, human, *in vitro* carcinogenesis model, 281
    metabolic cooperation assay, hepatocyte/liver epithelial (ARL) cell system, 171
  SHE cell assay, 189,197,198,242
13-*cis*-Retinoic acid (Accutane), gap junction disruption in teratogenesis, 115
  human embryonal palate mesenchyme, 120
Retinoids, 19
Retinoids, inhibition of tumor promotion, C_3H-10T^1/2 (clone 8) assay, 223–234
  colony size effects, 227–231
  4-hydroxyphenylretinamide, 226
  INIT C_3H-10T^1/2 cells, 226,227,229,230, 232,234
  intercellular communication model, 231–234
  MCA, 225,226,232
  retinoic acid, 231,232
  retinol, 232
  retinyl acetate, 225–227,234
  serial dilution effects, 230
  TPA, 224,226–227,232,233
  transformation frequency, 229
Retinol, 232
Retinyl acetate, 225–227,234
Retinyl, BALB/C-3T3 assay, 242
Rhodamine 6G, protein kinase C in tumor promotion, 347–348
Ribosylation, 102
  inhibitors, 82
Road dust bitumen, SHE cell transformation assay, 197,198
ros, 309,310
Rous sarcoma virus, 137,374
Roussin's red, C_3H-10T^1/2 assay, 241
RPA (12-O-retinoylphorbol-13-acetate), 318
  chromosomal aberrations, C_3H mouse keratinocytes, phorbol-ester-induced, 260, 261,264,265,270
  papilloma malignant conversion, mouse skin assay, 39–45,47,49,62
  protein kinase C in tumor promotion, 344

Saccharin, 80,374,426,438–439
  BALB/C-3T3 assay, 241,242
  metabolic cooperation assay, V79 cells, 153,154
Salmonella assay, 417–430,433,441
  genotoxic carcinogenesis, 417–425,428–430
    electrophilic theory, 420
    maximum tolerated dose, 418
    structure–activity relationships, 418,420, 425

summarized, 1983 cf. 1988, 428–429
  testing strategies, 426–427
  tumor promoters, 424–426
Sarcoma virus
  Kirsten, 374
  Rous, 137,374
Scarlet oil, 1
Second messengers, 331,332
SENCAR mice, 12,14,21,33–35,39,339
  susceptibility to skin tumor promotion, 52, 53,55–57,60–65
  tumor progression, 433,437
Sensitivity differences, cell strains, TCDD receptor, keratinocyte growth, 412–413
Serial dilution effects, retinoid inhibition of tumor promotion, C_3H-10T^1/2 (clone 8) assay, 230
Serum factor modulation, SHE cell transformation assay, 194–195
SHE cells. *See* Syrian hamster embryo (SHE) cell transformation assay
Signal transduction and protein phosphorylation in tumor promotion, 331–340
  calcium, 332,335,337
  calcium/calmodulin-dependent protein kinase, 338
  calcium ionophore A23187, 337
  cyclic-AMP, 332
  cyclic-GMP, 332
  diacylglycerol, 332–337
  EDTA, 334,335
  oncogenes, 332–333
    adenovirus E1A, 332
    myc, 332
  PDD, 338,339
  phorbol ester binding proteins, 339
  phospholipase C, 333
  protein kinase C, 333–340,396
    abnormal regulation by TPA, 334–339
    down regulation in tumor promotion, 337–339
Signal transduction, *pro* genes, 359
sis, 105,309,310
Skin. *See* Mouse skin multistage carcinogenesis assay
Sodium nitrilo-acetate, 81
Specificity, tumor promotion, summary, 443–444
  TPA, 443–444
Squamous cell carcinoma, TCDD effect, cf. keratinocytes, 407–409
Squamous differentiation, lung cells, *in vitro* carcinogenesis model, 278–280,282,286
Squamous metaplasia, lung, smokers, 278
src, 137,139
Stromal cells. *See* Endometrial stromal cells, human, MNNG-treated
Structure–activity relationships, *Salmonella* assay, carcinogen detection, 418,420,425

Superoxide dismutase, 18–19,21
Susceptibility. *See* Genetic factors and susceptibility to skin tumor promotion, mouse
Sutter strain mouse, tumor progression, promotion and, 433
SV40-T-antigen gene, 284,285
Syrian hamster embryo (SHE) cell transformation assay, 187–198
  gap junctions and transformation, 137
  immunologic modulation of initiated and promoted transformation, 179–185
  in vitro transformation–promotion assays compared, 238,239,242,243
  mechanisms of transformation, 191–194
    cell communication inhibition, 193,195
    chromosome changes, 191,192
    peroxisome proliferation, 191
  promoter identification, 195–198
  serum factor modulation, 194–195
  TPA, 188–193,195
  two-stage transformation experiments, 188–191,193

Tamoxifen and related triphenylethylenes, protein kinase C in tumor promotion, 345–347
TCDD, 80,139,374,376,445
  C_3H-10T^1/2 assay, 215–220,241
  genetic factors and susceptibility to skin tumor promotion, mouse, 61
  hepatocarcinogenesis, rat, receptor and DNA changes, 388,389,391–399,401,403
  Salmonella assay, 426,427
TCDD receptor, keratinocyte growth, 407–414
  calcium, 410
  carcinogenicity, 413–414
  cpidermal growth factor binding, 409,410,413
  epidermal growth factor receptor, 410–412
  genes, structural, 411,412
  sensitivity differences, cell strains, 412–413
  cf. squamous cell carcinoma, 407–409
  TPA, 413
Telocidin, 242,360
Teratogen disruption of gap junction, 115–116
  cf. carcinogenesis, 113
Testosterone, 374
Theophylline, 190,191
6-Thioguanine, metabolic cooperation assay
  hepatocyte/liver epithelial (ARL) cell system, tumor promoter detection, 162–165,167,169–171
  phosphoribosylation, 167
  V79 cells, 150–152
Thiourea, 426,427
TPA, 14–25,71,80,88,393

chromosomal aberrations, C_3H mouse keratinocytes, 259–262,264–270
C_3H-10T^1/2 (clone 8) *in vitro* transformation assay, 201–209,213–214,216–219
  regression of foci upon withdrawal, 214
  retinoid inhibition, 224,226–227,232,233
embryo fibroblasts, rat, 317–321
endometrial stromal cells, MNNG-treated, 289,290,294–300
  dichotomous effect, 300,301
gap junction effect, 101,103,133,135,136,140
human embryonal palate mesenchyme, 116,118
and transformation, 137,139
immunologic modulation of initiated and promoted transformation, 184,185
inhibitors, 35–36
in vitro transformation–promotion assays compared, 240–243
keratinocyte oncogenes, effects, 321–327
lung cells, human, *in vitro*, carcinogenesis model, 278,280,285
metabolic cooperation assay
  hepatocyte/liver epithelial (ARL) cell system, 162,171,172
  V79 cells, 152–154
mouse skin assay, 32–34
  distinct from conversion, 35–36
  genetic factors and susceptibility, 51–66
  papilloma malignant conversion, 39–49
  pro genes, 359,360,363,372–377
  promotion distinct from conversion, 35–36
  and protein kinase C, 334–339,345,346,348
receptors, 65
SHE cells, 188–193,195
specificity, 443–444
TCDD receptor, keratinocyte growth, 413
in teratogenesis, gap junction disruption, 115,116
tumor progression, promotion and, 433–435
Tracheal epithelial cells, rat, oncogene alteration during transformation, 305–314
  fms, 310–314
  MNNG, 305–307,314
  NMU, 308
  ras, 308–310
Transduction. *See* Signal transduction and protein phosphorylation in tumor promotion
Transformation frequency, and retinoid inhibition of tumor promotion, C_3H-10T^1/2 (clone 8) assay, 229
Transforming growth factor-β, 139,279–281
Tridentine, *Salmonella* assay, 420

Triphenylethylenes and protein kinase C in tumor promotion, 345–347

TRIS, *Salmonella* assay, 422

D(+)-Tryptophan, metabolic cooperation assay, V79 cells, 153,154

D,L-Tryptophan, 80

Tumor progression, promotion and, 431–439
  age, 436
  benign tumors, 435–436
  benzo(a)pyrene, 432
  calorie restriction, 437
  coal tar, 432,434
  croton oil, 432–437
  DMBA, 432,434,436
  inflammation/irritation, chronic, 431
  mouse skin, 435–437
  phenobarbital in liver, 438
  regression upon promoter removal, 434,436
  SENCAR mice, 433,437
  Sutter strain mice, 433
  TPA, 433–435
  turpentine, 434
  urinary bladder, 438–439

Tumor promoters
  effect on gap junctions, 133–136
  first cf. second stage, genetic factors and susceptibility to skin tumor promotion, mouse, 62,64
  identification, SHE cell transformation assay, 195–198
  inhibitors, gap junction effects, 134–135
  listed, 13,80–81
  receptors, 4,18
  Salmonella assay, 424–426
  see also specific promoters

Tumor promotion
  cell memory, 442–443
  definition, 442
  and hepatocarcinogenesis, 83–86,88,90
  history of study, 1–7
  human health and, 446–448
  in vitro systems, 441–444,447

in vivo systems, 444,446–447
  mouse skin multistage carcinogenesis assay, 11,12
  cf. papilloma conversion, mouse skin assay, 32–34,40–41
  full, 42–45
  two-stage vs. full, 42
  regression/reversibility, 443
  specificity, 443–444
  TPA, 443–444
  summary, 441–448

Turpentine, 434

Tyrosine kinase, EGF receptor, 411

Ultraviolet, 183–184,233

Unsaturated fat, 81

Uridine exchange, C_3H-10T^1/2 (clone 8) *in vitro* transformation assay, 215,216

Urinary bladder, tumor progression, promotion and, 438–439

U.S. Air Force study, Agent Orange, 414

U.S. National Toxicology Program, 418–430
  carcinogen database, 419,420

Vasopressin, *pro* genes, 359

V79 cells, 118,134–136,162,165,168,172; *see also* Metabolic cooperation assay, tumor promotion in V79 cells

Vinylcarbamate, oncogene activation, 307

Vitamin E, C_3H-10T^1/2 (clone 8) *in vitro* transformation assay, 206–209

Xanthine dehydrogenase, 22

Xanthine oxidase, 21–23

X chromosome, 56

Xenopus embryos, 132

X-rays, 187,227,229
  C_3H-10T^1/2 (clone 8) *in vitro* transformation assay, 203–204,206–209
  immunologic modulation of initiated and promoted transformation, 183–185